Fluids & Electrolytes made Incredibly Easy!

Sixth Edition

Clinical Editor
Laura M. Willis, MSN, APRN, FNP-C

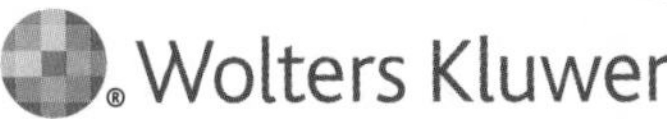

Philadelphia • Baltimore • New York • London
Buenos Aires • Hong Kong • Sydney • Tokyo

Acquisitions Editor: Shannon W. Magee
Product Development Editor: Maria M. McAvey
Senior Marketing Manager: Mark Wiragh
Editorial Assistant: Zachary Shapiro
Production Project Manager: Marian Bellus
Design Coordinator: Elaine Kasmer
Manufacturing Coordinator: Kathleen Brown
Prepress Vendor: Absolute Service, Inc.

Sixth Edition

Printed in China

Library of Congress Cataloging-in-Publication Data

Fluids & electrolytes made incredibly easy! / clinical editor, Laura Willis. — Sixth edition.
p. ; cm.
Fluids and electrolytes made incredibly easy!
Includes bibliographical references and index.
ISBN 978-1-4511-9396-1
I. Willis, Laura, 1969- editor. II. Lippincott Williams & Wilkins, issuing body. III. Title: Fluids and electrolytes made incredibly easy!
[DNLM: 1. Water-Electrolyte Imbalance—Nurses' Instruction. 2. Water-Electrolyte Balance—Nurses' Instruction. WD 220]
RC630
616.3'9920231—dc23
2014043245

LWW.com

9 8 7 6 5 4 3 2 1

Contents

Contributors

Cheryl Brady, MSN, RN, CNE
Nursing Faculty
Kent State University
Salem, OH

Shelba Durston, MSN, RN, CCRN
Nursing Instructor
San Joaquin Delta College
Stockton, CA

Laura Favand, MS, RN, CEN
Chief of Plans, Training Mobilization
U.S. Army Medical Department Activities
Fort Knox, KY

Margaret Gingrich, MSN, RN, CRNP
Professor of Nursing
Harrisburg Area Community College
Harrisburg, PA

Mary Jones, DNP, CNM, ENP-BC, FNP-BC
Family Nurse Practitioner
Doctor of Nursing Practice
MedQuest Health Center, Inc.
Mansfield, OH

Rexann Pickering, PhD, MS, RN, CIM, CIP
Director of Continuing Medical and Nursing Education
Methodist Le Bonheur Healthcare
Memphis, TN

Cherie Rebar, PhD, MBA, RN, FNP, COI
Director, Division of Nursing
Kettering College
Dayton, OH

Donna Scemons, PhD, FNP-BC, CNS
Assistant Professor
California State University
Los Angeles, CA

Allison Terry, PhD, MSN, RN
Assistant Dean of Clinical Practice
Auburn University
Montgomery, AL

Leigh Ann Trujillo, MSN, RN
Patient Care Manager
University of Chicago
Chicago, IL

Prior Contributors

Cheryl L. Brady, MSN, RN

Shelba Durston, MSN, RN, CCRN

Laura R. Favand, MS, RN, CEN

Margaret M. Gingrich, MSN, RN

Karla Jones, MS, RN

Patricia Lemelle-Wright, MS, RN

Linda Ludwig, BS, RN, MED

Rexann G. Pickering, PhD, MS, RN, CIP, CIM

Alexis Puglia, RN

Roseanne Hanlon Rafter, MSN, RN, GCNS-BC

Donna Scemons, PhD, RN, FNP-C, CNS

Vanessa M. Scheidt, RN, TNS, PHRN, FF2

Allison J. Terry, PhD, MSN, RN

Leigh Ann Trujillo, BSN, RN

Foreword

If you are like me, you are too busy to wade through a foreword that uses pretentious terms and umpteen dull paragraphs to get to the point. So let's cut right to the chase! Here is why this book is so terrific:

1. It will teach you all the important things you need to know about fluids and electrolytes. (It will leave out all the fluff that wastes your time.)
2. It will help you remember what you have learned.
3. It will make you smile as it enhances your knowledge and skills. Don't believe me? Try these recurring logos on for size:

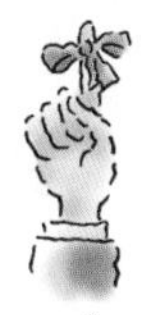

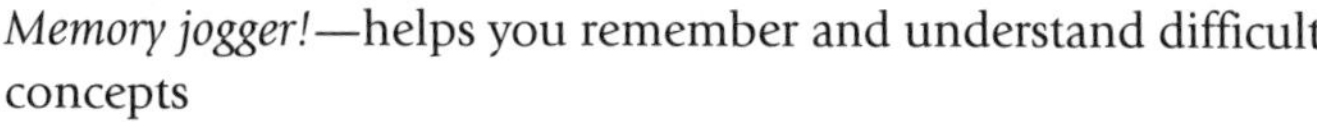

Memory jogger!—helps you remember and understand difficult concepts

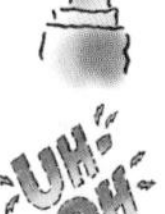

CAUTION!—lists dangerous signs and symptoms and enables you to quickly recognize trouble

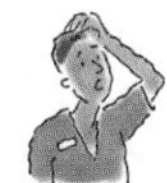

It's not working—helps you find alternative interventions when patient outcomes aren't what you expected

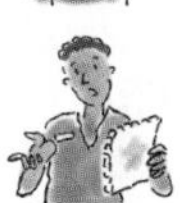

Chart smart—lists critical documentation elements that can keep you out of legal trouble

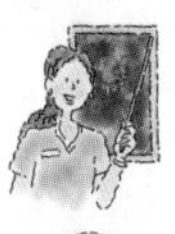

Teaching points—provides clear patient-teaching tips that you can use to help your patients prevent recurrence of the problem

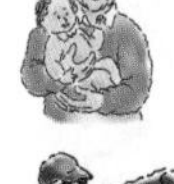

Ages and stages—identifies issues to watch for in your pediatric and geriatric patients

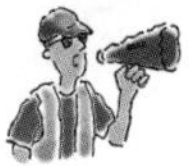

That's a wrap!—summarizes what you've learned in the chapter

See? I told you! And that's not all. Look for me and my friends in the margins throughout this book. We will be there to explain key concepts, provide important care reminders, and offer reassurance. Oh, and if you don't mind, we'll be spicing up the pages with a bit of humor along the way to teach and entertain in a way that no other resource can.

I hope you find this book helpful. Best of luck throughout your career!

Joy

Part I

Balancing basics

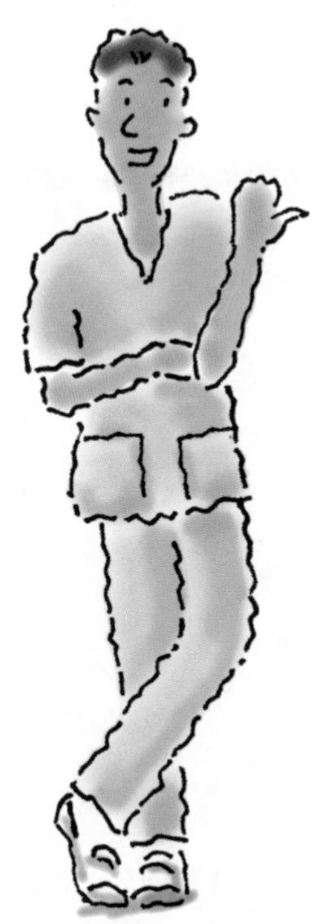

Chapter 1

Balancing fluids

Just the facts

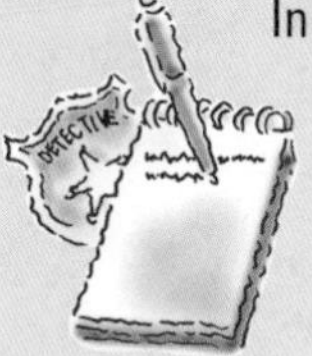

In this chapter, you'll learn:

- the process of fluid distribution throughout the body
- the meanings of certain fluid-related terms
- the different ways fluid moves through the body
- the roles that hormones and kidneys play in fluid balance.

A look at fluids

Where would we be without body fluids? Fluids are vital to all forms of life. They help maintain body temperature and cell shape, and they help transport nutrients, gases, and wastes. Let's take a close look at fluids and the way the body balances them.

Making gains equal losses

Just about all major organs work together to maintain the proper balance of fluid. To maintain that balance, the amount of fluid gained throughout the day must equal the amount lost. Some of those losses can be measured; others can't.

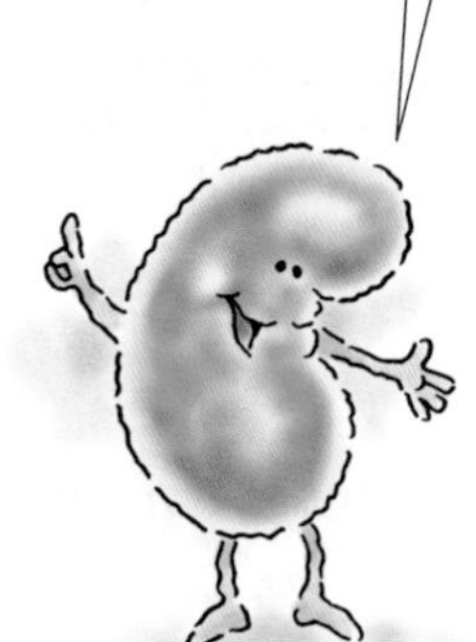
Major organs, including me, work together to maintain fluid balance.

How insensible

Fluid losses from the skin and lungs are referred to as *insensible losses* because they can't be measured or seen. Losses from evaporation of fluid through the skin are fairly constant but depend on a person's total body surface area. For example, the body surface area of an infant is greater than that of an adult relative to their respective weights. Because of this difference in body surface area—a higher metabolic rate, a larger percentage of extracellular body fluid, and immature kidney function—infants typically lose more water than adults do.

Changes in environmental humidity levels also affect the amount of fluid lost through the skin. Likewise, respiratory rate and depth affect the amount of fluid lost through the lungs. Tachypnea, for example, causes more water to be lost; bradypnea, less. Fever increases insensible losses of fluid from both the skin and lungs.

Now that's sensible

Fluid losses from urination, defecation, wounds, and other means are referred to as *sensible losses* because they can be measured.

A typical adult loses about 150 to 200 ml/day of fluid through defecation. In cases of severe diarrhea, losses may exceed 5,000 ml/day (Wait & Alouidor, 2011). (For more information about insensible and sensible losses, see *Sites involved in fluid loss*.)

Following the fluid

The body holds fluid in two basic areas, or compartments—inside the cells and outside the cells. Fluid found inside the cells is called *intracellular fluid (ICF)*; fluid found outside the cells, *extracellular fluid (ECF)*. Capillary walls and cell membranes separate the intracellular and extracellular compartments. (See *Fluid compartments*.)

Sites involved in fluid loss

Each day, the body gains and loses fluid through several different processes. This illustration shows the primary sites of fluid losses and gains as well as their average amounts. Gastric, intestinal, pancreatic, and biliary secretions are almost completely reabsorbed and aren't usually counted in daily fluid losses and gains.

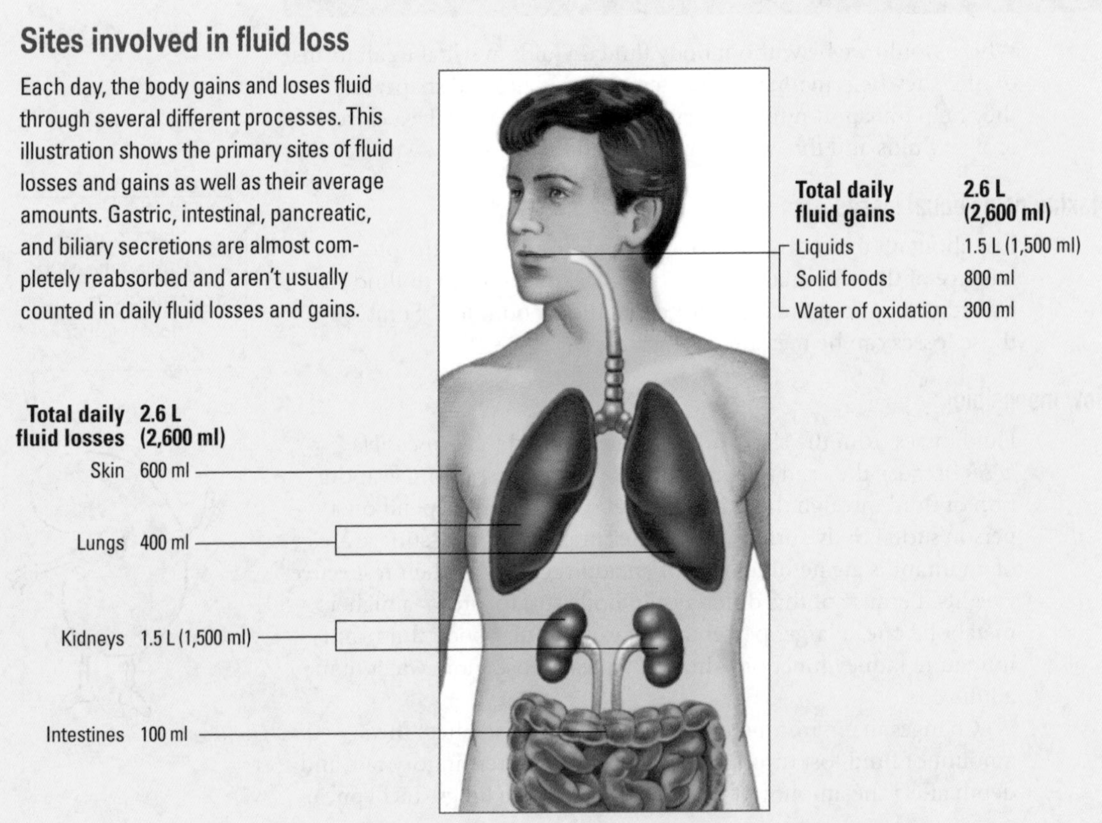

Fluid compartments

This illustration shows the primary fluid compartments in the body: intracellular and extracellular. Extracellular is further divided into interstitial and intravascular. Capillary walls and cell membranes separate ICFs from ECFs.

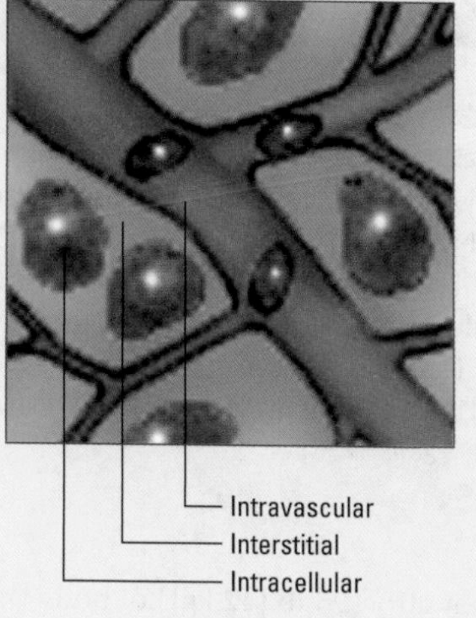

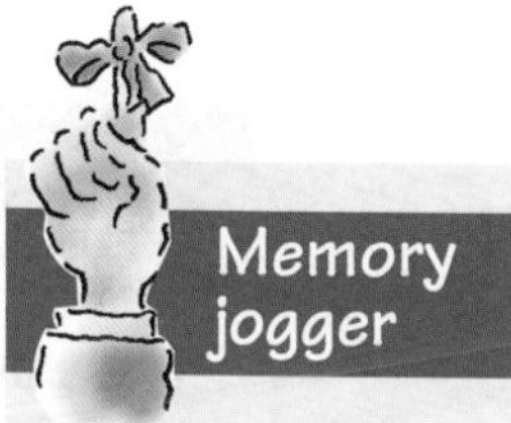

To help you remember which fluid belongs in which compartment, keep in mind that **inter** means between (as in **inter**val—between two events) and **intra** means within or inside (as in **intra**venous—inside a vein).

To maintain proper fluid balance, the distribution of fluid between the two compartments must remain relatively constant. In an average adult, the total amount of fluid is 42 L, with the total amount of ICF averaging 40% of the person's body weight, or about 28 L (Seager & Slaubaugh, 2011). The total amount of ECF averages 20% of the person's body weight, or about 14 L.

ECF can be broken down further into interstitial fluid, which surrounds the cells, and intravascular fluid or plasma, which is the liquid portion of blood. In an adult, interstitial fluid accounts for about 75% of the ECF. Plasma accounts for the remaining 25%.

The body contains other fluids, called *transcellular fluids*, in the cerebrospinal column, pleural cavity, lymph system, joints, and eyes. Transcellular fluids generally aren't subject to significant gains and losses throughout the day so they aren't discussed in detail here.

Water here, water there

The distribution of fluid within the body's compartments varies with age. Compared with adults, infants have a greater percentage of body water stored inside interstitial spaces. About 75% to 80% (40% ECF, 35% ICF) of the body weight of a full-term neonate is water. About 90% (60% ECF and 30% ICF) of the body weight of a premature (23 weeks gestation) infant is water (Ambalavanan & Rosenkrantz, 2012). The amount of water as a percentage of body weight decreases with age until puberty. In a typical 154-lb (70 kg)

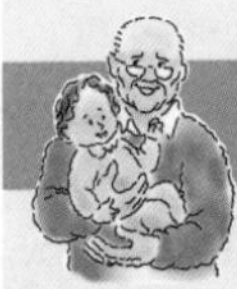

Ages and stages

The evaporation of time

The risk of suffering a fluid imbalance increases with age. Why? Skeletal muscle mass declines, and the proportion of fat within the body increases. After age 60 years, water content drops to about 45%.

Likewise, the distribution of fluid within the body changes with age. For instance, about 15% of a typical young adult's total body weight is made up of interstitial fluid. That percentage progressively decreases with age.

About 5% of the body's total fluid volume is made up of plasma. Plasma volume remains stable throughout life.

lean adult male, about 60% (93 lb [42 kg]) of body weight is water. (See *The evaporation of time*.)

Skeletal muscle cells hold much of that water; fat cells contain little of it. Women, who normally have a higher ratio of fat to skeletal muscle than men, typically have a somewhat lower relative water content. Likewise, an obese person may have a relative water content level as low as 45%. Accumulated body fat in these individuals increases weight without boosting the body's water content.

Understanding isotonic fluids

No net fluid shifts occur between isotonic solutions because the solutions are equally concentrated.

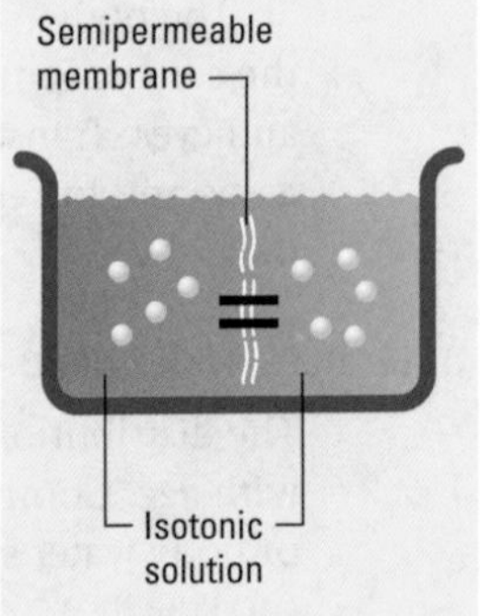

Fluid types

Fluids in the body generally aren't found in pure forms. They're usually found in three types of solutions: isotonic, hypotonic, and hypertonic.

Isotonic: Already at match point

An isotonic solution has the same solute (matter dissolved in solution) concentration as another solution. For instance, if two fluids in adjacent compartments are equally concentrated, they're already in balance, so the fluid inside each compartment stays put. No imbalance means no net fluid shift. (See *Understanding isotonic fluids*.)

For example, normal saline solution is considered isotonic because the concentration of sodium in the solution nearly equals the concentration of sodium in the blood.

Understanding hypotonic fluids

When a less concentrated, or hypotonic, solution is placed next to a more concentrated solution, fluid shifts from the hypotonic solution into the more concentrated compartment to equalize concentrations.

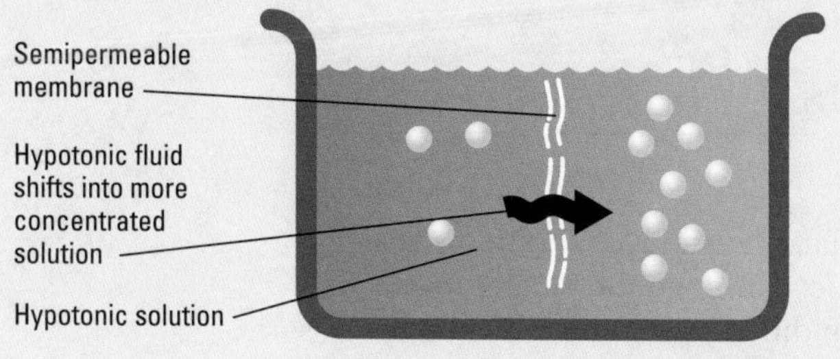

Understanding hypertonic fluids

If one solution has more solutes than an adjacent solution, it has less fluid relative to the adjacent solution. Fluid will move out of the less concentrated solution into the more concentrated, or hypertonic, solution until both solutions have the same amount of solutes and fluid.

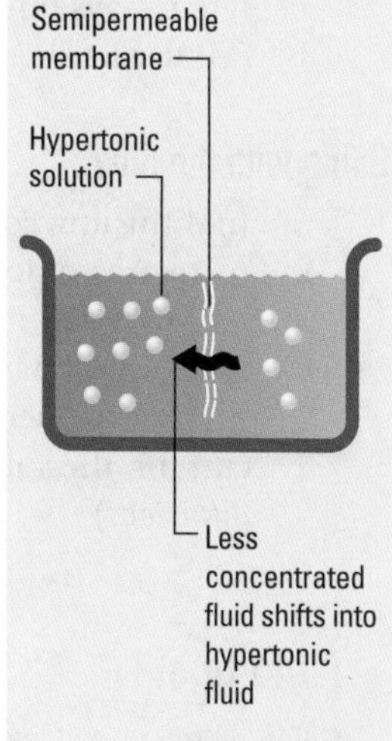

Hypotonic: Get the lowdown

A hypotonic solution has a lower solute concentration than another solution. For instance, say one solution contains only one part sodium and another solution contains two parts. The first solution is hypotonic compared with the second solution. As a result, fluid from the hypotonic solution would shift into the second solution until the two solutions had equal concentrations of sodium. Remember that the body constantly strives to maintain a state of balance, or equilibrium (also known as *homeostasis*). (See *Understanding hypotonic fluids*.)

Half-normal saline solution is considered hypotonic because the concentration of sodium in the solution is less than the concentration of sodium in the patient's blood.

Hypertonic: Just the highlights

A hypertonic solution has a higher solute concentration than another solution. For instance, say one solution contains a large amount of sodium and a second solution contains hardly any. The first solution is hypertonic compared with the second solution. As a result, fluid from the second solution would shift into the hypertonic solution until the two solutions had equal concentrations. Again, the body constantly strives to maintain a state of equilibrium (homeostasis). (See *Understanding hypertonic fluids*.)

For example, a solution of dextrose 5% in normal saline solution is considered hypertonic because the concentration of solutes in the solution is greater than the concentration of solutes in the patient's blood.

Fluid movement

Just as the heart constantly beats, fluids and solutes constantly move within the body. That movement allows the body to maintain homeostasis, the constant state of balance the body seeks. (See *Fluid tips*.)

Within the cells

Solutes within the intracellular, interstitial, and intravascular compartments of the body move through the membranes, separating those compartments in different ways. The membranes are semipermeable, meaning that they allow some solutes to pass through but not others. In this section, you'll learn the different ways fluids and solutes move through membranes at the cellular level.

Going with the flow

In diffusion, solutes move from an area of higher concentration to an area of lower concentration, which eventually results in an equal distribution of solutes within the two areas. Diffusion is a form of passive transport because no energy is required to make it happen; it just happens. Like fish swimming with the current, the solutes simply go with the flow. (See *Understanding diffusion*.)

Understanding diffusion

In diffusion, solutes move from areas of higher concentration to areas of lower concentration until the concentration is equal in both areas.

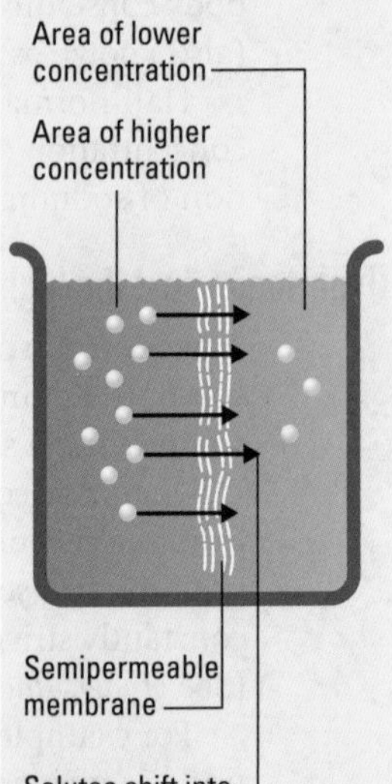

Fluid tips

Fluids, nutrients, and waste products constantly shift within the body's compartments—from the cells to the interstitial spaces, to the blood vessels, and back again. A change in one compartment can affect all of the others.

Keeping track of the shifts

That continuous shifting of fluids can have important implications for patient care. For instance, if a hypotonic fluid, such as half-normal saline solution, is given to a patient, it may cause too much fluid to move from the veins into the cells, and the cells can swell. On the other hand, if a hypertonic solution, such as dextrose 5% in normal saline solution, is given to a patient, it may cause too much fluid to be pulled from cells into the bloodstream, and the cells shrink.

For more information about I.V. solutions, see chapter 19, I.V. fluid replacement.

Understanding active transport

During active transport, energy from a molecule called *adenosine triphosphate (ATP)* moves solutes from an area of lower concentration to an area of higher concentration.

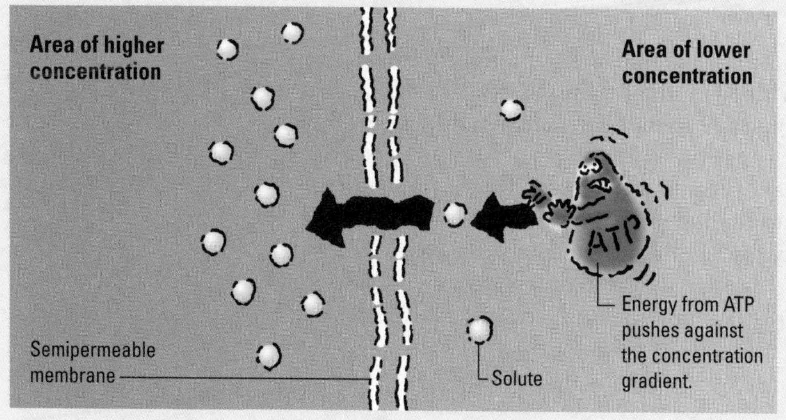

Understanding osmosis

In osmosis, fluid moves passively from areas with more fluid (and fewer solutes) to areas with less fluid (and more solutes). Remember that in osmosis, fluid moves, whereas in diffusion, solutes move.

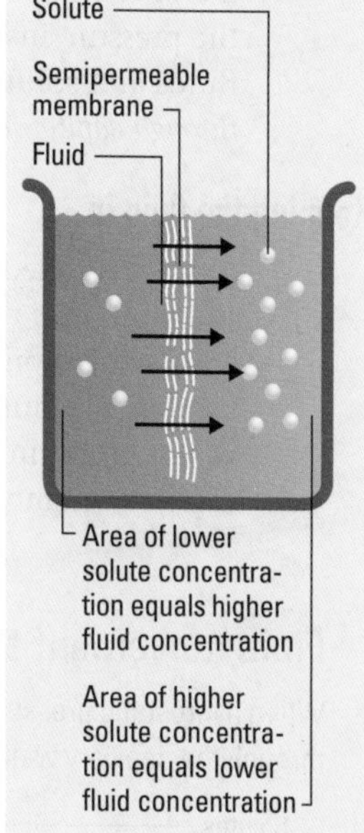

Giving that extra push

In active transport, solutes move from an area of lower concentration to an area of higher concentration. Like swimming against the current, active transport requires energy to make it happen.

The energy required for a solute to move against a concentration gradient comes from a substance called *adenosine triphosphate* or ATP. Stored in all cells, ATP supplies energy for solute movement in and out of cells. (See *Understanding active transport*.)

Some solutes, such as sodium and potassium, use ATP to move in and out of cells in a form of active transport called the *sodium-potassium pump*. (For more information on this physiologic pump, see chapter 5, *When sodium tips the balance*.) Other solutes that require active transport to cross cell membranes include calcium ions, hydrogen ions, amino acids, and certain sugars.

Letting fluids through

Osmosis refers to the passive movement of fluid across a membrane from an area of lower solute concentration and comparatively more fluid into an area of higher solute concentration and comparatively less fluid. Osmosis stops when enough fluid has moved through the membrane to equalize the solute concentration on both sides of the membrane. (See *Understanding osmosis*.)

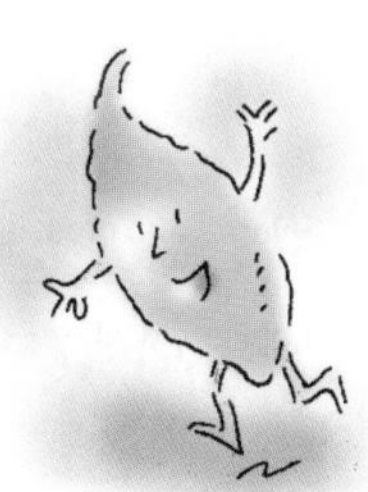

Within the vascular system

Within the vascular system, only capillaries have walls thin enough to let solutes pass through. The movement of fluids and solutes through capillary walls plays a critical role in the body's fluid balance.

The pressure is on

The movement of fluids through capillaries—a process called *capillary filtration*—results from blood pushing against the walls of the capillary. That pressure, called *hydrostatic pressure,* forces fluids and solutes through the capillary wall.

When the hydrostatic pressure inside a capillary is greater than the pressure in the surrounding interstitial space, fluids and solutes inside the capillary are forced out into the interstitial space. When the pressure inside the capillary is less than the pressure outside of it, fluids and solutes move back into the capillary. (See *Fluid movement through capillaries.*)

Keeping the fluid in

A process called *reabsorption* prevents too much fluid from leaving the capillaries no matter how much hydrostatic pressure exists within the capillaries. When fluid filters through a capillary, the protein albumin remains behind in the diminishing volume of water. Albumin is a large molecule that normally can't pass through capillary membranes. As the concentration of albumin inside a

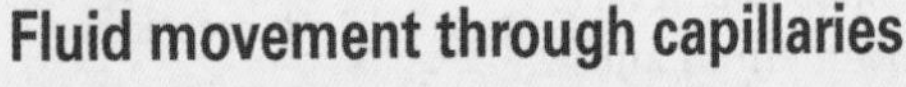

Fluid movement through capillaries

When hydrostatic pressure builds inside a capillary, it forces fluids and solutes out through the capillary walls into the interstitial fluid, as shown below.

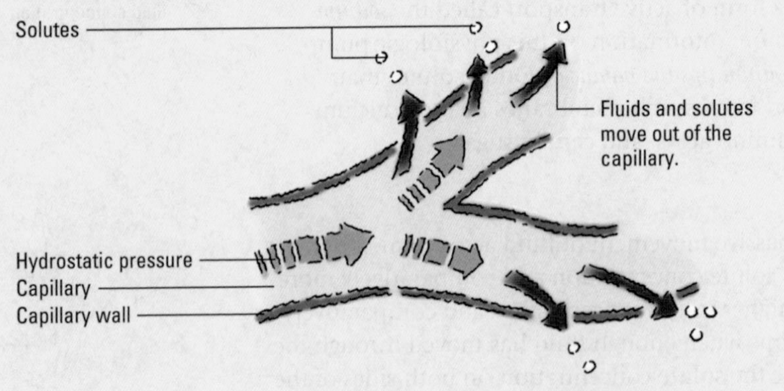
Solutes
Fluids and solutes move out of the capillary.
Hydrostatic pressure
Capillary
Capillary wall

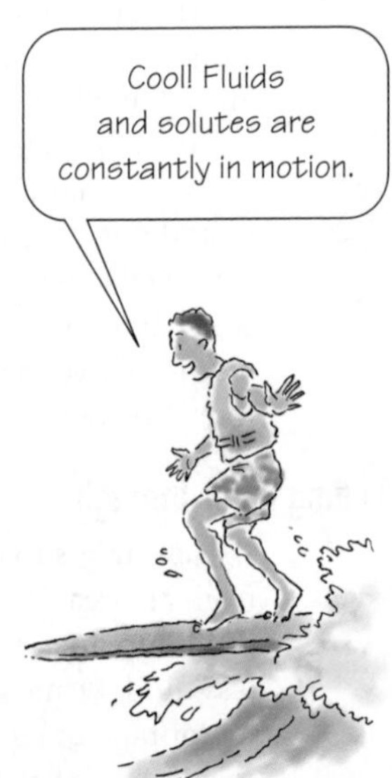
Cool! Fluids and solutes are constantly in motion.

capillary increases, fluid begins to move back into the capillaries through osmosis.

Think of albumin as a water magnet. The osmotic, or pulling, force of albumin in the intravascular space is called the *plasma colloid osmotic pressure*. The plasma colloid osmotic pressure in capillaries averages about 25 mm Hg. (See *Albumin magnetism*.)

As long as capillary blood pressure (the hydrostatic pressure) exceeds plasma colloid osmotic pressure, water and solutes can leave the capillaries and enter the interstitial fluid. When capillary blood pressure falls below plasma colloid osmotic pressure, water and diffusible solutes return to the capillaries.

Normally, blood pressure in a capillary exceeds plasma colloid osmotic pressure in the arteriole end and falls below it in the venule end. As a result, capillary filtration occurs along the first half of the vessel; reabsorption, along the second. As long as capillary blood pressure and plasma albumin levels remain normal, the amount of water that moves into the vessel equals the amount that moves out.

Albumin magnetism

Albumin, a large protein molecule, acts like a magnet to attract water and hold it inside the blood vessel.

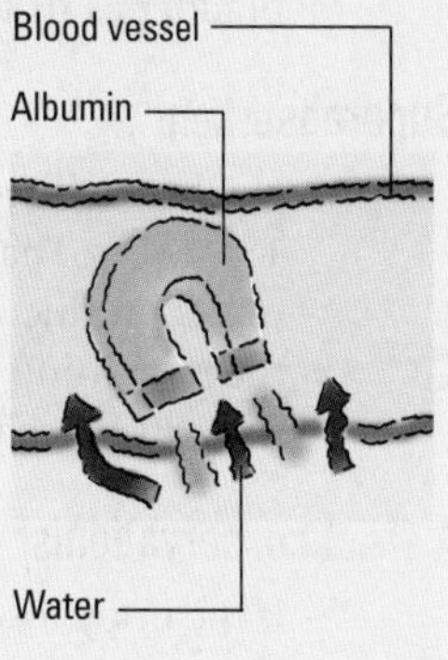
Blood vessel
Albumin
Water

Coming around again

Occasionally, extra fluid filters out of the capillary. When that happens, the excess fluid shifts into the lymphatic vessels located just outside the capillaries and eventually returns to the heart for recirculation.

Maintaining the balance

Many mechanisms in the body work together to maintain fluid balance. Because one problem can affect the entire fluid-maintenance system, it's important to keep all mechanisms in check. Here's a closer look at what makes this balancing act possible.

The kidneys

The kidneys play a vital role in fluid balance. If the kidneys don't work properly, the body has a hard time controlling fluid balance. The workhorse of the kidney is the nephron. The body puts the nephrons to work every day.

A nephron consists of a glomerulus and a tubule. The tubule, sometimes convoluted, ends in a collecting duct. The glomerulus is a cluster of capillaries that filters blood. Like a vascular cradle, Bowman's capsule surrounds the glomerulus.

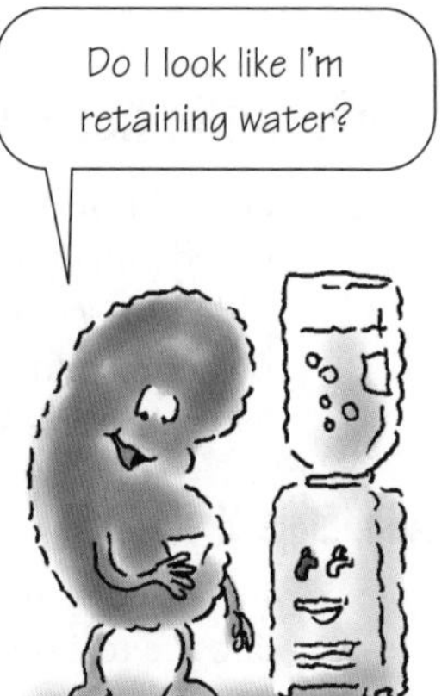
Do I look like I'm retaining water?

Capillary blood pressure forces fluid through the capillary walls and into Bowman's capsule at the proximal end of the tubule. Along the length of the tubule, water and electrolytes are either excreted or retained depending on the body's needs. If the body needs more fluid, for instance, it retains more. If it needs less fluid, less is reabsorbed and more is excreted. Electrolytes, such as sodium and potassium, are either filtered or reabsorbed throughout the same area. The resulting filtrate, which eventually becomes urine, flows through the tubule into the collecting ducts and eventually into the bladder as urine.

More than 30 oil changes a day would make me give up driving for good!

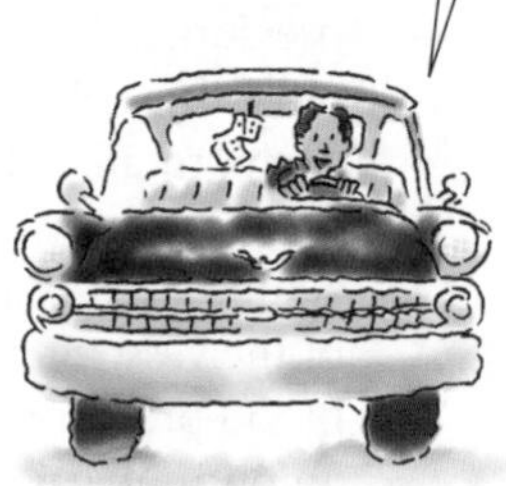

Superabsorbent

Nephrons filter about 125 ml of blood every minute, or about 180 L/day. That rate, called the *glomerular filtration rate,* usually leads to the production of 1 to 2 L of urine per day. The nephrons reabsorb the remaining 178 L or more of fluid, an amount equivalent to more than 30 oil changes for the family car!

A strict conservationist

If the body loses even 1% to 2% of its fluid, the kidneys take steps to conserve water. Perhaps the most important step involves reabsorbing more water from the filtrate, which produces a more concentrated urine.

The kidneys must continue to excrete at least 20 ml of urine every hour (about 500 ml/day) to eliminate body wastes. A urine excretion rate that's less than 20 ml/hour usually indicates renal disease and impending renal failure. The minimum excretion rate varies with age. (See *The higher the rate, the greater the waste.*)

The kidneys respond to fluid excesses by excreting urine that is more dilute, which rids the body of fluid and conserves electrolytes.

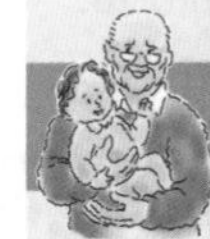

Ages and stages

The higher the rate, the greater the waste

Infants and young children excrete urine at a higher rate than adults because their higher metabolic rates produce more waste. Also, an infant's kidneys can't concentrate urine until about age 3 months, and they remain less efficient than an adult's kidneys until about age 2 years.

Antidiuretic hormone

Several hormones affect fluid balance, among them a water retainer called *antidiuretic hormone (ADH).* (You may also hear this hormone called *vasopressin.*) The hypothalamus produces ADH, but the posterior pituitary gland stores and releases it. (See *How antidiuretic hormone works.*)

Adaptable absorption

Increased serum osmolality, or decreased blood volume, can stimulate the release of ADH, which in turn increases the kidneys' reabsorption of water. The increased reabsorption of water results in more concentrated urine.

How antidiuretic hormone works

ADH regulates fluid balance in four steps.

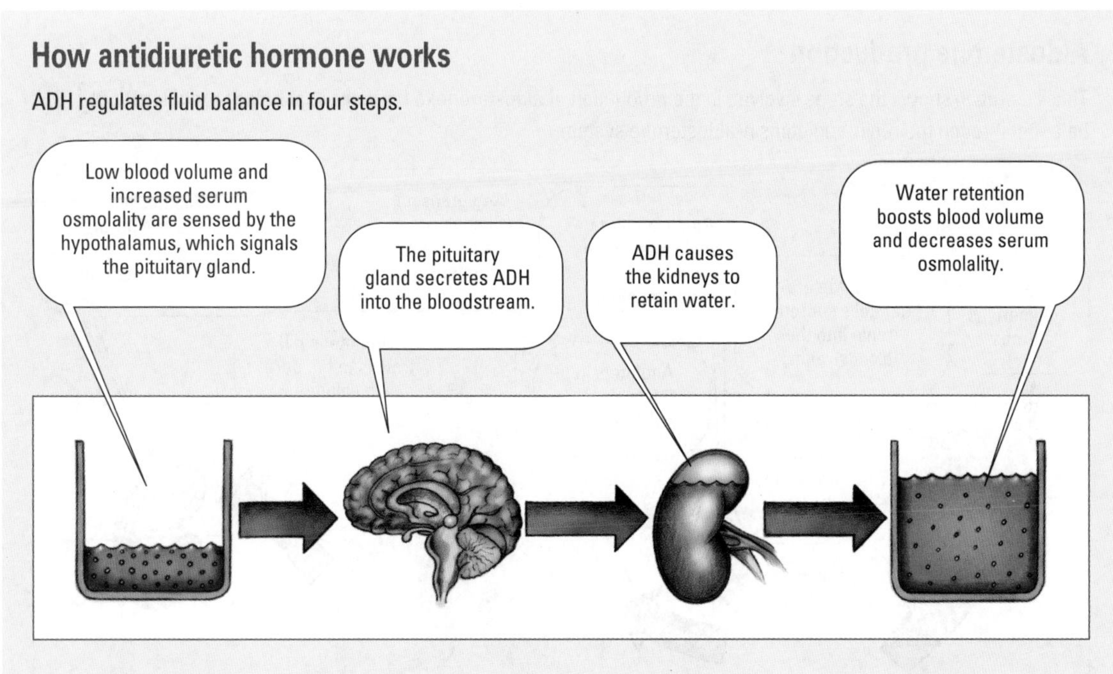

Low blood volume and increased serum osmolality are sensed by the hypothalamus, which signals the pituitary gland.
The pituitary gland secretes ADH into the bloodstream.
ADH causes the kidneys to retain water.
Water retention boosts blood volume and decreases serum osmolality.

Likewise, decreased serum osmolality, or increased blood volume, inhibits the release of ADH and causes less water to be reabsorbed, making the urine less concentrated. The amount of ADH released varies throughout the day, depending on the body's needs.

This up-and-down cycle of ADH release keeps fluid levels in balance all day long. Like a dam in a river, the body holds water when fluid levels drop and releases it when fluid levels rise.

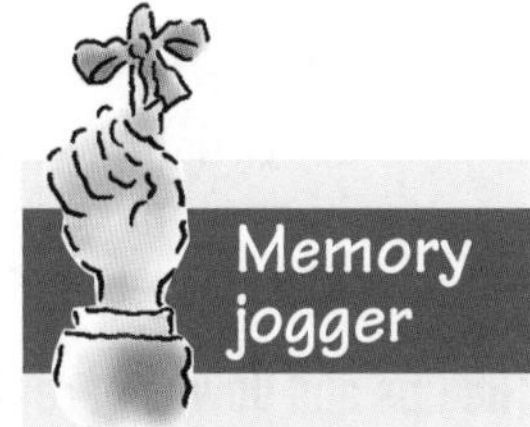

Remember what ADH stands for—antidiuretic hormone—and you'll remember its job: restoring blood volume by reducing diuresis and increasing water retention.

Renin-angiotensin-aldosterone system

To help the body maintain a balance of sodium and water as well as a healthy blood volume and blood pressure, special cells (called *juxtaglomerular cells*) near each glomerulus secrete an enzyme called *renin*. Through a complex series of steps, renin leads to the production of angiotensin II, a powerful vasoconstrictor.

Angiotensin II causes peripheral vasoconstriction and stimulates the production of aldosterone. Both actions raise blood pressure. (See *Aldosterone production*, page 14.)

Aldosterone production

This illustration shows the steps involved in the production of aldosterone (a hormone that helps to regulate fluid balance) through the renin-angiotensin-aldosterone system.

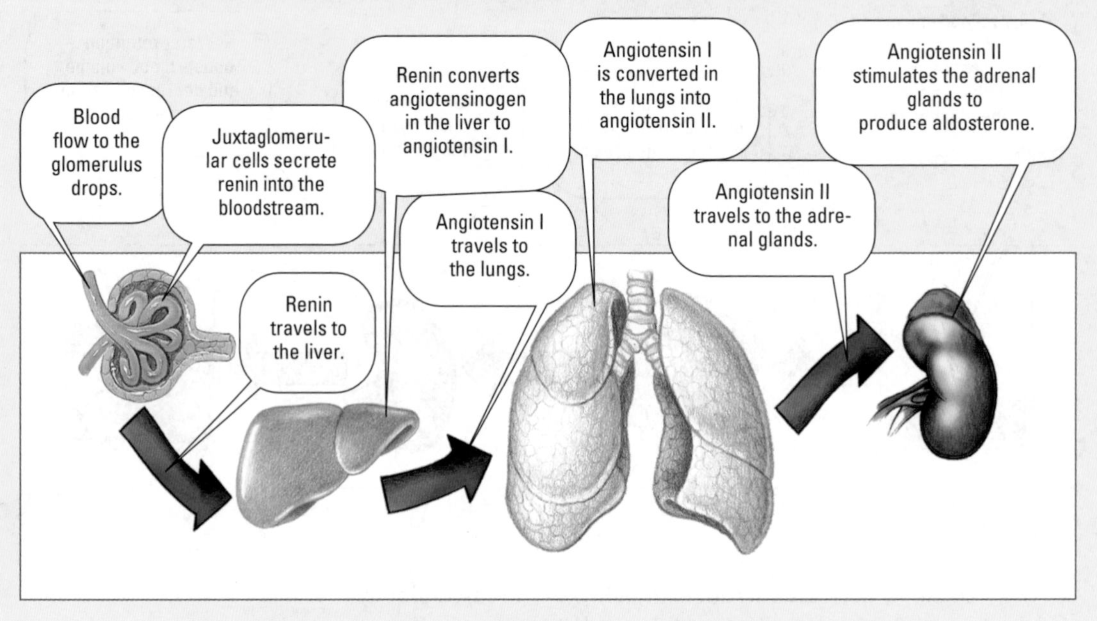

Usually, as soon as the blood pressure reaches a normal level, the body stops releasing renin, and this feedback cycle of renin to angiotensin to aldosterone stops.

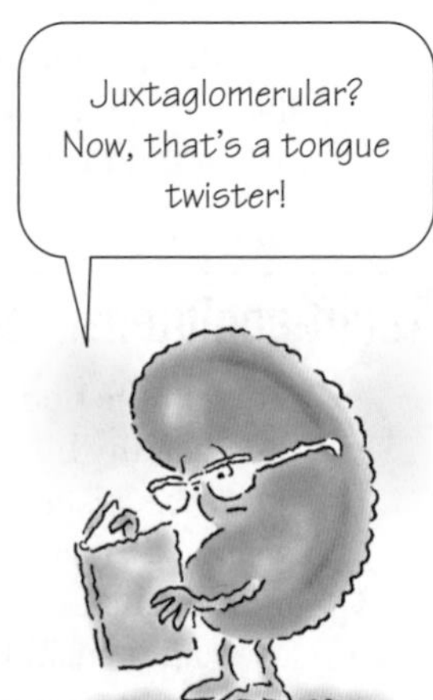

The ups and downs of renin

The amount of renin secreted depends on blood flow and the level of sodium in the bloodstream. If blood flow to the kidneys diminishes, as happens in a patient who is hemorrhaging, or if the amount of sodium reaching the glomerulus drops, the juxtaglomerular cells secrete more renin. The renin causes vasoconstriction and a subsequent increase in blood pressure.

Conversely, if blood flow to the kidneys increases, or if the amount of sodium reaching the glomerulus increases, juxtaglomerular cells secrete less renin. A drop-off in renin secretion reduces vasoconstriction and helps to normalize blood pressure.

How aldosterone works

Aldosterone, produced as a result of the renin-angiotensin mechanism, acts to regulate fluid volume as described below.

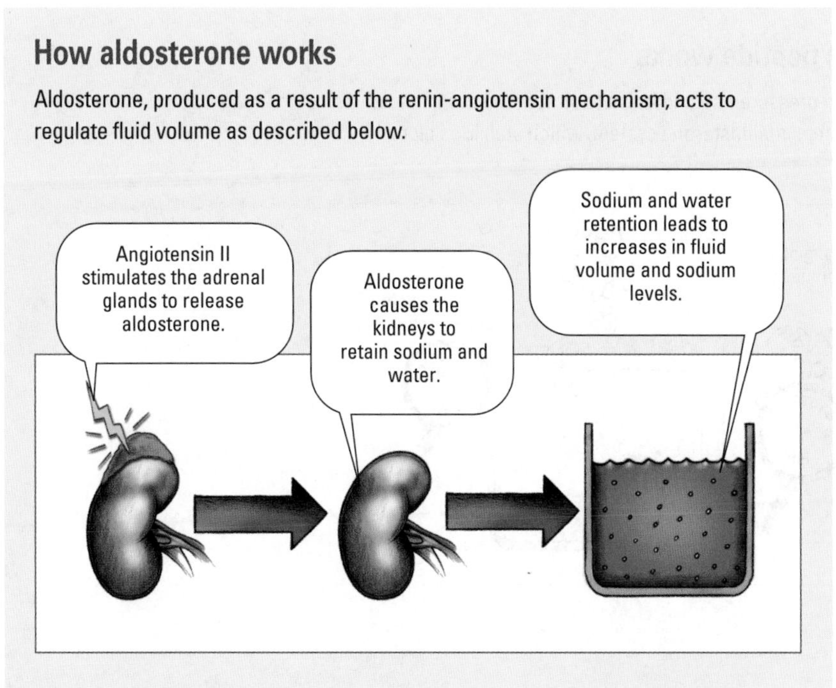

Angiotensin II stimulates the adrenal glands to release aldosterone.
Aldosterone causes the kidneys to retain sodium and water.
Sodium and water retention leads to increases in fluid volume and sodium levels.

Sodium and water regulator

The hormone aldosterone also plays a role in maintaining blood pressure and fluid balance. Secreted by the adrenal cortex, aldosterone regulates the reabsorption of sodium and water within the nephron. (See *How aldosterone works*.)

Triggering active transport

When blood volume drops, aldosterone initiates the active transport of sodium from the distal tubules and the collecting ducts into the bloodstream. When sodium is forced into the bloodstream, more water is reabsorbed and blood volume expands.

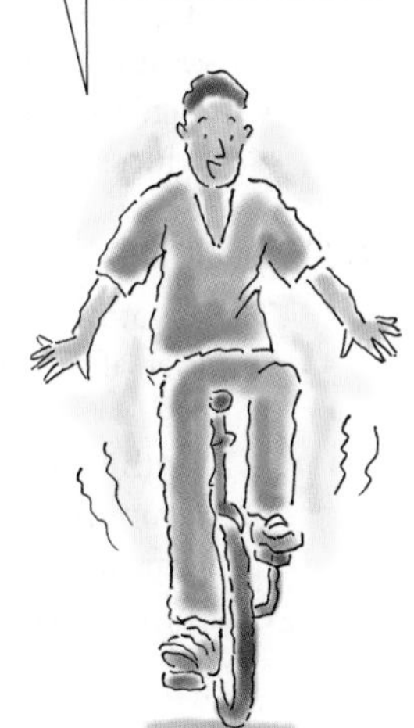

Maintaining body fluid levels is a real balancing act.

Atrial natriuretic peptide

The renin-angiotensin-aldosterone system isn't the only factor at work balancing fluids in the body. A cardiac hormone called *atrial natriuretic peptide* (ANP) also helps keep that balance. Stored in the cells of the atria, ANP is released when atrial pressure increases. The

How atrial natriuretic peptide works

When blood volume and blood pressure rise and begin to stretch the atria, the heart's ANP shuts off the renin-angiotensin-aldosterone system, which stabilizes blood volume and blood pressure.

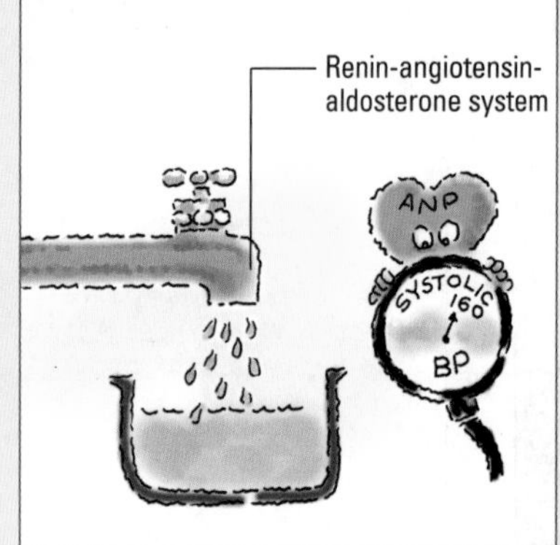

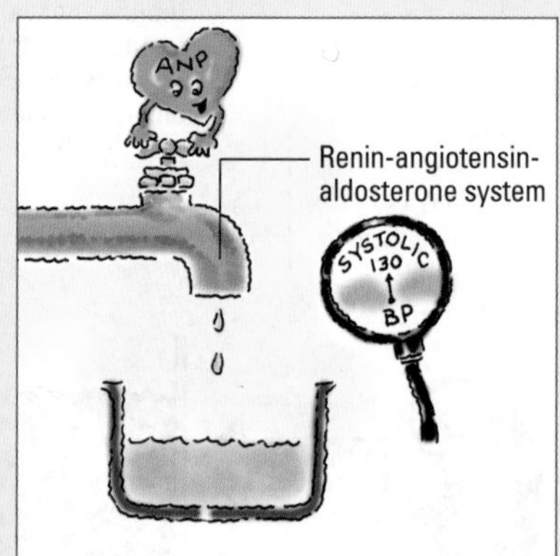

hormone counteracts the effects of the renin-angiotensin-aldosterone system by decreasing blood pressure and reducing intravascular blood volume. (See *How atrial natriuretic peptide works*.)

This powerful hormone:

- suppresses serum renin levels
- decreases aldosterone release from the adrenal glands
- increases glomerular filtration, which increases urine excretion of sodium and water
- decreases ADH release from the posterior pituitary gland
- reduces vascular resistance by causing vasodilation.

Stretch that atrium

The amount of ANP that the atria release rises in response to a number of conditions; for example, chronic renal failure and heart failure.

Anything that causes atrial stretching can also lead to increases in the amount of ANP released, including orthostatic changes, atrial tachycardia, high sodium intake, sodium chloride infusions, and use of drugs that cause vasoconstriction.

Thirst

Perhaps the simplest mechanism for maintaining fluid balance is the thirst mechanism. Thirst occurs as a result of even small losses of fluid. Losing body fluids or eating highly salty foods leads to an increase in ECF osmolality. This increase leads to drying of the mucous membranes in the mouth, which in turn stimulates the thirst center in the hypothalamus. In an elderly person, the thirst mechanism is less effective than it is in a younger person, leaving the older person more prone to dehydration. (See *Dehydration in elderly people*.)

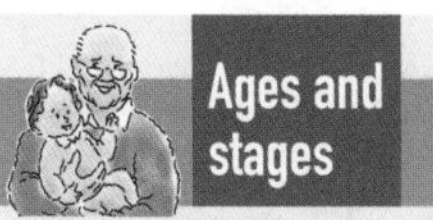

Dehydration in elderly people

The signs and symptoms of dehydration may be different in older adults. For example, they might include:

- confusion
- subnormal temperature
- tachycardia
- pinched facial expression.

Quench that thirst

Normally, when a person is thirsty, he drinks fluid. The ingested fluid is absorbed from the intestine into the bloodstream, where it moves freely between fluid compartments. This movement leads to an increase in the amount of fluid in the body and a decrease in the concentration of solutes, thus balancing fluid levels throughout the body.

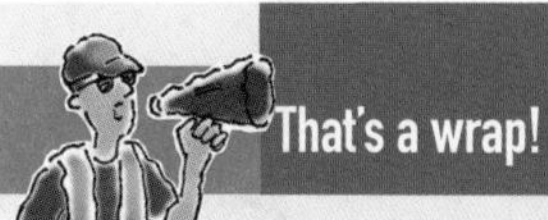

Balancing fluids review

Fluid balance basics

- Fluid movement throughout the body helps maintain body temperature and cell shape.
- Fluids help transport nutrients, gases, and wastes.
- Most of the body's major organs work together to maintain fluid balance.
- The amount of fluids gained through intake must equal the amount lost.

Fluid losses

- *Insensible losses*
  - Immeasurable
  - Examples: through the skin (affected by humidity and body surface area) and lungs (affected by respiratory rate and depth)
- *Sensible losses*
  - Measurable
  - Examples: from urination, defecation, and wounds

Understanding body fluids

- Different types of fluids are located in different compartments.
- Fluids move throughout the body by going back and forth across a cell's semipermeable membrane.
- Distribution of fluids varies with age.

Fluid compartments

- *ICF*—fluid inside the cell; must be balanced with ECF
- *ECF*—fluid outside the cell; must be balanced with ICF; made up of 75% interstitial fluid (fluid surrounding the cell) and 25% plasma (liquid portion of blood)
- *Transcellular fluid*—in the cerebrospinal column, pleural cavity, lymph system, joints, and eyes; remains relatively constant

Fluid types

- *Isotonic*—equally concentrated with other solutions

(continued)

Balancing fluids review *(continued)*

- *Hypotonic*—less concentrated than other solutions
- *Hypertonic*—more concentrated than other solutions

Fluid movement

- *Diffusion*—form of passive transport (no energy is required) that moves solutes from an area of higher concentration to an area of lower concentration, resulting in an equal distribution of solutes between the two areas
- *Active transport*—uses ATP to move solutes from an area of low concentration to an area of higher concentration; example: sodium-potassium pump
- *Osmosis*—passive movement of fluid across a membrane from an area of lower solute concentration to an area of higher solute concentration; stops when both sides have an equal solute concentration
- *Capillary filtration*—movement of fluid through capillary walls through hydrostatic pressure; balanced by plasma colloid osmotic pressure from albumin that causes reabsorption of fluid and solutes

Maintaining fluid balance

Kidneys

- Nephrons form urine by filtering blood.
- If the body needs more fluid, nephron tubules retain or reabsorb water and electrolytes.
- If the body needs less fluid, tubules absorb less, causing more fluids and electrolytes to be excreted.
- Kidneys also secrete renin, an enzyme that activates the renin-angiotensin-aldosterone system.
- Aldosterone secreted by the adrenal cortex regulates sodium and water reabsorption by the kidneys.

Hormones

- *ADH*—Also known as *vasopressin*, ADH is produced by the hypothalamus to reduce diuresis and increase water retention if serum osmolality increases or blood volume decreases.
- *Renin-angiotensin-aldosterone system*—If blood flow decreases, the juxtaglomerular cells in the kidneys secrete renin, which leads to the production of angiotensin II, a powerful vasoconstrictor; angiotensin II stimulates the production of aldosterone; aldosterone regulates the reabsorption of sodium and water in the nephron.
- *ANP*—This hormone, produced and stored in the atria of the heart, stops the action of the renin-angiotensin-aldosterone system; ANP decreases blood pressure by causing vasodilation and reduces fluid volume by increasing excretion of sodium and water.

Thirst

- Regulated by the hypothalamus
- Stimulated by an increase in ECF and drying of the mucous membranes
- Causes a person to drink fluids, which are absorbed by the intestines, moved to the bloodstream, and distributed between the compartments

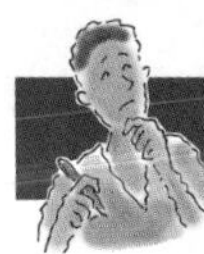

Quick quiz

1. If you were walking across the Sahara Desert with an empty canteen, the amount of ADH secreted would most likely:
   A. increase.
   B. decrease.
   C. stay the same.
   D. have no effect.

Answer: A. Because your body would probably be dehydrated, it would try to retain as much fluid as possible. To retain fluid, ADH secretion increases.

2. If you placed two containers next to each other, separated only by a semipermeable membrane, and the solution in one container was hypotonic relative to the other, fluid in the hypotonic container would:
   A. move out of the hypotonic container into the other.
   B. pull fluid from the other container into the hypotonic container.
   C. cause osmosis to occur.
   D. stay unchanged within the hypotonic container.

Answer: A. Fluid would move out of the hypotonic container into the other container to equalize the concentration of fluid within the two containers. Osmosis occurs when fluid moves from an area with more fluid to an area with less fluid.

3. Hydrostatic pressure, which pushes fluid out of the capillaries, is opposed by colloid osmotic pressure, which involves:
   A. reduced renin secretion.
   B. a decrease in aldosterone.
   C. the pulling power of albumin to reabsorb water.
   D. an increase in ADH secretion.

Answer: C. Albumin in capillaries draws water toward it, a process called *reabsorption*.

4. When a person's blood pressure drops, the kidneys respond by:
   A. secreting renin.
   B. producing aldosterone.
   C. slowing the release of ADH.
   D. secreting ANP.

Answer: A. Juxtaglomerular cells in the kidneys secrete renin in response to low blood flow or a low sodium level. The eventual effect of renin secretion is an increase in blood pressure.

5. Giving a hypertonic I.V. solution to a patient may cause too much fluid to be:

A. pulled from the cells into the bloodstream, which may cause the cells to shrink.
B. pulled out of the bloodstream into the cells.
C. pushed out of the bloodstream into the extravascular spaces.
D. pulled from the cells into the bloodstream, which may cause the cells to increase in size.

Answer: A. Because the concentration of solutes in the I.V. solution is greater than the concentration of solutes in the patient's blood, a hypertonic solution may cause fluid to be pulled from the cells into the bloodstream, causing the cells to shrink.

Scoring

☆☆☆ If you answered all five questions correctly, congratulations! You're a fluid whiz.

☆☆ If you answered four correctly, take a swig of water; you're just a little dry.

☆ If you answered fewer than four correctly, pour yourself a glass of sports drink and enjoy an invigorating burst of fluid refreshment!

References

Ambalavanan, N., & Rosenkrantz, T. (Eds.). (2012). *Fluid, electrolyte, and nutrition management of the newborn*. Retrieved from http://emedicine.medscape.com/article/976386-overview#aw2aab6b3

Seager, S. L., & Slaubaugh, M. L. (2011). *Organic and biochemistry for today* (7th ed., p. 412). Belmont, CA: Brooks/Cole Centage Learning.

Wait, R. B., & Alouidor, R. (2011). Fluids, electrolytes, and acid–base balance. In M. Mulholland et al. (Eds.), *Greenfield's surgery: Scientific principles & practice* (5th ed.). Philadelphia, PA: Lippincott Williams & Wilkins. Retrieved from http://books.google.com/books?id=KkJc0XYVc0IC&pg=PT483&lpg=PT483&dq=normal+24+hour+water+loss+in+stool&source=bl&ots=pIic8DvQj2&sig=65EaVLjtk2O5l0gNL6Wqav6-g4M&hl=en&sa=X&ei=z_XOUrXfFNTBoASSioGgCQ&ved=0CE0Q6AEwBzgK#v=onepage&q=normal%2024%20hour%20water%20loss%20in%20stool&f=false

Chapter 2

Balancing electrolytes

Just the facts

In this chapter, you'll learn:

- the difference between cations and anions
- the interpretation of normal and abnormal serum electrolyte results
- the role nephrons play in electrolyte balance
- the effect diuretics have on electrolytes in the kidneys
- the electrolyte concentration of selected I.V. fluids.

A look at electrolytes

Electrolytes work with fluids to maintain health and well-being. They're found in various concentrations, depending on whether they're inside or outside the cells. Electrolytes are crucial for nearly all cellular reactions and functions. Let's take a look at what electrolytes are, how they function, and what upsets their balance.

If you look closely, you can see that electrolytes are really just electrically charged particles.

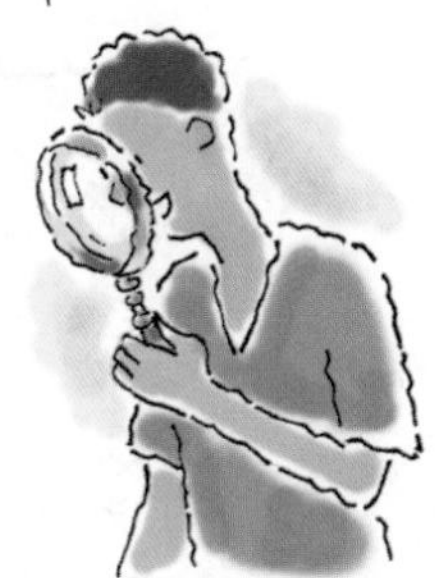

Ions

Electrolytes are substances that, when in solution, separate (or dissociate) into electrically charged particles called *ions*. Some ions are positively charged and others are negatively charged. Several pairs of oppositely charged ions are so closely linked that a problem with one ion causes a problem with the other. Sodium and chloride are linked that way, as are calcium and phosphorus.

A variety of diseases can disrupt the normal balance of electrolytes in the body. Understanding electrolytes and recognizing imbalances can make your patient assessment more accurate.

Anions and cations

Anions are electrolytes that generate a negative charge; cations are electrolytes that produce a positive charge. An electrical charge makes cells function normally. (See *Looking on the plus and minus sides.*)

The anion gap is a useful test for distinguishing types and causes of acid-base imbalances because it reflects serum anion-cation balance. (The anion gap is discussed in chapter 3, Balancing acids and bases.)

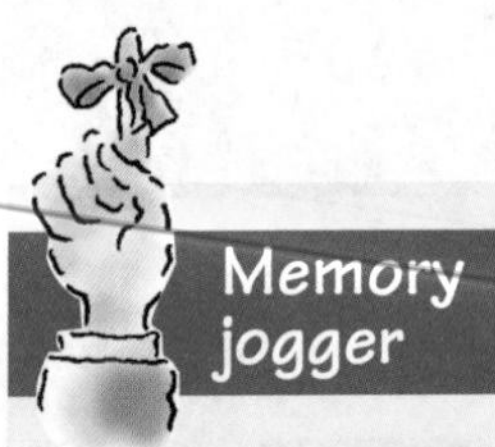

To remind yourself about the difference between anions and cations, remember that the *T* in "cation" looks like the positive symbol, "+."

Balancing the pluses and minuses

Electrolytes operate outside the cell in extracellular fluid compartments and inside the cell in intracellular fluid compartments. Individual electrolytes differ in concentration, but electrolyte totals balance to achieve a neutral electrical charge (positives and negatives balance each other). This balance is called *electroneutrality.*

Hooking up with hydrogen

Most electrolytes interact with hydrogen ions to maintain acid-base balance. The major electrolytes have specialized functions that contribute to metabolism and fluid and electrolyte balance.

Looking on the plus and minus sides

Electrolytes can be either anions or cations. Here's a list of anions (the negative charges) and cations (the positive charges).

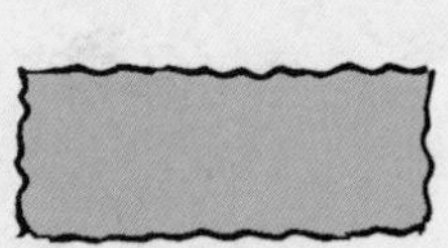

- Bicarbonate
- Chloride
- Phosphorus

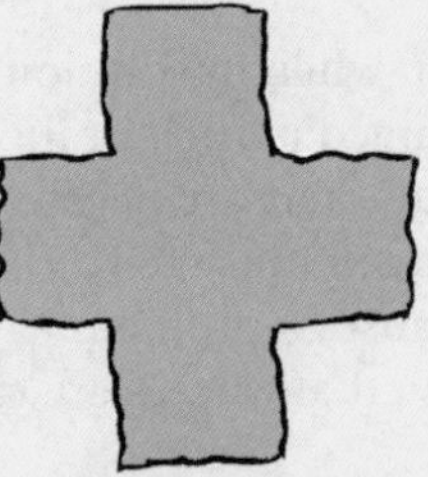

- Calcium
- Magnesium
- Potassium
- Sodium

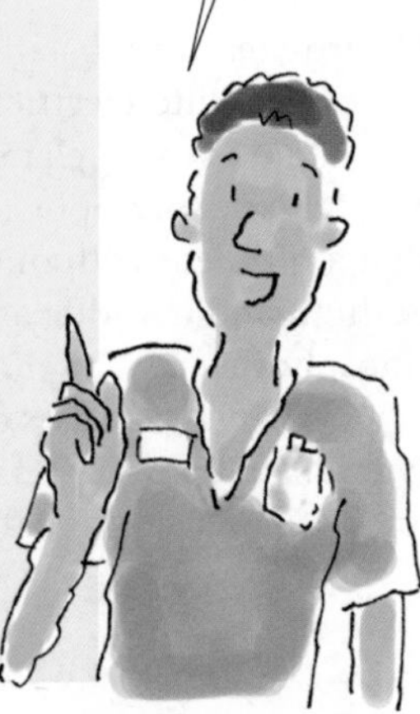

There's a positive and a negative to almost everything.

Major electrolytes outside the cell

Sodium and chloride, the major electrolytes in extracellular fluid, exert most of their influence outside the cell. Sodium concentration affects serum osmolality (solute concentration in 1 L of water) and extracellular fluid volume. Sodium also helps nerve and muscle cells interact. Chloride helps maintain osmotic pressure (water-pulling pressure). Gastric mucosal cells need chloride to produce hydrochloric acid, which breaks down food into absorbable components.

More outsiders

Calcium and bicarbonate are two other electrolytes found in extracellular fluid. Calcium is the major cation involved in the structure and function of bones and teeth. Calcium is needed to:

- stabilize the cell membrane and reduce its permeability to sodium
- transmit nerve impulses
- contract muscles
- coagulate blood
- form bone and teeth.

Bicarbonate plays a vital role in acid-base balance.

Major electrolytes inside the cell

Potassium, phosphorus, and magnesium are among the most abundant electrolytes inside the cell.

Potent potassium

Potassium plays an important role in:

- cell excitability regulation
- nerve impulse conduction
- resting membrane potential
- muscle contraction and myocardial membrane responsiveness
- intracellular osmolality control.

Fundamental phosphorus

The body contains phosphorus in the form of phosphate salts. Sometimes, the words *phosphorus* and *phosphate* are used interchangeably. Phosphate is essential for energy metabolism. Combined with calcium, phosphate plays a key role in bone and tooth mineralization. It also helps maintain acid-base balance.

Magnificent magnesium

Magnesium acts as a catalyst for enzyme reactions. It regulates neuromuscular contraction, promotes normal functioning of the nervous and cardiovascular systems, and aids in protein synthesis and sodium and potassium ion transportation.

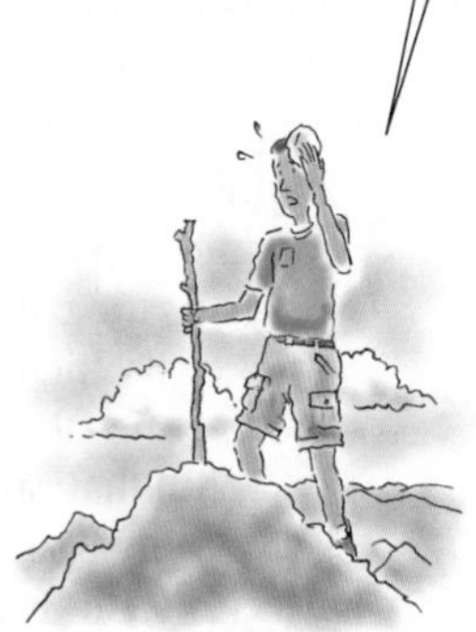

The body needs phosphorus to convert energy. I could use a little extra right now!

Electrolyte movement

When cells die (e.g., from trauma or chemotherapy), their contents spill into the extracellular area and upset the electrolyte balance. In this case, elevated levels of intracellular electrolytes are found in plasma.

Although electrolytes are generally concentrated in a specific compartment, they aren't confined to these areas. Like fluids, they move around trying to maintain balance and electroneutrality.

Electrolyte balance

Fluid intake and output, acid-base balance, hormone secretion, and normal cell function all influence electrolyte balance. Because electrolytes function both collaboratively, with other electrolytes, and individually, imbalances in one electrolyte can affect balance in others. (See *Understanding electrolytes*.)

Electrolyte levels

Even though electrolytes exist inside and outside the cell, only the levels outside the cell in the bloodstream are measured. Although serum levels remain fairly stable throughout a person's life span, understanding which levels are normal and which are abnormal is critical to reacting quickly and appropriately to a patient's electrolyte imbalance.

The patient's condition determines how often electrolyte levels are checked. Results for many laboratory tests are reported in milliequivalents per liter (mEq/L), which is a measure of the ion's chemical activity, or its power. (See *Interpreting serum electrolyte test results*, page 26, for a look at normal and abnormal electrolyte levels in the blood.)

See the whole picture

When you see an abnormal laboratory test result, consider what you know about the patient. For instance, a serum potassium level of 7 mEq/L for a patient with previously normal serum potassium levels and no apparent reason for the increase may be an inaccurate result. Perhaps the patient's blood sample was hemolyzed from trauma to the cells, which can occur when drawing the blood or during transport to the lab.

With that said, look at the whole picture before you act, including what you know about the patient, his signs and symptoms, and his electrolyte levels. (See *Documenting electrolyte imbalances*, page 27.)

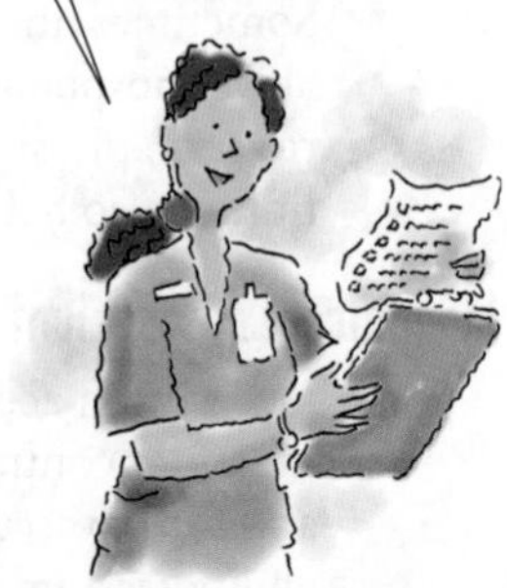
When you see abnormal test results, consider what you know about the patient.

Understanding electrolytes

Electrolytes help regulate water distribution, govern acid-base balance, and transmit nerve impulses. They also contribute to energy generation and blood clotting. This table summarizes the functions of each of the body's major electrolytes. Check the illustration below to see how electrolytes are distributed in and around the cell.

Potassium (K)
- Main intracellular fluid (ICF) cation
- Regulates cell excitability
- Permeates cell membranes, thereby affecting the cell's electrical status
- Helps to control ICF osmolality and, consequently, ICF osmotic pressure

Magnesium (Mg)
- A leading ICF cation
- Contributes to many enzymatic and metabolic processes, particularly protein synthesis
- Modifies nerve impulse transmission and skeletal muscle response (unbalanced Mg concentrations dramatically affect neuromuscular processes)
- Maintains cell membrane stability (Lobo, Lewington, & Allison, 2013)

Phosphorus (P)
- Main ICF anion
- Promotes energy storage and carbohydrate, protein, and fat metabolism
- Acts as a hydrogen buffer

Sodium (Na)
- Main extracellular fluid (ECF) cation
- Helps govern normal ECF osmolality (a shift in Na concentrations triggers a fluid volume change to restore normal solute and water ratios)
- Helps maintain acid-base balance
- Activates nerve and muscle cells
- Influences water distribution (with chloride)

Chloride (Cl)
- Main ECF anion
- Helps maintain normal ECF osmolality
- Affects body pH
- Plays a vital role in maintaining acid-base balance; combines with hydrogen ions to produce hydrochloric acid

Calcium (Ca)
- A major cation in teeth and bones; found in fairly equal concentrations in ICF and ECF
- Also found in cell membranes, where it helps cells adhere to one another and maintain their shape
- Acts as an enzyme activator within cells (muscles must have Ca to contract)
- Aids coagulation
- Affects cell membrane permeability and firing level

Bicarbonate (HCO_3^-)
- Present in ECF
- Regulates acid-base balance

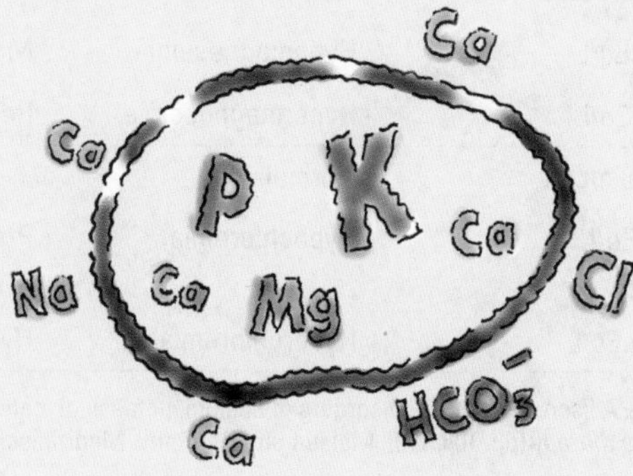

Interpreting serum electrolyte test results

Use the quick-reference chart below to interpret serum electrolyte test results in adult patients. This chart also lists disorders that can cause imbalances. Note: Always check your facility's norms, as they may differ slightly.

Electrolyte	Results	Implications	Common causes
Serum sodium	135 to 145 mEq/L	Normal	
	< 135 mEq/L	Hyponatremia	Syndrome of inappropriate antidiuretic hormone secretion
	> 145 mEq/L	Hypernatremia	Diabetes insipidus, diabetes mellitus, fluid loss, vomiting, and diarrhea
Serum potassium	3.5 to 5 mEq/L	Normal	
	< 3.5 mEq/L	Hypokalemia	Diarrhea, vomiting, diuretic therapy, excessive sweating, refeeding syndrome
	> 5 mEq/L	Hyperkalemia	Burns, renal failure, and response to injury
Total serum calcium	8.9 to 10.1 mg/dl	Normal	
	< 8.9 mg/dl	Hypocalcemia	Acute pancreatitis
	> 10.1 mg/dl	Hypercalcemia	Hyperparathyroidism
Ionized calcium	4.4 to 5.3 mg/dl	Normal	
	< 4.4 mg/dl	Hypocalcemia	Massive transfusion
	> 5.3 mg/dl	Hypercalcemia	Acidosis
Serum phosphates	2.5 to 4.5 mg/dl or 1.8 to 2.6 mEq/L	Normal	
	< 2.5 mg/dl or 1.8 mEq/L	Hypophosphatemia	Diabetic ketoacidosis
	> 4.5 mg/dl or 2.6 mEq/L	Hyperphosphatemia	Renal insufficiency
Serum magnesium	1.5 to 2.5 mEq/L	Normal	
	< 1.5 mEq/L	Hypomagnesemia	Malnutrition, chronic diarrhea
	> 2.5 mEq/L	Hypermagnesemia	Renal failure
Serum chloride	98 to 108 mEq/L	Normal	
	< 98 mEq/L	Hypochloremia	Prolonged vomiting or gastric aspiration
	> 108 mEq/L	Hyperchloremia	Hypernatremia

From Lobo, D. N., Lewington, A. J. P., & Allison, S. P. (2013). Disorders of sodium, potassium, calcium, magnesium, and phosphate. In *Basic concepts of fluid and electrolyte therapy* (pp. 105, 110). Melsungen, Germany: Medizinische Verlagsgesellschaft.

Fluid regulation

Many activities and factors are involved in regulating fluid and electrolyte balance. A quick review of some of the basics will help you understand this regulation better.

Fluid and solute movement

As discussed in chapter 1, active transport moves solutes upstream and requires pumps within the body to move the substances from areas of lower concentration to areas of higher concentration—against a concentration gradient. Adenosine triphosphate (ATP) is the energy that moves solutes upstream.

Pushing fluids

The sodium-potassium pump, an example of an active transport mechanism, moves sodium ions from intracellular fluid (an area of lower concentration) to extracellular fluid (an area of higher concentration). With potassium, the reverse happens: A large amount of potassium in intracellular fluid causes an electrical potential at the cell membrane. As ions rapidly shift in and out of the cell, electrical impulses are conducted. These impulses are essential for maintaining life.

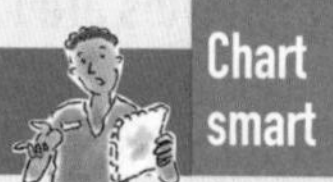

Documenting electrolyte imbalances

Be sure to include the following information in your documentation of a patient's electrolyte imbalance:

- assessment findings
- laboratory results pertaining to the imbalance
- related nursing diagnoses
- notification and response of the practitioner
- interventions and treatment for the electrolyte imbalance, including safety measures
- patient teaching
- patient's response to interventions.

Organ and gland involvement

Most major organs and glands in the body—the lungs, liver, adrenal glands, kidneys, heart, hypothalamus, pituitary gland, skin, gastrointestinal (GI) tract, and parathyroid and thyroid glands—help to regulate fluid and electrolyte balance.

As part of the renin-angiotensin-aldosterone system, the lungs and liver help regulate sodium and water balance as well as blood pressure. The adrenal glands secrete aldosterone, which influences sodium and potassium balance in the kidneys. These levels are affected because the kidneys excrete potassium, or hydrogen ions, in exchange for retained sodium.

The heart says no

The heart counteracts the renin-angiotensin-aldosterone system when it secretes atrial natriuretic peptide (ANP), causing sodium excretion. The hypothalamus and posterior pituitary gland produce and secrete an antidiuretic hormone that causes the body to retain water which, in turn, affects solute concentration in the blood.

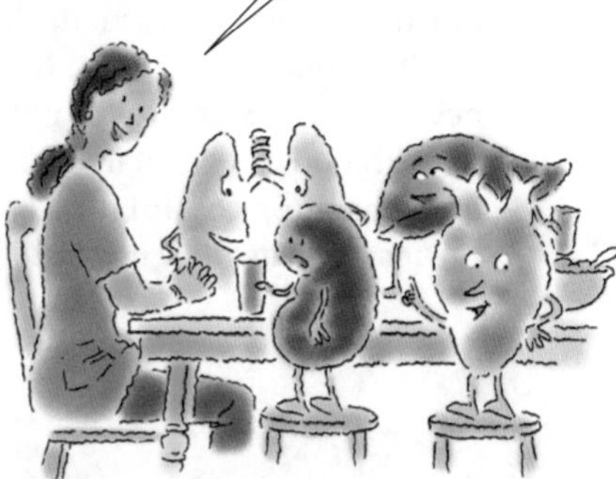
Most major organs in the body help to regulate fluid and electrolyte balance.

Where electrolytes are lost

Sodium, potassium, chloride, and water are lost in sweat and from the GI tract; however, electrolytes are also absorbed from the GI tract. Discussions of individual electrolytes in upcoming chapters explain how GI absorption of foods and fluids affects their balance.

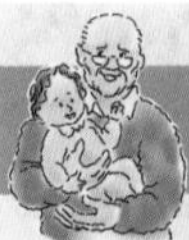

Ages and stages

Who's at risk?

The immature kidneys of an infant can't concentrate urine or reabsorb electrolytes the way the kidneys of an adult can, so infants are at a higher risk for electrolyte imbalances.

Older adults are also at risk for electrolyte imbalances. Their kidneys have fewer functional nephrons, a decreased glomerular filtration rate, and a diminished ability to concentrate urine.

The glands play on

The parathyroid glands also play a role in electrolyte balance, specifically the balance of calcium and phosphorus. The parathyroid glands (usually two pairs) are located behind and to the side of the thyroid gland. They secrete parathyroid hormone, which draws calcium into the blood from the bones, intestines, and kidneys and helps move phosphorus from the blood to the kidneys, where it's excreted in urine.

The thyroid gland is also involved in electrolyte balance by secreting calcitonin. This hormone lowers an elevated calcium level by preventing calcium release from bone. Calcitonin also decreases intestinal absorption and kidney reabsorption of calcium.

Kidney involvement

Remember filtration? It's the process of removing particles from a solution by allowing the liquid portion to pass through a membrane. Filtration occurs in the nephron (the anatomic and functional unit of the kidneys). As blood circulates through the glomerulus (a tuft of capillaries), fluids and electrolytes are filtered and collected in the nephron's tubule.

Some fluids and electrolytes are reabsorbed through capillaries at various points along the nephron; others are secreted. Age can play an important role in the way kidneys function—or malfunction. (See *Who's at risk?*)

I'm a master at juggling electrolyte levels.

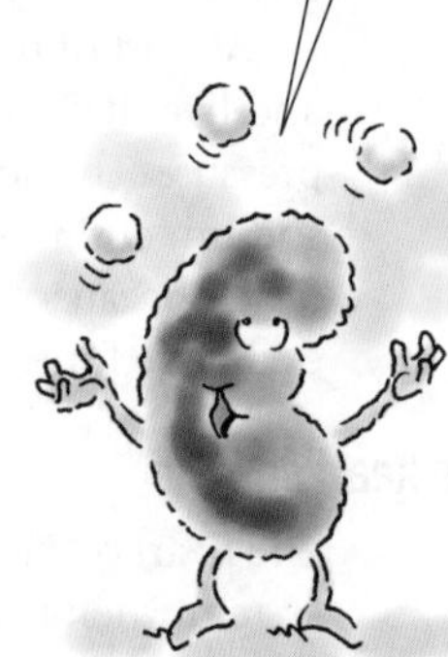

A juggling act

A vital part of the kidneys' job is to regulate electrolyte levels in the body. Normally functioning kidneys maintain the correct fluid level in the body. Sodium and fluid balance are closely related. When too much sodium is released, the body's fluid level drops.

The kidneys also rid the body of excess potassium. When the kidneys fail, potassium builds up in the body. High levels of potassium in the blood can be fatal. (For more information about which areas of the nephron control fluid and electrolyte balance, see *How the nephron regulates fluid and electrolyte balance.*)

How the nephron regulates fluid and electrolyte balance

In this illustration, the nephron has been stretched to show where and how fluids and electrolytes are regulated.

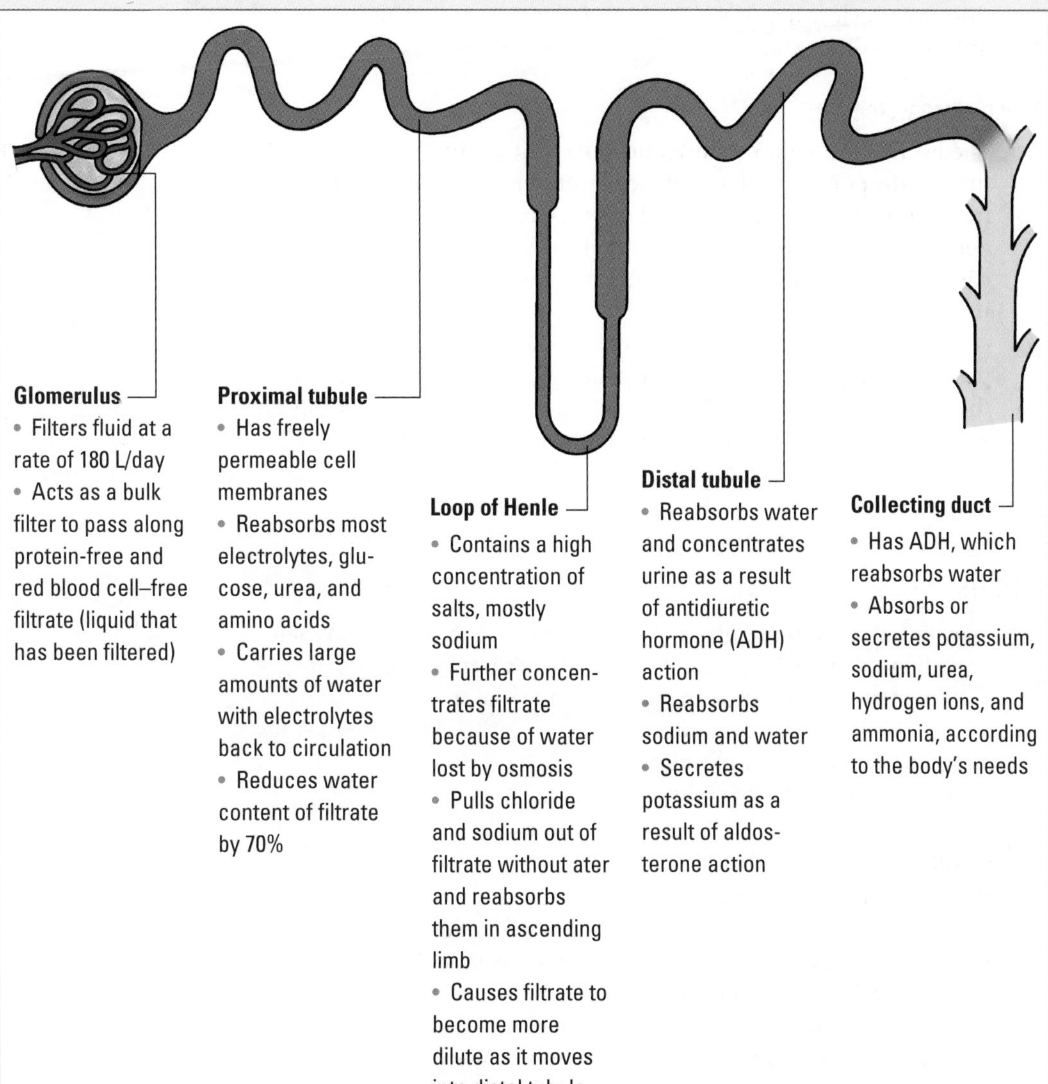
Glomerulus
• Filters fluid at a rate of 180 L/day
• Acts as a bulk filter to pass along protein-free and red blood cell–free filtrate (liquid that has been filtered)
Proximal tubule
• Has freely permeable cell membranes
• Reabsorbs most electrolytes, glucose, urea, and amino acids
• Carries large amounts of water with electrolytes back to circulation
• Reduces water content of filtrate by 70%
Loop of Henle
• Contains a high concentration of salts, mostly sodium
• Further concentrates filtrate because of water lost by osmosis
• Pulls chloride and sodium out of filtrate without ater and reabsorbs them in ascending limb
• Causes filtrate to become more dilute as it moves into distal tubule
Distal tubule
• Reabsorbs water and concentrates urine as a result of antidiuretic hormone (ADH) action
• Reabsorbs sodium and water
• Secretes potassium as a result of aldosterone action
Collecting duct
• Has ADH, which reabsorbs water
• Absorbs or secretes potassium, sodium, urea, hydrogen ions, and ammonia, according to the body's needs

How diuretics affect balance

Many patients—whether in a medical facility or at home—take a diuretic to increase urine production. Diuretics are used to treat many disorders, such as hypertension, heart failure, electrolyte imbalances, and kidney disease.

Keeping a close watch

The health care team monitors the effects of a diuretic, including its effect on electrolyte balance. A diuretic may cause electrolyte loss, whereas an I.V. fluid causes electrolyte gain. Older adults, who are at risk for fluid and electrolyte imbalances, need careful monitoring because a diuretic can worsen an existing imbalance.

When you know how the nephron functions normally, you can predict a diuretic's effects on your patient by knowing where along the nephron the drug acts. This knowledge and understanding can help you provide optimal care for a patient taking a diuretic. (See *How drugs affect nephron activity*.)

I.V. fluids

Like diuretics, I.V. fluids affect electrolyte balance in the body. When providing I.V. fluid, keep in mind the patient's normal electrolyte requirements. For instance, the patient may require:

- 1 to 2 mEq/kg/day of sodium
- 0.5 to 1 mEq/kg/day of potassium
- 1 to 2 mEq/kg/day of chloride.

Improving your I.V. IQ

To evaluate I.V. fluid treatment, ask:

- Is the I.V. fluid providing the correct amount of electrolytes?
- How long has the patient been receiving I.V. fluids?
- Is the patient receiving oral supplementation of electrolytes?

For more about I.V. fluids, see chapter 19, I.V. fluid replacement. (For the electrolyte content of some commonly used I.V. fluids, see *I.V. fluid components*, page 32.)

How drugs affect nephron activity

Here's a look at how certain diuretics and other drugs affect the nephron's regulation of fluid and electrolyte balance.

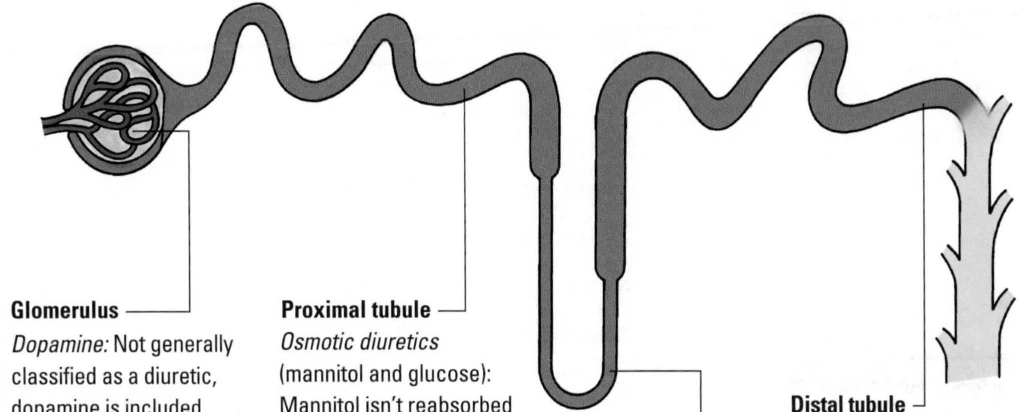

Glomerulus

Dopamine: Not generally classified as a diuretic, dopamine is included here because it may increase urine output. Dopaminergic receptor sites exist along the afferent arterioles (tiny vessels that bring blood to the glomerulus). In low doses (0.5 to 3 mcg/kg/minute), dopamine dilates these vessels in the glomerulus to increase blood flow to it. This, in turn, increases filtration in the nephron.

Proximal tubule

Osmotic diuretics (mannitol and glucose): Mannitol isn't reabsorbed in the tubule; it remains in high concentrations throughout its journey, increasing filtrate osmolality and hindering water, sodium, and chloride reabsorption, thereby increasing their excretion.

High blood glucose levels cause excess glucose to spill over into the tubules. The osmotic effect of glucose also results in increased urine output.

Carbonic anhydrase inhibitors (acetazolamide [Di-amox]): These drugs reduce hydrogen ion (acid) concentration in the tubule, which causes increased excretion of bicarbonate, water, sodium, and potassium.

Loop of Henle

Loop diuretics (furosemide [Lasix], bumetanide [Bumex], and ethacrynic acid [Edecrin]): Loop diuretics act on the ascending loop of Henle to prevent water and sodium reabsorption. As a result, volume in the tubules is increased and blood volume is decreased. Potassium and chloride are also excreted here.

Distal tubule

Thiazide diuretics (hydrochlorothiazide [HydroDIURIL] and metolazone [Zaroxolyn]): Thiazide diuretics act high in the distal tubule to prevent sodium reabsorption, which increases the amount of tubular fluid and electrolytes farther down the nephron. Blood volume decreases, aldosterone increases sodium reabsorption and, in exchange, potassium is lost from the body.

Potassium-sparing diuretics (spironolactone [Aldactone]): These diuretics interfere with sodium and chloride reabsorption in the tubule. Potassium is spared, and sodium, chloride, and water are excreted. Urine output increases, and the body retains potassium.

I.V. fluid components

This table lists the electrolyte content of some commonly used I.V. fluids.

I.V. solution	Electrolyte	Amount
Dextrose	None	—
Sodium chloride		
5%	Sodium chloride	855 mEq/L
3%	Sodium chloride	513 mEq/L
0.9%	Sodium chloride	154 mEq/L
0.45%	Sodium chloride	77 mEq/L
Dextrose and sodium chloride		
5% dextrose and 0.9% sodium chloride	Sodium chloride	154 mEq/L
5% dextrose and 0.45% sodium chloride	Sodium chloride	77 mEq/L
Ringer's solution (plain)		
	Chloride	156 mEq/L
	Sodium	147 mEq/L
	Calcium	4.5 mEq/L
	Potassium	4 mEq/L
Lactated Ringer's solution		
	Sodium	130 mEq/L
	Chloride	109 mEq/L
	Lactate	28 mEq/L
	Potassium	4 mEq/L
	Calcium	3 mEq/L

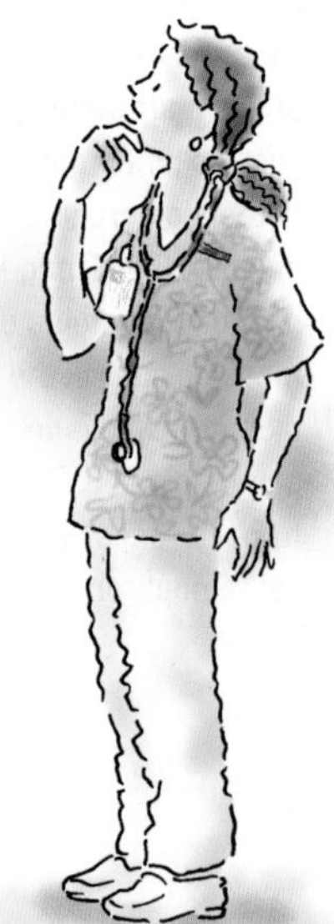

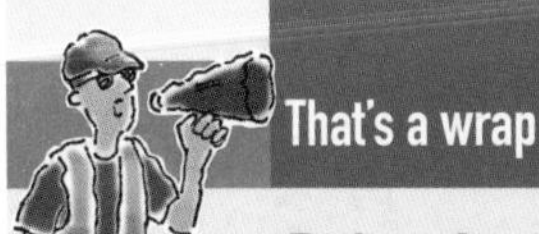

That's a wrap!

Balancing electrolytes review

Electrolyte basics
- Found throughout the body in various concentrations
- Critical to cell function

Ions, anions, cations
- *Ions*—electrically charged particles created when electrolytes separate in a solution; may be positively or negatively charged
- *Anions*—negatively charged electrolytes; include chloride, phosphorus, and bicarbonate
- *Cations*—positively charged electrolytes; include sodium, potassium, calcium, and magnesium
- *Electroneutrality*—positive and negative ions balance each other out, achieving a neutral electrical charge

Major extracellular electrolytes
- *Sodium*—helps nerve cells and muscle cells interact
- *Chloride*—maintains osmotic pressure and helps gastric mucosal cells produce hydrochloric acid
- *Calcium*—stabilizes cell membrane, reducing its permeability; transmits nerve impulses; contracts muscles; coagulates blood; and forms bones and teeth
- *Bicarbonate*—regulates acid-base balance

Major intracellular electrolytes
- *Potassium*—regulates cell excitability, nerve impulse conduction, resting membrane potential, muscle contraction, myocardial membrane responsiveness, and intracellular osmolality
- *Phosphate*—controls energy metabolism
- *Magnesium*—influences enzyme reactions, neuromuscular contractions, normal functioning of nervous and cardiovascular system, protein synthesis, and sodium and potassium ion transportation

Influences on electrolyte balance
- Normal cell function
- Fluid intake and output
- Acid-base balance
- Hormone secretion

Maintaining electrolyte balance
- Most major organs and glands in the body help regulate fluid and electrolyte balance.

The role of organs and glands
- *Kidneys*—regulate sodium and potassium balance (excrete potassium in exchange for sodium retention)
- *Lungs and liver*—regulate sodium and water balance and blood pressure
- *Heart*—secretes ANP, causing sodium excretion
- *Sweat glands*—excrete sodium, potassium, chloride, and water in sweat
- *GI tract*—absorbs and excretes fluids and electrolytes
- *Parathyroid glands*—secrete parathyroid hormone, which draws calcium into the blood and helps move phosphorous to the kidneys for excretion
- *Thyroid gland*—secretes calcitonin, which prevents calcium release from the bone

• *Hypothalamus and posterior pituitary*—produce and secrete antidiuretic hormone causing water retention, which affects solute concentration
• *Adrenal glands*—secrete aldosterone, which influences sodium and potassium balance in the kidneys

The effect of diuretics
• Treat hypertension, heart failure, electrolyte imbalances, and kidney disease
• Increase urine production
• Cause loss of electrolytes, particularly potassium
• Require careful monitoring of electrolytes

Key issues in I.V. fluid treatment
• Patient's normal electrolyte requirements
• Correct amount of electrolytes prescribed and given
• Length of treatment
• Concomitant oral electrolyte supplementation

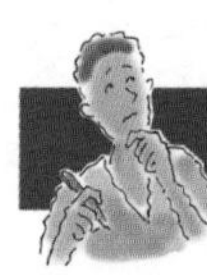

Quick quiz

1. When a burn damages cells, you would expect the cells to release the major electrolyte:
   A. potassium.
   B. chloride.
   C. calcium.
   D. sodium.

Answer: A. Potassium is one of the major electrolytes inside the cell that leaks out into extracellular fluid after a major trauma, such as a burn. This puts the patient at risk for hyperkalemia.

2. Diuretics affect the kidneys by altering the reabsorption and excretion of:
   A. water only.
   B. electrolytes only.
   C. water and electrolytes.
   D. other drugs.

Answer: C. Diuretics generally affect how much water and sodium the body excretes. At the same time, other electrolytes such as potassium can also be excreted in urine.

3. The main extracellular cation is:
   A. calcium.
   B. potassium.
   C. bicarbonate.
   D. sodium.

Answer: D. Sodium is the main extracellular cation. In addition to other functions, it helps regulate fluid balance in the body.

4. In the nephron, most electrolytes are reabsorbed in the:
   A. proximal tubule.
   B. glomerulus.
   C. loop of Henle.
   D. distal tubule.

Answer: A. The proximal tubule reabsorbs most electrolytes from the filtrate. It also reabsorbs glucose, urea, amino acids, and water.

5. Potassium is essential for conducting electrical impulses because it causes ions to:
   A. clump together to generate a current.
   B. shift in and out of the cell to conduct a current.
   C. trap sodium inside the cell to maintain a current.
   D. adhere to each other to create a current.

Answer: B. Potassium in the intracellular fluid causes ions to shift in and out of the cell, which allows electrical impulses to be conducted from cell to cell.

6. Older adults are at increased risk for electrolyte imbalances because, with age, the kidneys have:
   A. increased glomerular filtration rate.
   B. fewer functioning nephrons.
   C. increased ability to concentrate urine.
   D. increased blood flow.

Answer: B. Older adults are at increased risk for electrolyte imbalances because their kidneys have fewer functioning nephrons, a decreased glomerular filtration rate, and a diminished ability to concentrate urine.

Scoring

☆☆☆ If you answered all six questions correctly, congratulations! You understand balance so well, you're ready to walk the high wire.

☆☆ If you answered four or five correctly, great! You still have all the qualities of a well-balanced individual!

☆ If you answered fewer than four correctly, no need to feel too unbalanced! Just review the chapter and you'll be fine.

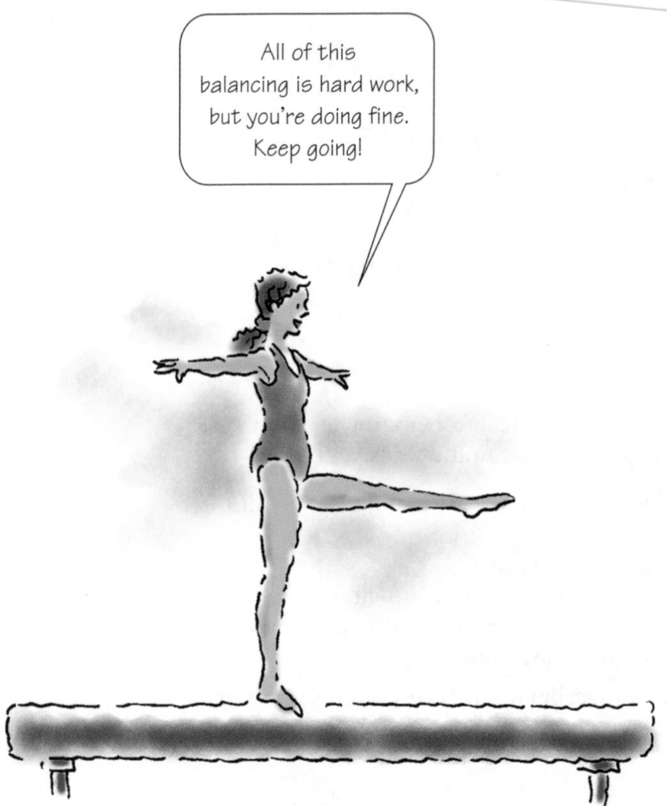
All of this
balancing is hard work,
but you're doing fine.
Keep going!

Reference

Lobo, D. N., Lewington, A. J. P., & Allison, S. P. (2013). Disorders of sodium, potassium, calcium, magnesium, and phosphate. In *Basic concepts of fluid and electrolyte therapy* (pp. 105, 110). Melsungen, Germany: Medizinische Verlagsgesellschaft.

Chapter 3

Balancing acids and bases

Just the facts

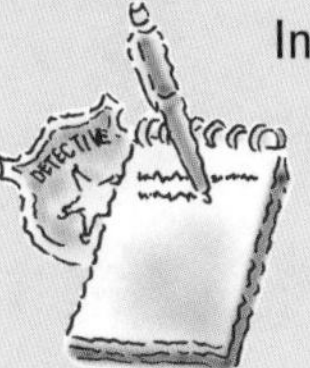

In this chapter, you'll learn:

- the definitions of acids and bases
- the role pH plays in metabolism
- regulation of acid-base balance in the body
- essential diagnostic tests for assessing acid-base balance.

A look at acids and bases

The chemical reactions that sustain life depend on a delicate balance—or homeostasis—between acids and bases in the body. Even a slight imbalance can profoundly affect metabolism and essential body functions. Several conditions, such as infection or trauma, and medications can affect acid-base balance. However, to understand this balance, you need to understand some basic chemistry.

Understanding pH

Understanding acids and bases requires an understanding of pH, a calculation based on the percentage of hydrogen ions in a solution as well as the amount of acids and bases.

Acids consist of molecules that can give up, or donate, hydrogen ions to other molecules. Carbonic acid is an acid that occurs naturally in the body. Bases consist of molecules that can accept hydrogen ions; bicarbonate is one example of a base.

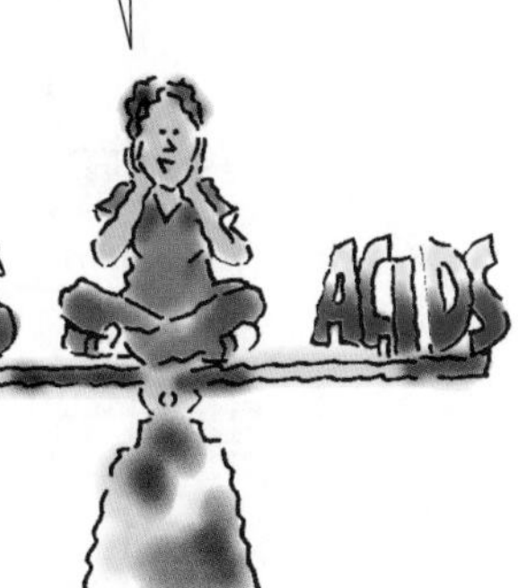

To understand acid-base balance, you must understand a little chemistry. Think I can learn it by osmosis?
BASES
ACIDS

A solution that contains more base than acid has fewer hydrogen ions, so it has a higher pH. A solution with a pH above 7 is a base, or alkaline. A solution that contains more acid than base has more hydrogen ions, so it has a lower pH. A solution with a pH below 7 is an acid, or acidotic.

Getting your PhD in pH

You can assess a patient's acid-base balance if you know the pH of his blood. Because arterial blood is usually used to measure pH, this discussion focuses on arterial samples.

Arterial blood is normally slightly alkaline, ranging from 7.35 to 7.45. A pH level within that range represents a balance between the percentage of hydrogen ions and bicarbonate ions. Generally, pH is maintained in a ratio of 20 parts bicarbonate to 1 part carbonic acid. A pH below 6.8 or above 7.8 is usually fatal. (See *Understanding normal pH*.)

Too low

Under certain conditions, the pH of arterial blood may deviate significantly from its normal narrow range. If the blood's hydrogen ion concentration increases or bicarbonate level decreases, pH may decrease. In either case, a decrease in pH below 7.35 signals acidosis. (See *Understanding acidosis*.)

Understanding normal pH

This illustration shows that blood pH normally stays slightly alkaline, between 7.35 and 7.45. At that point, the amount of acid (H+) is balanced with the amount of base (represented here as bicarbonate). A pH below 7.35 is abnormally acidic; a pH above 7.45 is abnormally alkaline.

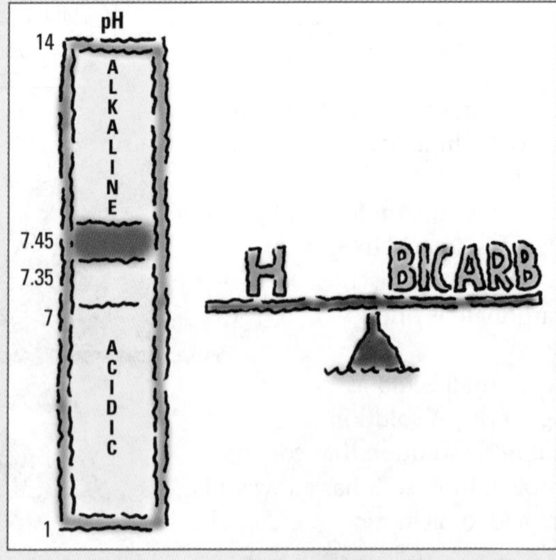

Understanding acidosis

Acidosis, a condition in which pH is below 7.35, occurs when acids (H+) accumulate or bases, such as bicarbonate, are lost.

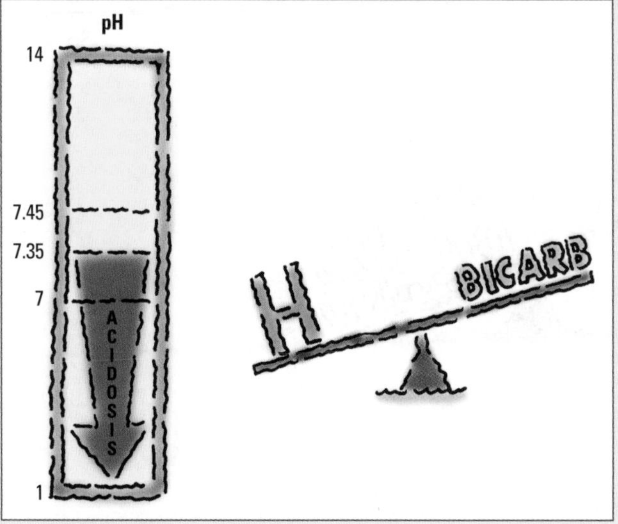

Too high

If the blood's bicarbonate level increases or hydrogen ion concentration decreases—the opposite effect of a low pH—pH may increase. In either case, an increase in pH above 7.45 signals alkalosis. (See *Understanding alkalosis,* page 40.)

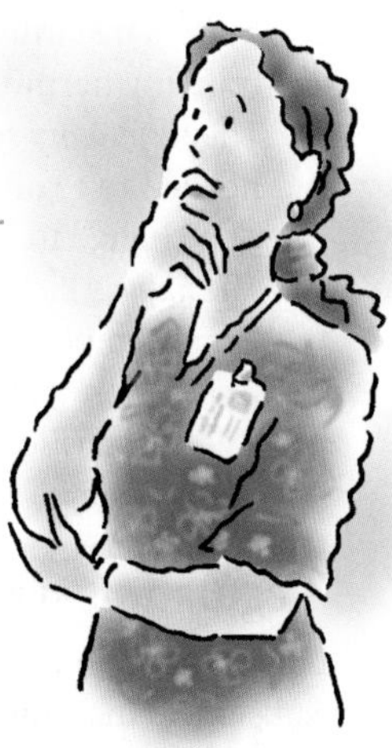

Regulating acids and bases

A person's well-being depends on his ability to maintain a normal pH. A deviation in pH can compromise essential body processes, including electrolyte balance, activity of critical enzymes, muscle contraction, and basic cellular function. The body normally maintains pH within a narrow range by carefully balancing acidic and alkaline elements. When one aspect of that balancing act breaks down, the body can't maintain a healthy pH as easily, and problems arise.

Understanding alkalosis

Alkalosis, a condition in which pH is higher than 7.45, occurs when bases, such as bicarbonate, accumulate or acids (H+) are lost.

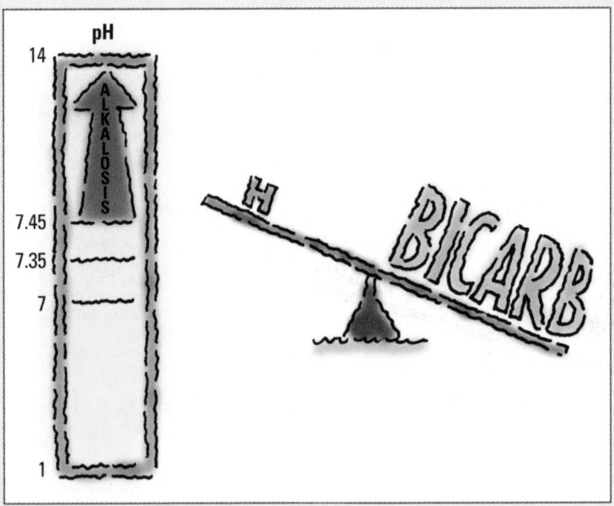

The big three

The body regulates acids and bases to avoid potentially serious consequences. Therefore, when pH rises or falls, three regulatory systems come into play:

- *Chemical buffers* act immediately to protect tissues and cells. These buffers instantly combine with the offending acid or base, neutralizing harmful effects until other regulators take over.
- The *respiratory system* uses hypoventilation or hyperventilation as needed to regulate excretion or retention of acids within minutes of a change in pH.
- The *kidneys* kick in by excreting or retaining acids and bases as needed. Renal compensation kicks in after the aforementioned systems fail to restore normal pH levels, typically after approximately 6 hours of alkalosis or acidosis (Appel & Downs, 2008). Renal regulation can take hours or days to restore normal hydrogen ion concentration.

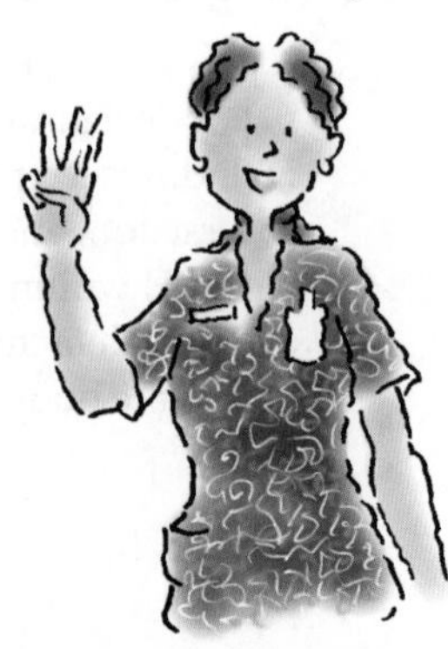
When pH rises or falls, the body uses three regulatory systems: chemical buffers, the respiratory system, and the kidneys.

Regulation system 1: Buffers

The body maintains a healthy pH in part through chemical buffers, substances that minimize changes in pH by combining with excess acids or bases. Chemical buffers in the blood, intracellular fluid, and interstitial fluid serve as the body's most efficient pH-balancing weapon. The main chemical buffers are bicarbonate, phosphate, and protein.

Bring on the bicarbonate

The bicarbonate buffer system is the body's primary buffer system. It's mainly responsible for buffering blood and interstitial fluid. This system relies on a series of chemical reactions in which pairs of weak acids and bases (such as carbonic acid and bicarbonate) combine with stronger acids (such as hydrochloric acid) and bases to weaken them.

Decreasing the strength of potentially damaging acids and bases reduces the danger those chemicals pose to pH balance. The kidneys assist the bicarbonate buffer system by regulating production of bicarbonate. The lungs assist by regulating the production of carbonic acid, which results from combining carbon dioxide and water.

Feeling better with phosphate

Like the bicarbonate buffer system, the phosphate buffer system depends on a series of chemical reactions to minimize pH changes. Phosphate buffers react with either acids or bases to form compounds that slightly alter pH, which can provide extremely effective buffering. This system proves especially effective in renal tubules, where phosphates exist in greater concentrations.

Plenty of protein

Protein buffers, the most plentiful buffers in the body, work inside and outside cells. They're made up of hemoglobin as well as other proteins. Behaving chemically like bicarbonate buffers, protein buffers bind with acids and bases to neutralize them. In red blood cells, for instance, hemoglobin combines with hydrogen ions to act as a buffer.

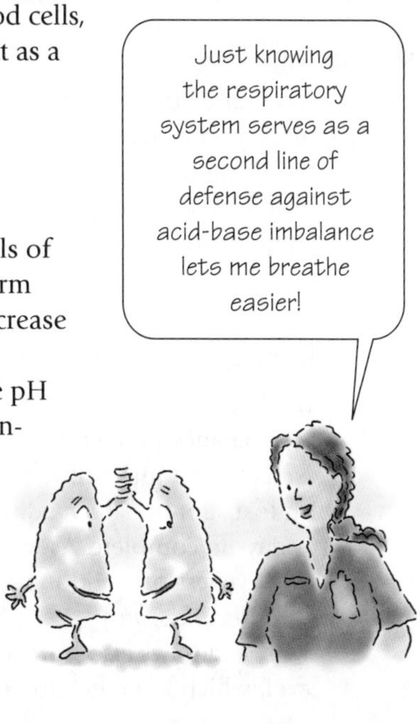

Regulation system 2: Respiration

The respiratory system serves as the second line of defense against acid-base imbalances. The lungs regulate blood levels of carbon dioxide (CO_2), a gas that combines with water to form carbonic acid. Increased levels of carbonic acid lead to a decrease in pH.

Chemoreceptors in the medulla of the brain sense those pH changes and vary the rate and depth of breathing to compensate. Breathing faster or deeper eliminates more carbon dioxide from the lungs. The more carbon dioxide that is lost, the less carbonic acid that is made and, as a result, pH rises. The body detects that pH change and reduces carbon dioxide excretion by breathing slower or less deeply. (See *Carbon dioxide and hyperventilation,* page 42.)

Just knowing the respiratory system serves as a second line of defense against acid-base imbalance lets me breathe easier!

Carbon dioxide and hyperventilation

When a patient's rate of breathing increases, the body blows off carbon dioxide, and carbon dioxide level drops.

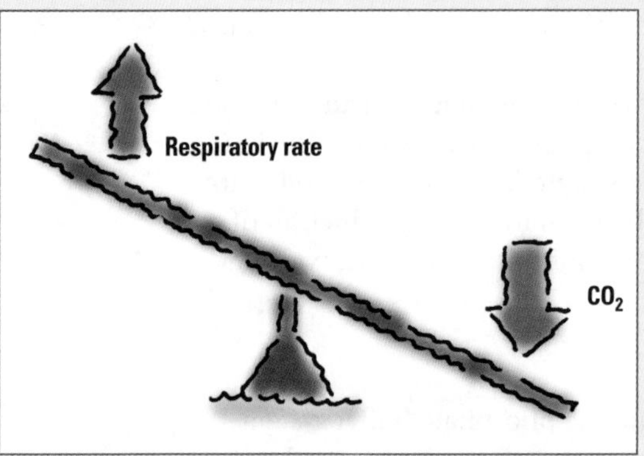

Check for success

To assess the effectiveness of ventilation, look at the partial pressure of carbon dioxide in arterial blood ($PaCO_2$). A normal $PaCO_2$ level in the body is 35 to 45 mm Hg. $PaCO_2$ values reflect carbon dioxide levels in the blood. As those levels increase, so does $PaCO_2$.

Twice as good

As a buffer, the respiratory system can maintain acid-base balance twice as effectively as chemical buffers because it can handle twice the amount of acids and bases. Although the respiratory system responds to pH changes within minutes, it can restore normal pH only temporarily. The kidneys are responsible for long-term adjustments to pH.

Regulation system 3: Kidneys

The kidneys serve as yet another mechanism for maintaining acid-base balance in the body. They can reabsorb acids and bases or excrete them into urine. They can also produce bicarbonate to replenish lost supplies. Such adjustments to pH can take the kidneys hours or days to complete. As with other acid-base regulatory systems, the effectiveness of the kidneys changes with age. (See *Acid-base balance across the life span.*)

The kidneys also have a part in the regulation of the bicarbonate level, which is a reflection of the metabolic component of acid-base

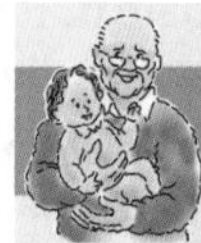

Ages and stages

Acid-base balance across the life span

The effectiveness of the systems that regulate acid-base balance vary with age. For example, an infant's kidneys can't acidify urine as well as an adult's can. Also, the respiratory system of an older adult may be compromised and, therefore, less able to regulate acid-base balance.
In addition, because ammonia production decreases with age, the kidneys of an older adult can't handle excess acid as well as the kidneys of a younger adult.

balance. Normally, the bicarbonate level is reported with arterial blood gas (ABG) results. The normal bicarbonate level is 22 to 26 mEq/L.

The kidneys keep working

If the blood contains too much acid or not enough base, pH drops and the kidneys reabsorb sodium bicarbonate. The kidneys also excrete hydrogen along with phosphate or ammonia. Although urine tends to be acidic because the body usually produces slightly more acids than bases, in such situations, urine becomes more acidic than normal.

The reabsorption of bicarbonate and the increased excretion of hydrogen causes more bicarbonate to be formed in the renal tubules and eventually retained in the body. The bicarbonate level in the blood then rises to a more normal level, increasing pH.

Ups and downs of acids and bases

If the blood contains more base and less acid, pH rises. The kidneys compensate by excreting bicarbonate and retaining more hydrogen ions. As a result, urine becomes more alkaline and blood bicarbonate level drops. Conversely, if the blood contains less bicarbonate and more acid, pH drops.

Altogether now

The body responds to acid-base imbalances by activating compensatory mechanisms that minimize pH changes. Returning the pH to a normal or near-normal level mainly involves changes in the component—metabolic or respiratory—not primarily affected by the imbalance.

If the body compensates only partially for an imbalance, pH remains outside the normal range. If the body compensates fully or completely, pH returns to normal.

Respiratory helps metabolic . . .

If metabolic disturbance is the primary cause of an acid-base imbalance, the lungs compensate in one of two ways. When a lack of bicarbonate causes acidosis, the lungs increase the rate of breathing, which blows off carbon dioxide and helps raise the pH to normal. When an excess of bicarbonate causes alkalosis, the lungs decrease the rate of breathing, which retains carbon dioxide and helps lower pH.

When a lack of bicarbonate causes acidosis, the lungs increase the rate of breathing, which blows off carbon dioxide. Want some excess carbon dioxide, cheap?

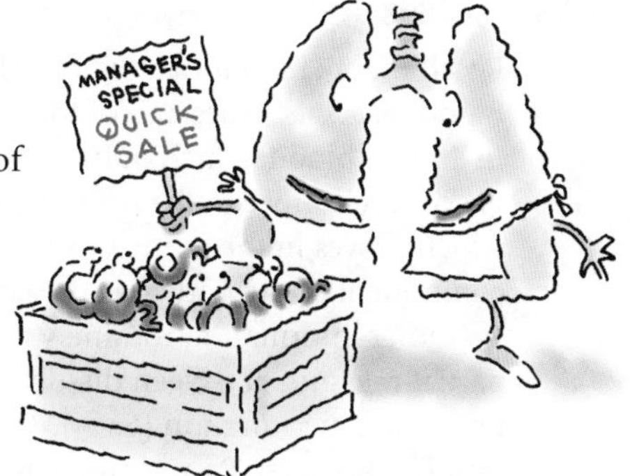

. . . And vice versa

If the respiratory system disturbs the acid-base balance, the kidneys compensate by altering levels of bicarbonate and hydrogen ions. When $Paco_2$ is high (a state of acidosis), the kidneys retain bicarbonate and excrete more acid to raise the pH. When $Paco_2$ is low (a state of alkalosis), the kidneys excrete bicarbonate and hold on to more acid to lower the pH.

Memory jogger

Remember, $Paco_2$ and pH move in opposite directions. If $Paco_2$ rises, then pH falls, and vice versa.

Diagnosing imbalances

A number of tests are used to diagnose acid-base disturbances. Here's a look at the most commonly used tests.

Arterial blood gas analysis

An ABG analysis is a diagnostic test in which a sample of blood obtained from an arterial puncture can be used to assess the effectiveness of breathing and overall acid-base balance. In addition to helping you identify problems with oxygenation and acid-base imbalances, the test can help you monitor a patient's response to treatment. (See *Taking an ABG sample*.)

Keep in mind that ABG analysis should be used only in conjunction with a full patient assessment. Only by assessing all information can you gain a clear picture of what's happening.

An ABG analysis involves several separate test results, only three of which relate to acid-base balance: pH, $Paco_2$, and bicarbonate level. The normal ranges for adults are:

- pH—7.35 to 7.45
- $Paco_2$—35 to 45 mm Hg
- bicarbonate—22 to 26 mEq/L.

The ABCs of ABGs

Recall that pH is a measure of the hydrogen ion concentration of blood; $Paco_2$ is a measure of the partial pressure of carbon dioxide in arterial blood, which indicates the effectiveness of breathing. $Paco_2$ levels move in the opposite direction of pH levels. Bicarbonate, which moves in the same direction of pH, represents the metabolic component of the body's acid-base balance.

Other information routinely reported with ABG results includes partial pressure of oxygen dissolved in arterial blood (Pao_2) and arterial oxygen saturation (Sao_2). The normal Pao_2 range is 80 to 100 mm Hg; however, Pao_2 varies with age. After age 60 years, the Pao_2 may drop below 80 mm Hg without signs and symptoms of hypoxia. The normal Sao_2 range is 95% to 100%.

Taking an ABG sample

When a needle puncture is needed to obtain an ABG sample, the radial, brachial, or femoral arteries may be used. However, the angle of penetration varies.

For the radial artery (the artery most commonly used), the needle should enter bevel up at a 45-degree angle, as shown below. For the brachial artery, the angle should be 60 degrees; for the femoral artery, 90 degrees.

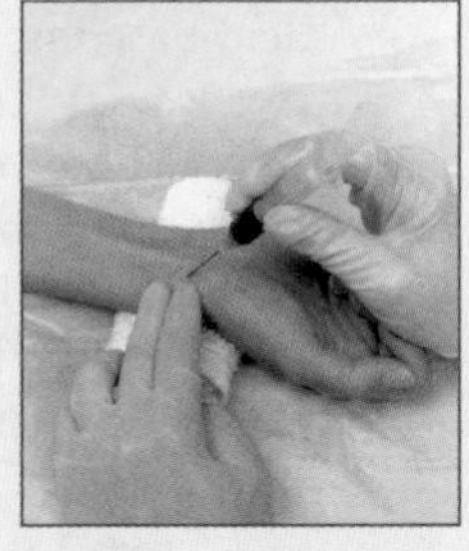

Interpreting ABG results

When interpreting results from an ABG analysis, follow a consistent sequence to analyze the information. Here's one step-by-step process you can use. (See *Quick look at ABG results*.)

Step 1: Check the pH

First, check the pH level. This figure forms the basis for understanding most other figures.

If pH is abnormal, determine whether it reflects acidosis (below 7.35) or alkalosis (above 7.45). Then figure out whether the cause is respiratory or metabolic.

Step 2: Determine the $Paco_2$

Remember that the $Paco_2$ level provides information about the respiratory component of acid-base balance.

If $Paco_2$ is abnormal, determine whether it's low (less than 35 mm Hg) or high (greater than 45 mm Hg). Then determine whether the abnormal result corresponds with a change in pH. For example, if the pH is high, you would expect the $Paco_2$ to be low (hypocapnia), indicating that the problem is respiratory alkalosis. Respiratory alkalosis is caused by hyperventilation, mechanical overventilation, pregnancy, stroke, high altitudes, and septicemia (Appel & Downs, 2008; Rogers & McCutcheon, 2013). Conversely, if the pH is low, you would expect the $Paco_2$ to be high (hypercapnia), indicating that the problem is respiratory acidosis caused by hypoventilation. Causes of respiratory acidosis may be acute or chronic and are linked to chronic diseases such as chronic bronchitis, asthma, pneumonia, and airway obstruction (Rogers & McCutcheon, 2013).

Step 3: Watch the bicarbonate

Next, examine the bicarbonate level. This value provides information about the metabolic aspect of acid-base balance.

If the bicarbonate level is abnormal, determine whether it's low (less than 22 mEq/L) or high (greater than 26 mEq/L). Then determine whether the abnormal result corresponds with the change in pH. For example, if pH is high, you would expect the bicarbonate level to be high, indicating that the problem is metabolic alkalosis. Causes of metabolic alkalosis include the use of diuretics, vomiting, hyperaldosteronism, excessive use of alkaline medications such as antacids, and Cushing's syndrome (Appel & Downs, 2008; Rogers & McCutcheon, 2013). Conversely, if pH is low, you would expect the bicarbonate level to be low, indicating that the problem is metabolic acidosis. Causes of metabolic acidosis include diabetic ketoacidosis,

Quick look at ABG results

Here's a quick look at how to interpret ABG results:

- Check the pH. Is it normal (7.35 to 7.45), acidotic (below 7.35), or alkalotic (above 7.45)?
- Check $Paco_2$. Is it normal (35 to 45 mm Hg), low, or high?
- Check the bicarbonate level. Is it normal (22 to 26 mEq/L), low, or high?
- Check for signs of compensation. Which value ($Paco_2$ or bicarbonate) more closely corresponds to the change in pH?
- Check Pao_2 and Sao_2. Is the Pao_2 normal (80 to 100 mm Hg), low, or high? Is the Sao_2 normal (95% to 100%), low, or high?

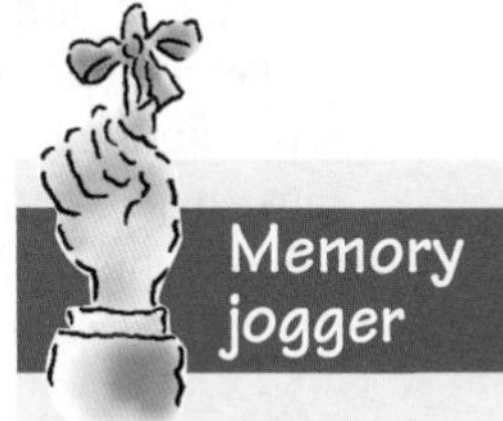

Remember, bicarbonate and pH increase or decrease together. When one rises or falls, so does the other.

lactic acidosis, and severe diarrhea that lead to a loss of bicarbonate (Appel & Downs, 2008; Rogers & McCutcheon, 2013).

Step 4: Look for compensation

Sometimes you'll see a change in both the $Paco_2$ and the bicarbonate level. One value indicates the primary source of the pH change; the other, the body's effort to compensate for the disturbance.

Complete compensation occurs when the body's ability to compensate is so effective that pH falls within the normal range. Partial compensation, on the other hand, occurs when pH remains outside the normal range.

Compensation involves opposites. For instance, if results indicate primary metabolic acidosis, compensation will come in the form of respiratory alkalosis. For example, the following ABG results indicate metabolic acidosis with compensatory respiratory alkalosis:

- pH—7.29
- $Paco_2$—17 mm Hg
- bicarbonate—19 mEq/L.

The low pH indicates acidosis. However, the $Paco_2$ is low, which normally leads to alkalosis, and the bicarbonate level is low, which normally leads to acidosis. The bicarbonate level, then, more closely corresponds with the pH, making the primary cause of the problem metabolic. The resultant decrease in $Paco_2$ reflects partial respiratory compensation.

Normal values for pH, $Paco_2$, and bicarbonate would indicate that the patient's acid-base balance is normal.

Inaccurate ABG results

To avoid altering ABG results, be sure to use proper technique when drawing a sample of arterial blood. Remember:

- A delay in getting the sample to the laboratory or drawing blood for ABG analysis within 15 to 20 minutes of a procedure, such as suctioning or administering a respiratory treatment, could alter results.
- Air bubbles in the syringe could affect the oxygen level.
- Venous blood in the syringe could alter carbon dioxide and oxygen levels and pH.

Step 5: Determine Pao_2 and Sao_2

Last, check Pao_2 and Sao_2, which yield information about the patient's oxygenation status. If the values are abnormal, determine whether they're high (Pao_2 greater than 100 mm Hg) or low (Pao_2 less than 80 mm Hg and Sao_2 less than 95%).

Remember that Pao_2 reflects the body's ability to pick up oxygen from the lungs. A low Pao_2 represents hypoxemia and can cause hyperventilation. The Pao_2 value also indicates when to make adjustments in the concentration of oxygen being administered to a patient. (See *Inaccurate ABG results*.)

Anion gap

You may also come across a test result called the *anion gap*. (See *Crossing the great anion gap*.) Earlier chapters discuss how the strength of cations (positively charged ions) and anions (negatively charged ions) must be equal in the blood to maintain a proper balance of electrical charges. The anion gap result helps you differentiate among various acidotic conditions.

Crossing the great anion gap

This illustration represents the normal anion gap. The gap is calculated by adding the chloride level and the bicarbonate level and then subtracting that total from the sodium level. The value normally ranges from 8 to 14 mEq/L and represents the level of unmeasured anions in extracellular fluid.

In the example below, the chloride level is 105 mEq/L, the bicarbonate level is 25 mEq/L, and the sodium level is 140 mEq/L. To find the anion gap, first add the chloride and bicarbonate levels to get a total of 130 mEq/L. Then subtract that total from the sodium level of 140 mEq/L, which leaves 10 mEq/L—the anion gap.

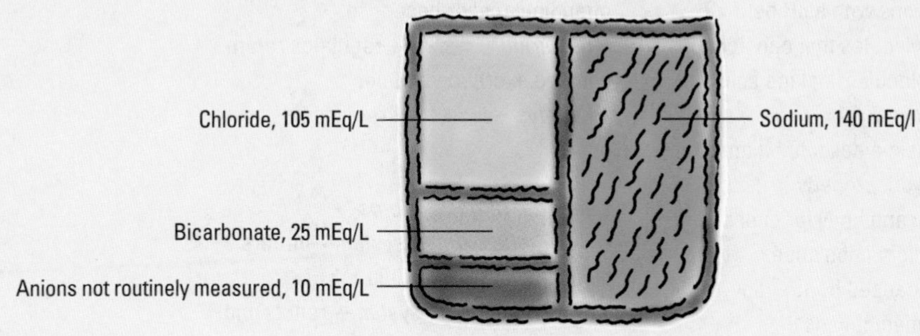

Identifying the gap

The anion gap refers to the relationship among the body's cations and anions. Sodium accounts for more than 90% of the circulating cations. Chloride and bicarbonate together account for 85% of the counterbalancing anions. (Potassium is generally omitted because it occurs in such low, stable amounts.)

The gap between the two measurements represents the anions not routinely measured, including sulfates, phosphates, proteins, and organic acids such as lactic acid and ketone acids. Because these anions aren't measured in routine laboratory tests, the anion gap is a way of determining their presence.

Gazing into the gap

An increase in the anion gap that's greater than 14 mEq/L indicates an increase in the percentage of one or more unmeasured anions in the bloodstream. Increases can occur with acidotic conditions characterized by higher than normal amounts of organic acids. Such conditions include lactic acidosis and ketoacidosis.

The anion gap remains normal for certain other conditions, including hyperchloremic acidosis, renal tubular acidosis, and severe bicarbonate-wasting conditions, such as biliary or pancreatic fistulas and poorly functioning ileal loops.

A decreased anion gap is rare but may occur with hypermagnesemia and paraprotein anemia states, such as multiple myeloma and Waldenström's macroglobulinemia.

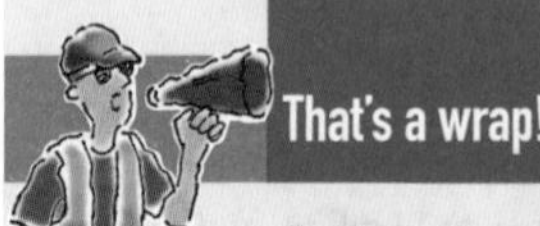

That's a wrap!

Balancing acids and bases review

Acid-base basics
- *Acids*—molecules that can give hydrogen molecules to other molecules; include solutions with a pH below 7
- *Bases*—molecules that can accept hydrogen molecules; include solutions with a pH above 7
- Must maintain a delicate balance for the body to work properly
- Metabolism and body functions affected by slight imbalances
- Imbalance caused by infection, trauma, and medications

Understanding pH
- *pH*—calculation based on the percentage of hydrogen ions and the amount of acids and bases in a solution
- *Normal blood pH*—7.35 to 7.45, which represents the balance between hydrogen ions and bicarbonate ions

Deviation from normal pH
- *Acidosis*—blood pH is below 7.35 and either the hydrogen ion concentration has increased or the bicarbonate level has decreased.
- *Alkalosis*—blood pH is above 7.45 and either the hydrogen ion concentration has decreased or the bicarbonate level has increased.
- A pH below 6.8 or above 7.8 is generally fatal.
- Deviation compromises well-being, electrolyte balance, activity of critical enzymes, muscle contraction, and basic cellular function.

Maintaining acid-base balance
Three systems regulate acids and bases:
- *Chemical buffers*—neutralize the offending acid or base
- *Respiratory system*—regulates retention and excretion of acids
- *Kidneys*—excrete or retain acids or bases

Chemical buffer systems
- *Bicarbonate buffer system*—buffers blood and interstitial fluid
- *Phosphate buffer system*—reacts with acids and bases to form compounds that alter pH; especially effective in the renal tubules
- *Protein buffer system*—acts inside and outside the cell; binds with acids and bases to neutralize them

Respiratory system
- Functions as the second line of defense
- Responds to pH changes in minutes
- Makes temporary adjustments to pH
- Regulates carbon dioxide levels in the blood by varying the rate and depth of breathing
- Compensates with quick and deep breathing so more carbon dioxide is lost when bicarbonate levels are low
- Compensates with slow, shallow breathing so more carbon dioxide is retained when bicarbonate levels are high
- Regulates carbonic acid production

(continued)

Balancing acids and bases review *(continued)*

Kidneys

- Kick in when the first two systems fail to reverse the acidosis or alkalosis
- Make long-term adjustments to pH
- Reabsorb acids and bases or excrete them into urine
- Produce bicarbonate to replenish lost supply
- Regulate bicarbonate production
- Compensate with bicarbonate retention and increased acid excretion when $Paco_2$ level is high
- Respond with bicarbonate excretion and increased acid retention when $Paco_2$ level is low

Anion gap

- Represents the level of unmeasured anions in extracellular fluid
- Normally ranges from 8 to 14 mEq/L
- Helps differentiate acidotic conditions

Interpreting acid-base imbalances

- Step 1: Check pH. Acidosis or alkalosis?
- Step 2: Determine $Paco_2$. Is it normal, high, or low?
- Step 3: Watch bicarbonate for information about metabolic condition.
- Step 4: Look for compensation. For example, metabolic acidosis can lead to compensation by respiratory alkalosis.
- Step 5: Determine Pao_2 and Sao_2. Together they yield information about oxygen status.

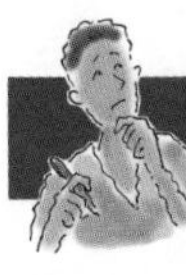

Quick quiz

1. $Paco_2$ level indicates the effectiveness of:
   A. kidney function.
   B. lung ventilation.
   C. phosphate buffers.
   D. bicarbonate buffers.

Answer: B. $Paco_2$ reflects how well the respiratory system is helping to maintain acid-base balance.

2. The kidneys respond to acid-base disturbances by:
   A. adjusting $Paco_2$ levels.
   B. producing phosphate buffers.
   C. producing protein buffers.
   D. excreting or reabsorbing hydrogen or bicarbonate.

Answer: D. The kidneys respond to particular acid-base imbalances by excreting or reabsorbing hydrogen or bicarbonate, according to the body's needs.

3. If your patient is breathing rapidly, his body is attempting to:
   A. retain carbon dioxide.
   B. get rid of excess carbon dioxide.
   C. improve the buffering ability of bicarbonate.
   D. produce more carbonic acid.

Answer: B. High carbon dioxide levels in the blood, measured as $PaCO_2$, cause a drop in pH. Chemoreceptors in the brain sense this decrease and stimulate the lungs to hyperventilate, causing the body to eliminate more carbon dioxide.

4. If your patient has a higher than normal pH (alkalosis), you would expect to also see:
   A. high $PaCO_2$ and high bicarbonate.
   B. low $PaCO_2$ and high bicarbonate.
   C. low bicarbonate and high $PaCO_2$.
   D. low $PaCO_2$ and low bicarbonate.

Answer: B. A low $PaCO_2$ means less carbon dioxide (acid) is in the blood, which raises pH. When pH is raised, the bicarbonate level also increases.

5. The laboratory reports the following ABG results for your patient: pH, 7.33; $PaCO_2$, 40 mm Hg; and bicarbonate, 20 mEq/L. You interpret these results as:
   A. respiratory acidosis.
   B. metabolic acidosis.
   C. respiratory alkalosis.
   D. metabolic alkalosis.

Answer: B. The patient's pH is low, which indicates acidosis. Because $PaCO_2$ is normal and bicarbonate is low (matching the pH), the primary cause of the problem is metabolic.

6. A colleague hands you these ABG results: pH, 7.52; $PaCO_2$, 47 mm Hg; and bicarbonate, 36 mEq/L. You interpret these results as:
   A. normal.
   B. respiratory acidosis.
   C. respiratory alkalosis with respiratory compensation.
   D. metabolic alkalosis with respiratory compensation.

Answer: D. The pH is alkalotic. Although both $PaCO_2$ and bicarbonate have changed, the bicarbonate matches the pH. The elevated $PaCO_2$ represents the efforts of the respiratory system to compensate for the alkalosis by retaining carbon dioxide.

Scoring

☆☆☆ If you answered all six questions correctly, congratulations! You did a great job covering all the bases (and acids)!

☆☆ If you answered four or five correctly, great! You certainly didn't hydrogen bomb!

☆ If you answered fewer than four correctly, don't worry! It's never too late to get your PhD in pH!

References

Appel, S. J., & Downs, C. A. (2008). Understanding acid-base balance. Find out how to interpret values and steady a disturbed equilibrium in an acutely ill patient. *Nursing 2014*, *38*, 9–11.

Rogers, K. M., & McCutcheon, K. (2013). Understanding arterial blood gases. *Journal of Perioperative Practice*, *23*(9), 191–197.

Part II

Fluid and electrolyte imbalances

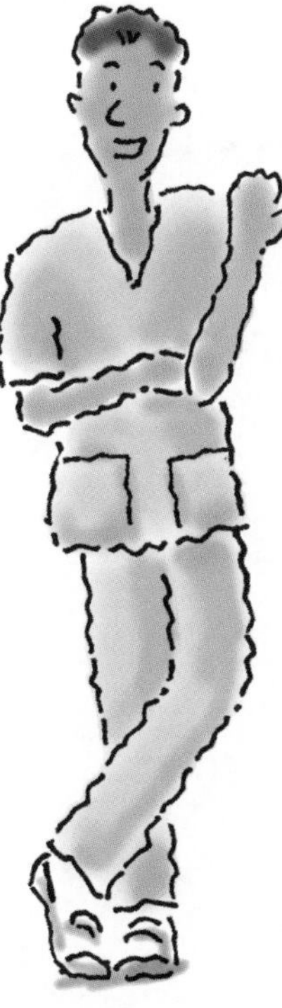

Chapter 4

When fluids tip the balance

Just the facts

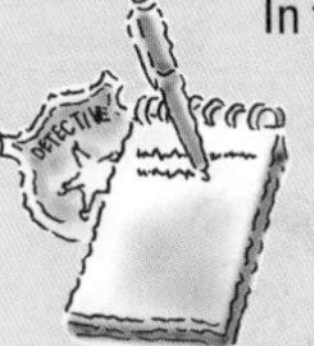

In this chapter, you'll learn:

- ways to assess a patient's fluid status
- ways to identify patients at risk for fluid imbalances
- signs and symptoms of fluid imbalances
- teaching tips for patients with fluid imbalances
- tips for ensuring proper documentation of fluid imbalances.

A look at fluid volume

Blood pressure is related to the amount of blood the heart pumps and the extent of vasoconstriction present. Fluid volume affects these elements, making blood pressure measurement key in assessing a patient's fluid status. Certain types of pressure, such as pulmonary artery pressure (PAP) and central venous pressure (CVP), are measured through specialized catheters. These measurements also help assess fluid volume status.

To maintain the accuracy of whatever blood pressure measurement system you use, periodically compare the readings of automated and direct measurement systems with manual readings.

Cuff measurements

A simple blood pressure measurement, taken with a stethoscope and a sphygmomanometer, is still one of the best tools for assessing fluid volume. It's quick and easy and carries little risk for the patient. Direct and indirect blood pressure measurements are generally related to the amount of blood flowing through the patient's circulatory system.

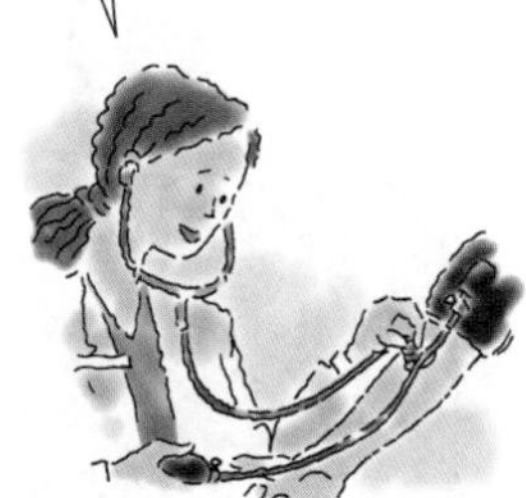
A simple blood pressure measurement is still one of the best tools for assessing fluid volume.

A sizeable task

To measure blood pressure accurately, you must first make sure the cuff is the correct size. The bladder of the cuff should have a length that's 80% and a width that's at least 40% of the upper arm circumference.

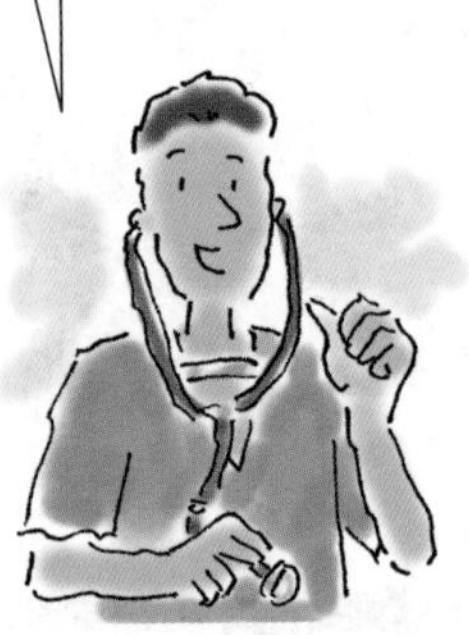
Size matters! The blood pressure cuff bladder should have a length that's 80% and width that's at least 40% of the upper arm circumference.

In position

Position the arm so that the brachial artery is at heart level. To position the blood pressure cuff properly, wrap it snugly around the upper arm. For adults, place the lower border of the cuff about 1″ (2.5 cm) above the antecubital fossa. For children, place the lower border closer to the antecubital fossa.

Place the center of the cuff's bladder directly over the medial aspect of the arm, over the brachial artery. Most cuffs have a reference mark to help you position the bladder. After positioning the cuff, palpate the brachial artery using your index finger, and place the bell of the stethoscope directly over the point where you can feel the strongest pulsations. (See *Positioning a blood pressure cuff.*) Once the patient is properly positioned, he or she should be allowed a 5-minute rest period before blood pressure measurement (Garcia, Ang, Ahmad, & Lim, 2012).

Listen up

Once you have the stethoscope and cuff in place, use the thumb and index finger of your other hand to turn the screw on the rubber bulb of the air pump and close the valve. Then pump air into the cuff while auscultating over the brachial artery and continue

Positioning a blood pressure cuff

This photograph shows how to properly position a blood pressure cuff and stethoscope bell.

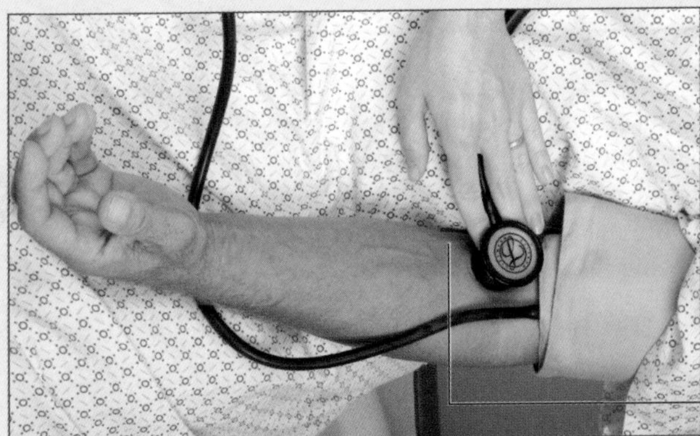

pumping air until the gauge registers at least 10 mm Hg above the level of the last audible sound. Next, carefully open the air pump valve and slowly deflate the cuff. While releasing air, watch the gauge and auscultate over the artery. When you hear the first beat, note the pressure on the gauge; this is the systolic pressure. Continue gradually releasing air, watching the gauge, and auscultating. Note the diastolic reading when the tone becomes soft and muffled. If you suspect a false-high or false-low reading, take steps to correct the problem. (See *Correcting problems of blood pressure measurement*.)

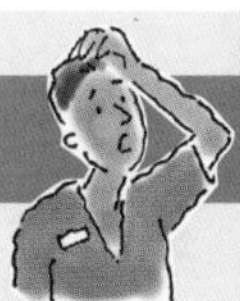

It's not working!

Correcting problems of blood pressure measurement

Use this chart to figure out what to do for each possible cause of a false-high or false-low blood pressure reading.

Problem and possible cause	What to do
False-high reading	
Cuff too small	Make sure the cuff bladder is long enough to completely encircle the extremity.
Cuff wrapped too loosely, reducing its effective width	Tighten the cuff.
Slow cuff deflation, causing venous congestion in the arm or leg	Never deflate the cuff slower than 2 mm Hg per heartbeat.
Poorly timed measurement (after the patient has eaten, ambulated, appeared anxious, or flexed his arm muscles)	Postpone blood pressure measurement or help the patient relax before taking pressures.
Multiple attempts at reading blood pressure in the same arm, causing venous congestion	Don't attempt to measure blood pressure more than twice in the same arm; wait several minutes between attempts.
False-low reading	
Incorrect position of the arm or leg	Make sure the arm or leg is level with the patient's heart.
Failure to notice auscultatory gap (sound fades out for 10 to 15 mm Hg, then returns)	Estimate systolic pressure using palpation before actually measuring it. Then check the palpable pressure against the measured pressure.
Inaudible or low-volume sounds	Before reinflating the cuff, instruct the patient to raise his arm or leg to decrease venous pressure and amplify low-volume sounds. After inflating the cuff, tell the patient to lower his arm or leg. Then deflate the cuff and listen. If you still fail to detect low-volume sounds, chart the palpable systolic pressure.

It's all automatic

You may also have access to an automated blood pressure unit. This unit is designed to take blood pressure measurements repeatedly, which is helpful when you're caring for a patient whose blood pressure is expected to change frequently (for example, a patient with a fluid imbalance). The unit automatically computes and digitally records blood pressure readings.

The cuff automatically inflates to check the blood pressure and deflates immediately afterward. You can program the monitor to inflate the cuff as often as needed and set alarms for high, low, and mean blood pressures. Most monitors display each blood pressure reading until the next reading is taken.

Palpable pressures

If you have trouble hearing the patient's blood pressure, which is common when a patient is hypotensive, palpate the blood pressure to estimate systolic pressure.

To palpate blood pressure, place a cuff on the upper arm and palpate the brachial pulse or the radial pulse. Inflate the cuff until you no longer feel the pulse. Then slowly deflate the cuff, noting the point at which you feel the pulse again—the systolic pressure. If you palpate a patient's blood pressure at 90 mm Hg, for example, chart it as "90/P" (the P stands for *palpable*).

The Doppler difference

What should you do if your patient's arm is swollen or his blood pressure is so low you can't feel his pulse? First, palpate his carotid artery to make sure he has a pulse. Then, use a Doppler device to obtain a reading of his systolic pressure. (See *How to take a Doppler blood pressure.*)

The Doppler probe uses ultrasound waves directed at the blood vessel to detect blood flow. Through the Doppler unit, you'll be able to hear the patient's blood flow with each pulse.

To obtain a Doppler blood pressure, take these steps:

- Place a blood pressure cuff on the arm as you normally would.
- Apply lubricant to the antecubital area where you would expect to find the brachial pulse.
- Turn the unit on and place the probe lightly on the arm over the brachial artery.
- Adjust the volume control and the placement of the probe until you hear the pulse clearly.
- Inflate the blood pressure cuff until the pulse sound disappears.
- Slowly deflate the cuff and note the point at which the pulse sound returns—the systolic pressure. If you hear the pulse at 80 mm Hg, for instance, record it as "80/D" (the D stands for *Doppler*).

How to take a Doppler blood pressure

When you can't hear or feel a patient's blood pressure, try using a Doppler ultrasound device, as shown below.

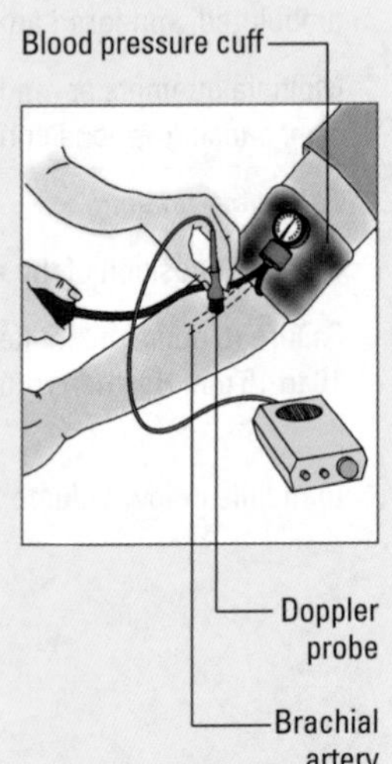

Direct measurements

Direct measurement is an invasive method of obtaining blood pressure readings using arterial catheters. Direct measurement is used when highly accurate or frequent blood pressure measurements are required, such as with severe fluid imbalances.

Arterial lines

Arterial lines, or A-lines, are inserted into the radial or the brachial artery (or the femoral artery, if needed). A-lines continuously monitor blood pressure and can also be used to sample arterial blood for blood gas analysis or other laboratory tests. Because A-lines require a certain level of technology and staff training, patients who have them are usually placed in intermediate or critical care units.

Lines under pressure

The catheter is connected to a continuous flush system—a bag of normal saline solution (which may contain heparin) inside a pressurized cuff. This system maintains the patency of the A-line.

The A-line is connected to a transducer and then to a bedside monitor. The transducer converts fluid-pressure waves from the catheter into an electronic signal that can be analyzed and displayed on the monitor. Because the patient's blood pressure is displayed continuously, you can instantly note changes in the measurements and respond quickly.

A PA catheter provides a clear picture of fluid volume status, including the status of left-sided heart function. You're looking good to me!

Pulmonary artery catheters

An A-line directly measures blood pressure, whereas a pulmonary artery (PA) catheter directly measures other pressures. PA catheters are usually inserted into the subclavian vein or the internal jugular vein, although the lines are sometimes inserted into a vein in the arm (brachial vein) or the leg (femoral vein).

The tip of the catheter is advanced through the vein into the right atrium, then into the right ventricle, and finally into the pulmonary artery. The hubs of the catheter are then connected to a pressurized transducer system that's similar to the system used for an A-line. (See *Pulmonary artery catheter ports*, page 60.)

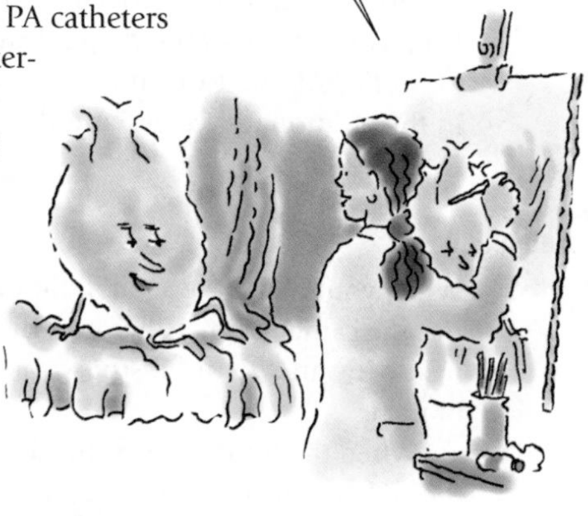

Getting a clearer picture

A PA catheter provides a clearer picture of the patient's fluid volume status than other measurement techniques. The catheter allows for measurement of PAP, pulmonary artery wedge pressure (PAWP),

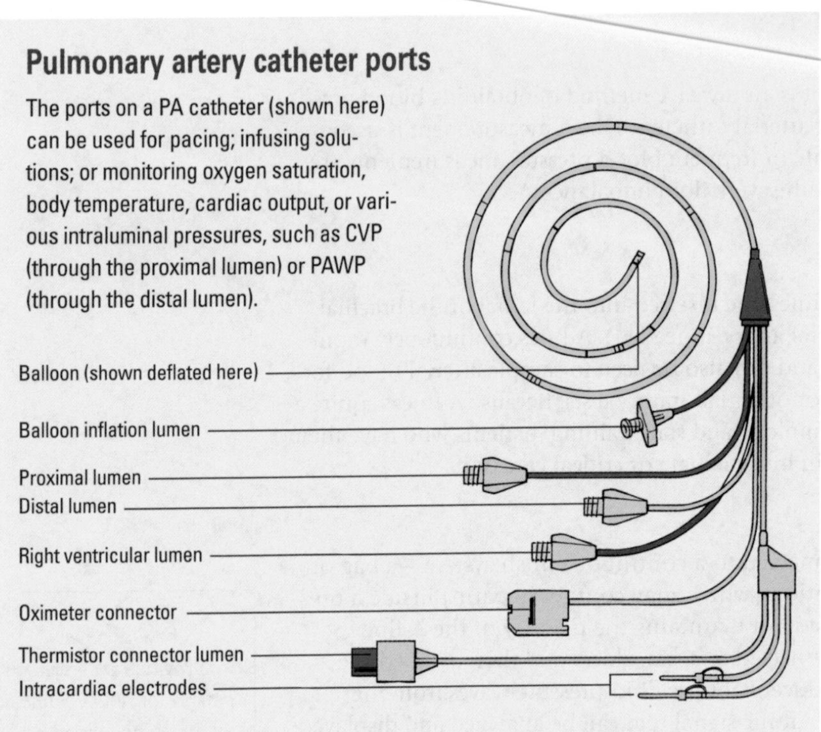

Pulmonary artery catheter ports

The ports on a PA catheter (shown here) can be used for pacing; infusing solutions; or monitoring oxygen saturation, body temperature, cardiac output, or various intraluminal pressures, such as CVP (through the proximal lumen) or PAWP (through the distal lumen).

cardiac output, and CVP—all of which provide information about how the left side of the heart is functioning, including its pumping ability, filling pressures, and vascular volume.

The PAP is the pressure routinely displayed on the monitor. A normal systolic PAP is 15 to 25 mm Hg and reflects pressure from contraction of the right atrium (Muralidhar, 2002). A normal diastolic PAP is 8 to 15 mm Hg and reflects the lowest pressure in the pulmonary vessels, and the mean PAP is 10 to 20 mm Hg (Muralidhar, 2002).

Wedged in

When you inflate the small balloon at the catheter tip, blood carries the catheter tip farther into the pulmonary artery. The tip floats inside the artery until it stops—or becomes wedged—in a smaller branch.

When the tip is wedged in a branch of the pulmonary artery, the catheter measures pressures coming from the left side of the heart, which is a measurement that may prove useful in gauging changes in blood volume. A normal PAWP is 4 to 12 mm Hg (Muralidhar, 2002).

PAP and PAWP are generally increased in cases of fluid overload and decreased in cases of fluid volume deficit, explaining why a PA catheter is useful when assessing and treating an acutely ill patient with a fluid imbalance (Muralidhar, 2002).

Multiple measurements

PA catheters also measure cardiac output, either continuously or after injections of I.V. fluid through the proximal lumen. Cardiac output is the amount of blood that the heart pumps in 1 minute and is calculated by multiplying the heart rate by the stroke volume. (Conveniently, the monitor makes that calculation for you.)

The stroke volume is the amount of blood the ventricle pumps out with each beat, and it's also calculated by the bedside monitor. Normal cardiac output is 4 to 8 L/minute. If a person lacks adequate blood volume, cardiac output is low (assuming the heart can pump normally otherwise). If the person is overloaded with fluid, cardiac output is high.

Central venous pressure

A central venous catheter can measure CVP, another useful indication of a patient's fluid status. The term *CVP* refers to the pressure of the blood inside the central venous circulation. The CVP catheter is typically inserted in one of the jugular veins in the neck or in a subclavian vein in the chest, with the tip of the catheter positioned above the right atrium in the superior vena cava.

Normal CVP ranges from 2 to 8 mm Hg (2 to 6 cm H_2O). If CVP is high, it usually means the patient is overloaded with fluid. If it's low, it usually means the patient is low on fluid. (To calculate CVP by yourself, see *Estimating CVP*, page 62.)

Maintaining balance

Most of the time, the body adequately compensates for minor fluid imbalances and keeps blood pressure readings and other measurements fairly normal. Sometimes, however, the body can't compensate for fluid deficits or excesses. When that happens, any of several problems may result, including dehydration, hypovolemia, hypervolemia, and water intoxication.

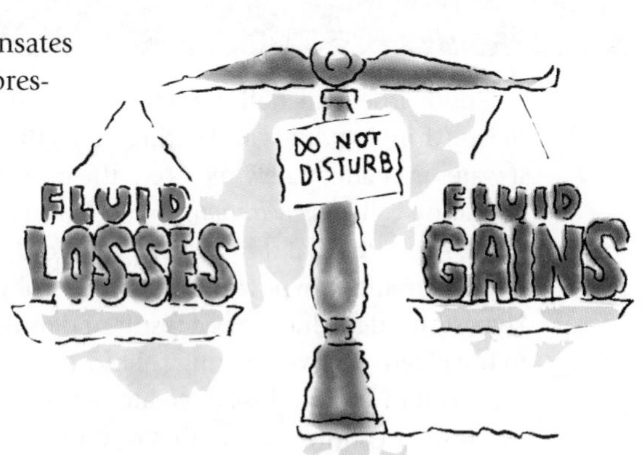

Estimating CVP

To estimate a patient's CVP, follow these steps:

1. Place the patient at a 45- to 60-degree angle.
2. Use tangential lighting to observe the internal jugular vein.
3. Note the highest level of visible pulsation.
4. Next, locate the angle of Louis or sternal notch. To do this, first palpate the point at which the clavicles join the sternum to find the suprasternal notch.
5. Then place two fingers on the patient's suprasternal notch and slide them down the sternum until they reach a bony protuberance—the angle of Louis. The right atrium lies about 2″ (5 cm) below this point.
6. Measure the distance between the angle of Louis and the highest level of visible pulsation. Normally, this distance is less than 1.2″ (3 cm).
7. Add 2″ to this figure to estimate the distance between the highest level of pulsation and the right atrium. A distance greater than 4″ (10 cm) may indicate elevated CVP.

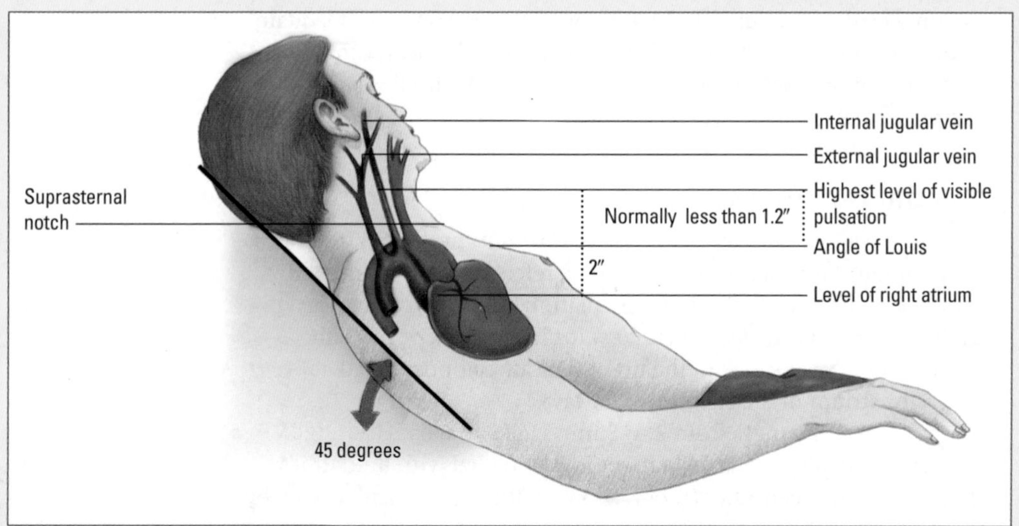

Dehydration

The body loses water all the time. A person responds to the thirst reflex by drinking fluids and eating foods that contain water. However, if water isn't adequately replaced, the body's cells can lose water, a condition called *dehydration*. Dehydration can be classified as isotonic, hypertonic, and hypotonic (Ashford, 2008). Isotonic dehydration is a result of hypovolemia or fluid volume loss (Ashford, 2008). Hypertonic dehydration is a result of deprivation of fluids often seen in the elderly and very young (Ashford, 2008). Hypotonic dehydration is a result of sodium loss in greater amounts than free water often seen as a result of a low-sodium diet or diuretic overuse (Ashford, 2008).

How it happens

Loss of body fluids causes blood solute concentration to increase (increased osmolality) and serum sodium levels to rise. In an attempt to regain fluid balance between intracellular and extracellular spaces, water molecules shift out of cells into more concentrated blood. This process, combined with increased water intake and increased water retention in the kidneys, usually restores the body's fluid volume.

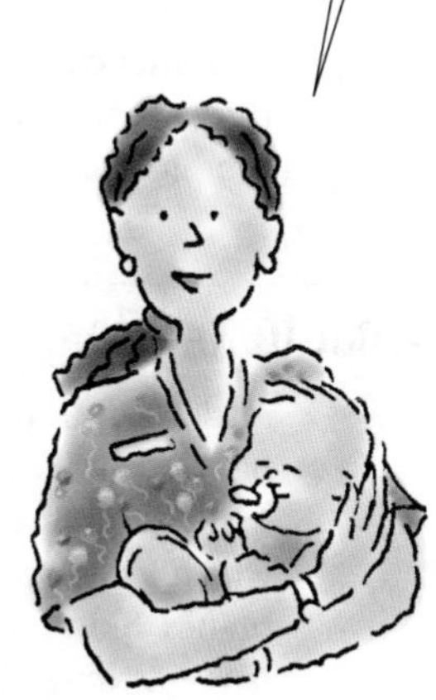
Infants are at risk for dehydration because they have immature kidneys and can't drink fluid on their own.

Incredibly shrinking cells

Without an adequate supply of water in the extracellular space, fluid continues to shift out of the cells into that space. The cells begin to shrink as the process continues. Because water is essential for obtaining nutrients, expelling wastes, and maintaining cell shape, cells can't function properly without adequate fluid.

Who is at risk?

Failure to respond adequately to the thirst stimulus increases the risk of dehydration. Confused, comatose, and bedridden patients are particularly vulnerable, as are infants, who can't drink fluid on their own and who have immature kidneys that can't concentrate urine efficiently.

Older patients are also prone to dehydration because they have a lower body water content, diminished kidney function, and a reduced ability to sense thirst, so they can't correct fluid volume deficits as easily as younger adults. A patient may also become dehydrated if he's receiving highly concentrated tube feedings without enough supplemental water. (See *Different but the same.*)

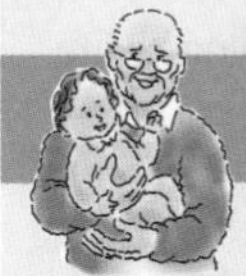

Ages and stages

Different but the same

Elderly and very young patients are highly susceptible to fluid and electrolyte imbalances. Despite the significant age difference, the contributing factors for these imbalances are the same in many cases:

- inability to obtain fluid without help
- inability to express feelings of thirst
- inaccurate assessment of output—for example, if the patient must wear a diaper
- loss of fluid through perspiration because of fever
- loss of fluid through diarrhea and vomiting.

What brings it on?

Any situation that accelerates fluid loss can lead to dehydration. For instance, in diabetes insipidus, the brain fails to secrete antidiuretic hormone (ADH). If the brain doesn't secrete enough ADH, the result is greater-than-normal diuresis. A patient with diabetes insipidus produces large amounts of highly diluted urine—as much as 30 L/day. The patient is also thirsty and tends to drink large amounts of fluids, although he generally can't keep up with the diuresis.

Other causes of dehydration include prolonged fever, watery diarrhea, renal failure, and hyperglycemia (which causes the person to produce large amounts of diluted urine).

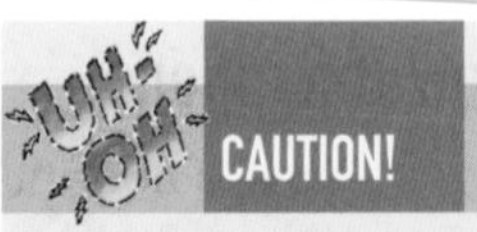

Danger signs of dehydration

Begin emergency treatment for dehydration if a patient with a suspected fluid imbalance develops any of these conditions:

- impaired mental status
- seizure
- coma.

What to look for

As dehydration progresses, watch for changes in mental status. The patient may complain of dizziness, weakness, or extreme thirst. He may have a fever (because less fluid is available for perspiration, which lowers body temperature), dry skin, or dry mucous membranes. Skin turgor may be poor. Because an older patient's skin may lack elasticity, checking skin turgor may be an unreliable indicator of dehydration.

The patient's heart rate may go up, and his blood pressure may fall. In severe cases, seizures and coma may result. Also, urine output may fall because less fluid is circulating in the body. The patient's urine will be more concentrated unless he has diabetes insipidus, in which case the urine will probably be pale and produced in large volume. (See *Danger signs of dehydration*.)

If a patient receives a hypotonic solution too quickly, the fluid moves from the veins into the cells, causing them to swell.

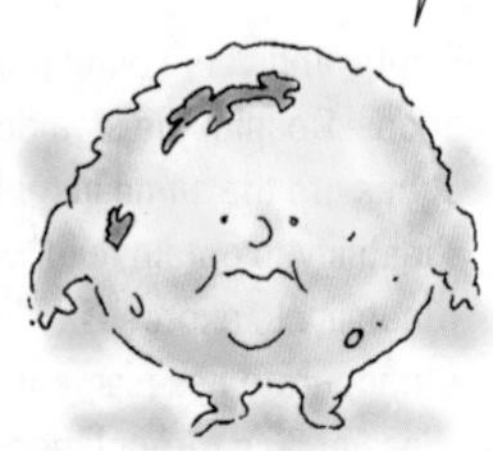

What tests show

Diagnostic test results may include:

- elevated hematocrit (HCT)
- elevated serum osmolality (above 300 mOsm/kg)
- elevated serum sodium level (above 145 mEq/L)
- urine specific gravity above 1.030.

Because patients with diabetes insipidus have more diluted urine, specific gravity is usually less than 1.005; osmolality, 50 to 200 mOsm/kg.

How it's treated

Treatment for dehydration aims to replace missing fluids. Because a dehydrated patient's blood is concentrated, avoid hypertonic solutions. If the patient can handle oral fluids, encourage them; however, because the serum sodium level is elevated, make sure the fluids given are salt-free.

A severely dehydrated patient should receive I.V. fluids to replace lost fluids. Most patients receive hypotonic, low-sodium fluids, such as dextrose 5% in water (D_5W). Remember, if you give a hypotonic solution too quickly, the fluid moves from the veins into the cells, causing them to become edematous. Swelling of cells in the brain can create cerebral edema. To avoid such potentially devastating problems, give fluids gradually, over a period of about 48 hours.

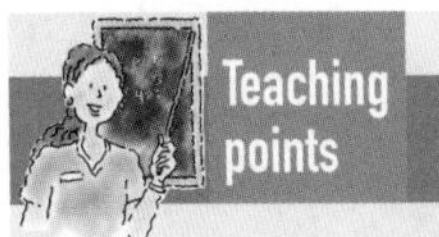

Teaching about dehydration

When teaching a patient with dehydration, be sure to cover the following topics and then evaluate your patient's learning:
- explanation of dehydration and its treatment
- warning signs and symptoms
- prescribed medications
- importance of complying with therapy.

How you intervene

Monitor at-risk patients closely to detect impending dehydration. If a patient becomes dehydrated, here are some steps you'll want to take:

- Monitor symptoms and vital signs closely so you can intervene quickly.
- Accurately record the patient's intake and output, including urine and stool.
- Maintain I.V. access as ordered. Monitor I.V. infusions. Watch for signs and symptoms of cerebral edema when your patient is receiving hypotonic fluids. These include headache, confusion, irritability, lethargy, nausea, vomiting, widening pulse pressure, decreased pulse rate, and seizures. (See *Teaching about dehydration*.)
- Keep in mind that vasopressin may be ordered for patients with diabetes insipidus.
- Monitor serum sodium levels, urine osmolality, and urine specific gravity to assess fluid balance.
- Insert a urinary catheter as ordered to accurately monitor output.
- Provide a safe environment for any patient who is confused, dizzy, or at risk for a seizure, and teach his family to do the same.
- Obtain daily weights (same scale, same time of day) to evaluate treatment progress. (See *Documenting dehydration*, page 66.)
- Provide skin and mouth care to maintain the integrity of the skin surface and oral mucous membranes.
- Assess the patient for diaphoresis—it can be the source of major water loss.

Hypovolemia

Hypovolemia refers to isotonic fluid loss (which includes loss of fluids and solutes) from the extracellular space. Children and older patients are especially vulnerable to hypovolemia. Some of the initial signs

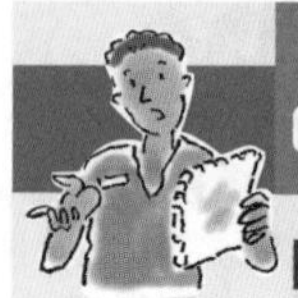

Chart smart

Documenting dehydration

When your patient is dehydrated, you should document:
- assessment findings
- intake, output, and daily weight
- I.V. therapy
- patient's response to interventions
- associated diagnostic test results
- patient teaching performed and the patient's understanding.

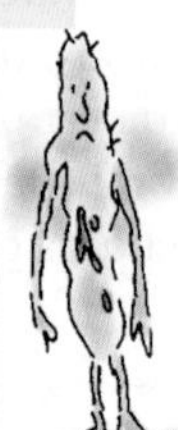

and symptoms of hypovolemia can be subtle as the body tries to compensate for the loss of circulating blood volume. Subtle signs can become more serious and, if not detected early and treated properly, can progress to hypovolemic shock, a common form of shock.

How it happens

Excessive fluid loss (bleeding, for instance) is a risk factor for hypovolemia, especially when combined with reduced fluid intake. Another risk factor is a third-space fluid shift, which occurs when fluid moves out of intravascular spaces but not into intracellular spaces. For instance, fluid may shift into the abdominal cavity (ascites), the pleural cavity, or the pericardial sac. These third-space fluid shifts may occur as a result of increased permeability of the capillary membrane or decreased plasma colloid osmotic pressure.

Fluid loss from the extracellular compartment can stem from several causes, including excessive sweating. Could someone please turn down the heat?

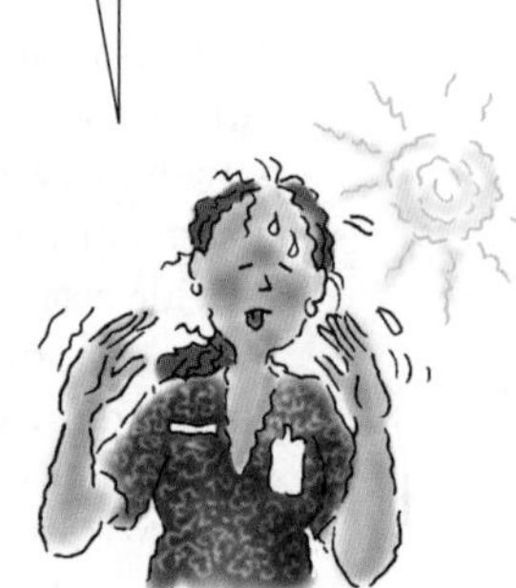

A cluster of causes

Fluid loss from the extracellular compartment can result from many different causes, including:
- abdominal surgery
- diabetes mellitus (with increased urination)
- excessive diuretic therapy
- excessive laxative use
- excessive sweating
- fever
- fistulas
- hemorrhage (bleeding may be frank [obvious] or occult [hidden])
- nasogastric drainage
- renal failure with increased urination
- vomiting and diarrhea.

Trading spaces

Third-space fluid shifts also can result from any number of conditions, including:

- acute intestinal obstruction
- acute peritonitis
- burns (during the initial phase)
- crush injuries
- heart failure
- hip fracture
- hypoalbuminemia
- liver failure
- pleural effusion.

What to look for

If volume loss is minimal (10% to 15% of total circulating blood volume), the body tries to compensate for its lack of circulating volume by increasing its heart rate. You may also note orthostatic hypotension, restlessness, or anxiety. The patient will probably produce more than 30 ml of urine per hour, but he may have delayed capillary refill and cool, pale skin over the arms and legs. (See *Danger signs of hypovolemia,* page 68.)

Weighty evidence

A patient with hypovolemia may also lose weight. Acute weight loss can indicate rapid fluid changes. A drop in weight of 5% to 10% can indicate mild to moderate loss; more than 10%, severe loss. As hypovolemia progresses, the patient's signs and symptoms worsen. CVP and PAWP may fall as well. Monitor your patient for subtle signs, including orthostatic hypotension.

Dazed and confused

With moderate intravascular volume loss (about 25%), the patient may become more confused and irritable and may complain of dizziness, nausea, or extreme thirst. The pulse usually becomes rapid and thready, and the blood pressure drops. The patient's skin may feel cool and clammy, and urine output may drop to 10 to 30 ml/hour.

Shock!

Severe hypovolemia (40% or more of intravascular volume loss) may lead to hypovolemic shock. In a patient with this condition, cardiac output drops and mental status can deteriorate to unconsciousness. Signs may progress to marked tachycardia and hypotension with weak or absent peripheral pulses. The skin may become cool and mottled or even cyanotic. Urine output drops to less than 10 ml/hour.

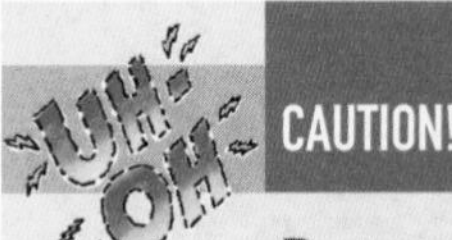

CAUTION!

Danger signs of hypovolemia

Avoid surprises. Watch for these signs and symptoms of hypovolemia and impending hypovolemic shock:

- deterioration in mental status (from restlessness and anxiety to unconsciousness)
- thirst
- dizziness
- nausea
- tachycardia
- delayed capillary refill
- orthostatic hypotension progressing to marked hypotension
- urine output initially more than 30 ml/hour, then urine output drops below 10 ml/hour
- cool, pale skin over the arms and legs
- weight loss
- flat jugular veins
- decreased CVP
- weak or absent peripheral pulses.

What tests show

No single diagnostic finding can confirm hypovolemia. Laboratory test values can vary, depending on the underlying cause and other factors. Laboratory values usually suggest an increased concentration of blood. Typical laboratory findings include:

- normal or high serum sodium level (>145 mEq/L), depending on the amount of fluid and sodium lost
- decreased hemoglobin levels and HCT with hemorrhage
- elevated blood urea nitrogen (BUN) and creatinine ratio
- increased urine specific gravity, as the kidneys try to conserve fluid
- increased serum osmolality.

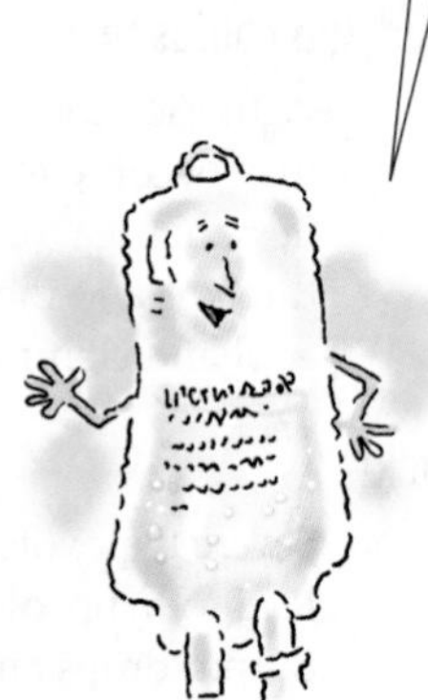
In cases of hypovolemic shock, the patient needs large amounts of I.V. fluids in a short amount of time.

How it's treated

Treatment for hypovolemia includes replacing lost fluids with fluids of the same concentration. Such replacement helps normalize blood pressure and restore blood volume. Oral fluids generally aren't enough to adequately treat hypovolemia. Isotonic fluids, such as normal saline solution or lactated Ringer's solution, are given I.V. to expand circulating volume.

A flood of fluid

Fluids may initially be administered as a fluid bolus in which the patient receives large amounts of I.V. fluids in a short amount of time. For hypovolemic shock, an emergency condition, multiple fluid boluses are essential. Numerous I.V. infusions should be started with the shortest, largest bore catheters possible because they offer less resistance to fluid flow than long, skinny catheters.

Pumping it in

Infusions of normal saline solution or lactated Ringer's solution are given rapidly, commonly followed by an infusion of plasma proteins such as albumin. If a patient is hemorrhaging, he'll need a blood transfusion. He may also need a vasopressor, such as dopamine, to support his blood pressure until his fluid levels are back to normal.

Oxygen therapy should be initiated to ensure sufficient tissue perfusion. Surgery may be required to control bleeding.

How you intervene

Nursing responsibilities for a hypovolemic patient include those listed here:

- Make sure the patient has a patent airway.
- Apply and adjust oxygen therapy as ordered.
- Lower the head of the bed to slow a declining blood pressure.
- If the patient is bleeding, apply direct, continuous pressure to the area and elevate it if possible. Assist with other interventions to stop bleeding.
- If the patient's blood pressure doesn't respond to interventions as expected, look again for a site of bleeding that might have been missed. Remember, a patient can lose a large amount of blood internally from a fractured hip or pelvis. Furthermore, fluids alone may not be enough to correct hypotension associated with a hypovolemic condition. A vasopressor may be needed to raise blood pressure.
- Maintain patent I.V. access. Use short, large-bore catheters to allow for faster infusion rates. Typically, this patient should have two large-bore I.V. catheters.
- Administer I.V. fluid, a vasopressor, and blood as prescribed. An autotransfuser, which allows for reinfusion of the patient's own blood, may be required.
- Draw blood for typing and crossmatching as ordered to prepare for transfusion.

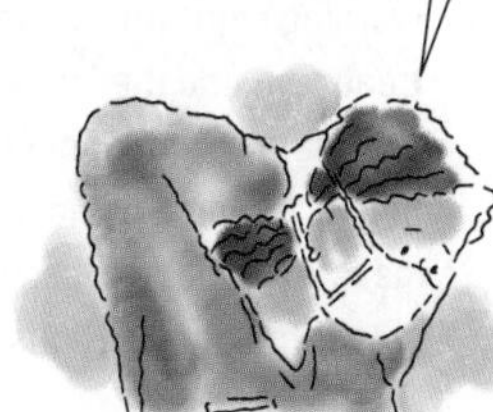

The patient may need surgery to control bleeding.

- Closely monitor the patient's mental status and vital signs, including orthostatic blood pressure measurements, when appropriate. Watch for arrhythmias.
- If available, monitor hemodynamics (cardiac output, CVP, PAP, and PAWP) using a PA catheter to judge how well the patient is responding to treatment. (See *Hemodynamic values in hypovolemic shock.*)
- Monitor the quality of peripheral pulses and skin temperature and appearance to assess for continued peripheral vascular constriction.
- Obtain and record results from diagnostic tests, such as a complete blood count, electrolyte levels, arterial blood gas (ABG) analyses, a 12-lead electrocardiogram, and chest X-rays.
- Offer emotional support to the patient and his family. (See *Teaching about hypovolemia.*)
- Encourage the patient to drink fluids as appropriate.
- Insert a urinary catheter as ordered, and measure urine output hourly if indicated. (See *Documenting hypovolemia.*)
- Auscultate the patient's breath sounds to monitor for signs of fluid overload, a potential complication of I.V. therapy. Excess fluid in the lungs may cause crackles on auscultation.
- Monitor the patient for increased oxygen requirements, a sign of fluid overload.
- Observe the patient for development of such complications as disseminated intravascular coagulation, myocardial infarction, or adult respiratory distress syndrome.
- Weigh the patient daily to monitor the progress of treatment.
- Provide effective skin care to prevent skin breakdown.

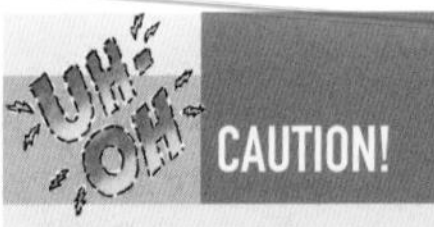

CAUTION!

Hemodynamic values in hypovolemic shock

Hemodynamic monitoring helps you evaluate the patient's cardiovascular status in hypovolemic shock. Look for these values:

- CVP below the normal range of 2 to 6 cm H_2O
- PAP below the normal mean of 10 to 20 mm Hg
- PAWP below the normal mean of 4 to 12 mm Hg
- cardiac output below the normal range of 4 to 8 L/minute.

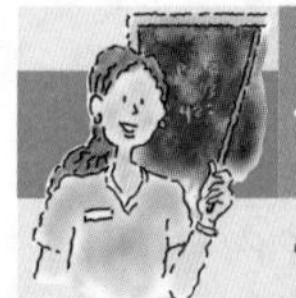

Teaching points

Teaching about hypovolemia

When teaching a patient with hypovolemia, be sure to cover the following topics and then evaluate the patient's learning:

- nature of the condition and its causes
- warning signs and symptoms and when they should be reported
- treatment and the importance of compliance
- importance of changing positions slowly, especially when going from a supine position to a standing position, to avoid orthostatic hypotension
- measuring blood pressure and pulse rate
- prescribed medications.

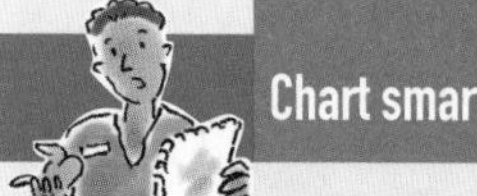

Chart smart

Documenting hypovolemia

For a patient who is hypovolemic, you should document:

- mental status
- vital signs
- strength of peripheral pulses
- appearance and temperature of skin
- I.V. therapy administered
- blood products infused
- doses of vasopressors (if necessary)
- breath sounds and oxygen therapy used
- hourly urine output
- laboratory results
- daily weight
- interventions and the patient's response
- patient teaching.

Hypervolemia

Hypervolemia is an excess of isotonic fluid (water and sodium) in the extracellular compartment. Osmolality is usually unaffected because fluid and solutes are gained in equal proportion. The body has compensatory mechanisms to deal with hypervolemia, but when they fail, signs and symptoms of hypervolemia develop.

How it happens

Extracellular fluid volume may increase in either the interstitial or intravascular compartments. Usually, the body can compensate and restore fluid balance by fine-tuning circulating levels of aldosterone, ADH, and atrial natriuretic peptide (a hormone produced by the atrial muscle of the heart), causing the kidneys to release additional water and sodium.

However, if hypervolemia is prolonged or severe or the patient has poor heart function, the body can't compensate for the extra volume. Heart failure and pulmonary edema may result. Fluid is forced out of the blood vessels and moves into the interstitial space, causing edema of the tissues.

Elderly patients and patients with impaired renal or cardiovascular function are especially prone to developing hypervolemia.

The rising tide

Hypervolemia results from excessive sodium or fluid intake, fluid or sodium retention, or a shift in fluid from the interstitial space into the intravascular space. It may also result from acute or chronic renal failure with low urine output.

Factors that cause excessive sodium or fluid intake include:
- I.V. replacement therapy using normal saline solution or lactated Ringer's solution
- blood or plasma replacement
- high intake of dietary sodium.

Factors that cause fluid and sodium retention include:
- heart failure
- cirrhosis of the liver
- nephrotic syndrome
- corticosteroid therapy
- hyperaldosteronism
- low intake of dietary protein.

Factors that cause fluids to shift into the intravascular space include:
- remobilization of fluids after burn treatment
- administration of hypertonic fluids, such as mannitol or hypertonic saline solution
- use of plasma proteins such as albumin.

What to look for

Because no single diagnostic test confirms hypervolemia, signs and symptoms are key to diagnosis. Cardiac output increases as the body tries to compensate for the excess volume. The pulse becomes rapid and bounding. Blood pressure, CVP, PAP, and PAWP rise. As the heart fails, blood pressure and cardiac output drop. A third heart sound (S_3) gallop develops with heart failure. You'll see distended veins, especially in the hands and neck. When the patient raises his hand above the level of his heart, his hand veins remain distended for more than 5 seconds.

Edema's many faces

Edema results as hydrostatic (fluid-pushing) pressure builds in the vessels, forcing fluid into the tissues. Edema may first be visible only in dependent areas, such as the sacrum and buttocks when the patient is lying down or in the legs and feet when the patient is standing. (See *Evaluating pitting edema*.) Later, the edema may become generalized. *Anasarca* refers to severe, generalized edema. Edematous skin looks puffy, even around the eyes, and feels cool and pits when touched. The patient gains weight as a result of fluid retention (each 17 oz [0.5 L] of fluid gained translates to a 1-lb [0.45 kg] weight gain). An increase in weight of 5% to 10% indicates mild to moderate fluid gain; an increase of more than 10%, a more severe fluid gain.

Overload!

Edema may also occur in the lungs. As the left side of the heart becomes overloaded and pump efficiency declines, fluid backs up into the lungs.

Hydrostatic pressure forces fluid out of the pulmonary blood vessels (just as in other blood vessels) and into the interstitial and alveolar areas. Pulmonary edema results. In a patient with this condition, you'll hear crackles on auscultation. The patient becomes short of breath and tachypneic with a frequent, sometimes frothy, cough. Pink, frothy sputum is a hallmark of pulmonary edema. (See *How pulmonary edema develops*, page 74.)

What tests show

Typical laboratory findings for a patient with hypervolemia include:

- low HCT due to hemodilution
- normal serum sodium level
- low serum potassium and BUN levels due to hemodilution (higher levels may indicate renal failure or impaired renal perfusion)
- decreased serum osmolality

Evaluating pitting edema

You can evaluate edema using a scale of +1 to +4. Press your fingertip firmly into the skin over a bony surface for a few seconds. Then note the depth of the imprint your finger leaves on the skin. The imprint should disappear within 10 to 30 seconds depending on the severity of the edema. According to Dix (2012), 1+ edema is characterized by a 2-mm indentation into the swollen tissue, 2+ edema is characterized by a 4-mm indentation, 3+ edema is characterized by a 6-mm indentation, and 4+ edema is characterized by an 8-mm indentation into the swollen tissue.

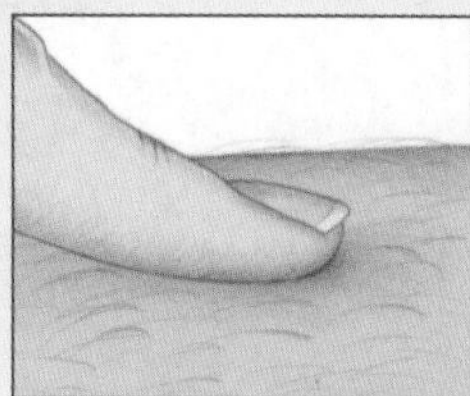

A slight imprint indicates +1 pitting edema.

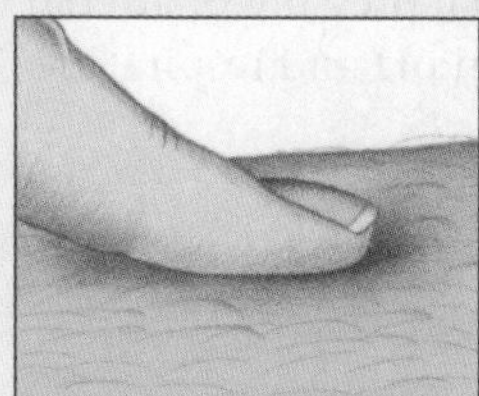

A deep imprint, with the skin slow to return to its original contour, indicates +4 pitting edema.

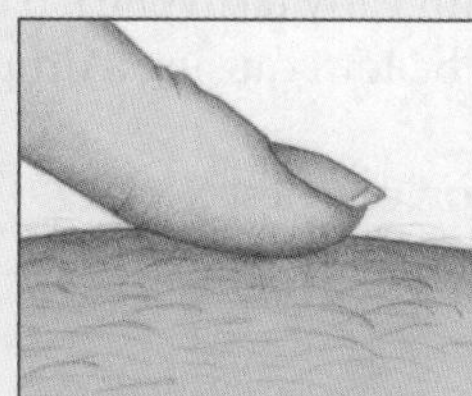

When the skin resists pressure but appears distended, the condition is called *brawny edema*. In brawny edema, the skin swells so much that fluid can't be displaced.

How pulmonary edema develops

Excess fluid volume that lasts a long time can cause pulmonary edema. These illustrations show how that process occurs.

Normal

Normal pulmonary fluid movement depends on the equal force of two opposing pressures—hydrostatic pressure and plasma oncotic pressure from protein molecules in the blood.

Congestion

Abnormally high pulmonary hydrostatic pressure (indicated by increased PAWP) forces fluid out of the capillaries and into the interstitial space, causing pulmonary congestion.

Edema

When the amount of interstitial fluid becomes excessive, fluid is forced into the alveoli. Pulmonary edema results. Fluid fills the alveoli and prevents the exchange of gases.

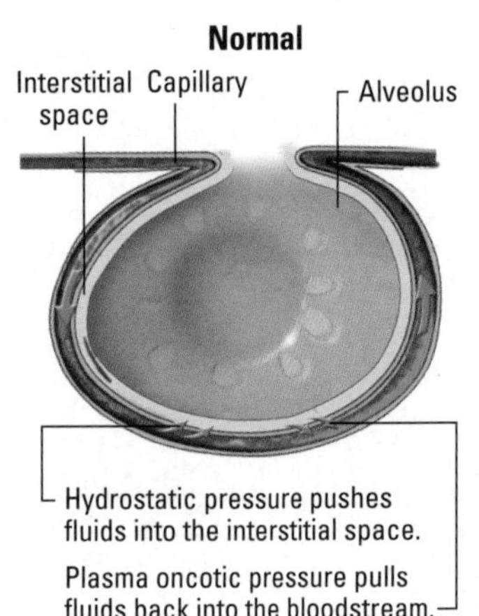

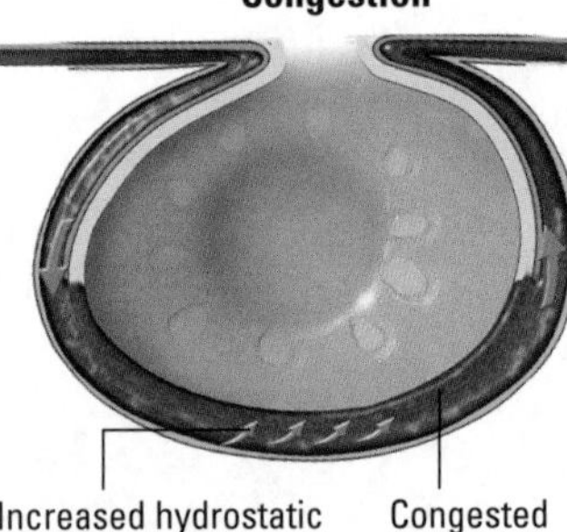

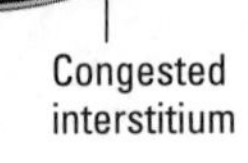

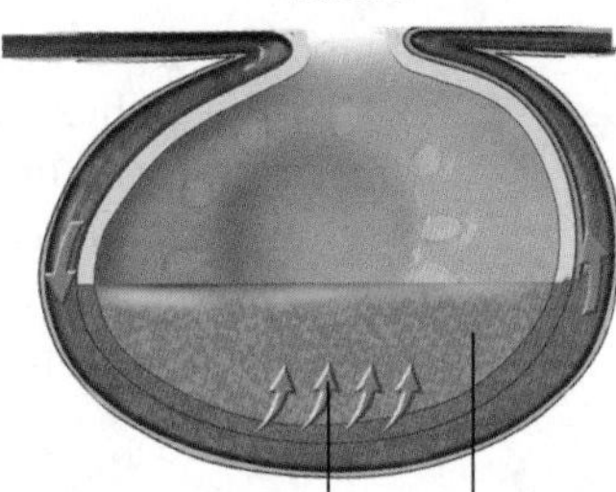

- low oxygen level (with early tachypnea, partial pressure of arterial carbon dioxide may be low, causing a drop in pH and respiratory alkalosis)
- pulmonary congestion on chest X-rays.

How it's treated

Treatment for hypervolemia includes restriction of sodium and fluid intake and administration of medications to prevent such complications as heart failure and pulmonary edema. The cause of the hypervolemia should also be treated. The patient receives diuretics to promote the loss of excess fluid.

If the patient has pulmonary edema, he may receive additional drugs, such as morphine and nitroglycerin, to dilate blood vessels, which in turn reduces pulmonary congestion and the amount of blood returning to the heart. Heart failure is treated with digoxin, which strengthens cardiac contractions and slows the heart rate. Oxygen and bed rest help support the patient.

When the kidneys aren't working properly, diuretics may not be enough to rid the body of extra fluid. The patient may require hemodialysis or continuous renal replacement therapy (CRRT). (See *Understanding CRRT.*)

Understanding CRRT

CRRT is used to manage fluid and electrolyte imbalances in hemodynamically unstable patients with multiple organ failure or renal failure who can't tolerate hemodialysis (Gaspar, Moreira, Moutinho, Pinto, & Lima, 2002). In CRRT, a dual-lumen venous catheter provides access to the patient's blood and propels it through a tubing circuit.

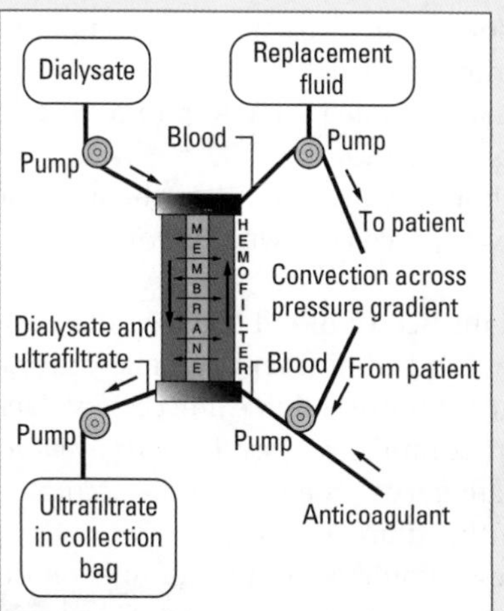

How it works

The illustration at the right shows the standard setup for one type of CRRT called *continuous venovenous hemofiltration.* The patient's blood enters the hemofilter from a line connected to one lumen of the venous catheter, flows through the hemofilter, and returns to the patient through the second lumen of the catheter.

At the first pump, an anticoagulant may be added to the blood. A second pump moves dialysate through the hemofilter. A third pump adds replacement fluid if needed. The ultrafiltrate (plasma water and toxins) removed from the blood drains into a collection bag.

Advantages

- Allows immediate access to the patient's blood via a dual-lumen venous catheter
- Conserves cellular and protein components of blood
- Doesn't create dramatic changes in the patient's blood pressure, which often occurs with hemodialysis
- Offers precise control of fluid volume

Disadvantages

- Must be performed by a specially trained critical care or nephrology nurse
- Must take place on a critical care unit
- Requires CRRT equipment and supplies
- May pose issues of staff competency if CRRT is rarely used
- Is time consuming and expensive
- May cause hypothermia

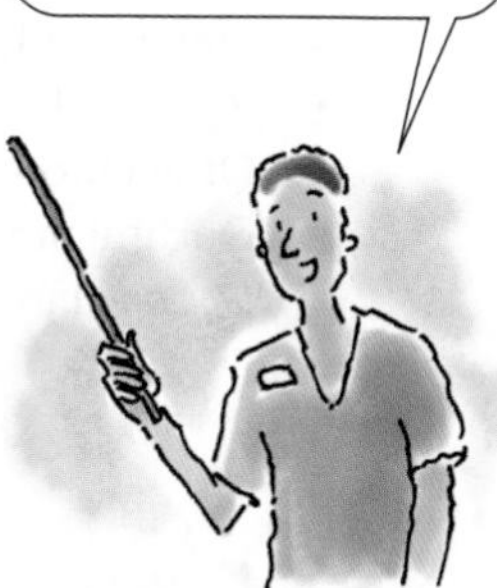
For a patient who can't tolerate dialysis, CRRT may be the solution.

How you intervene

Caring for a patient with hypervolemia requires a number of nursing actions. Here are some of them:

- Assess the patient's vital signs and hemodynamic status, noting his response to therapy. Watch for signs of hypovolemia due to overcorrection. Remember that elderly, pediatric, and otherwise compromised patients are at higher risk for complications.
- Monitor respiratory patterns for worsening distress, such as increased tachypnea or dyspnea.
- Watch for distended veins in the hands or neck.
- Record intake and output hourly.
- Listen to breath sounds regularly to assess for pulmonary edema. Note crackles or rhonchi.
- Follow ABG results and watch for a drop in oxygen level or changes in acid-base balance.
- Monitor other laboratory test results for changes, including potassium levels (decreased with use of most diuretics) and HCT.
- Raise the head of the bed (if blood pressure allows) to help the patient's breathing, and administer oxygen as ordered.
- Make sure the patient restricts fluids if necessary. Alert the family and staff to ensure compliance. (See *Teaching about hypervolemia.*)
- Insert a urinary catheter as ordered to more accurately monitor output before starting diuretic therapy.
- Maintain I.V. access as ordered for the administration of medications such as diuretics. If the patient is prone to hypervolemia, use an infusion pump with any infusions to prevent administering too much fluid.
- Give prescribed diuretics and other medications and monitor the patient for effectiveness and adverse reactions.
- Watch for edema, especially in dependent areas.
- Check for an S_3, audible when the ventricles are volume overloaded. S_3 is best heard over the heart's apex over the mitral area.
- Provide frequent mouth care.
- Obtain daily weight and evaluate trends.
- Provide skin care because edematous skin is prone to break down.
- Offer emotional support to the patient and his family.
- Document your assessment findings and interventions. (See *Documenting hypervolemia.*)

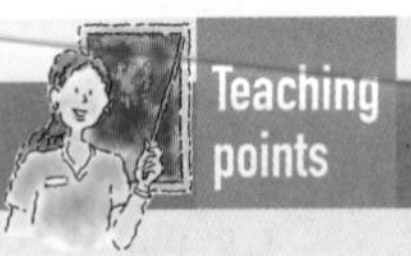

Teaching about hypervolemia

When teaching a patient with hypervolemia, be sure to cover the following topics and then evaluate the patient's learning:

- nature of the condition and its causes
- warning signs and symptoms and when they should be reported
- treatment and the importance of compliance
- measurement of blood pressure and pulse rate
- restriction of sodium and fluids
- importance of being weighed regularly
- prescribed medications
- referral to dietitian, if appropriate.

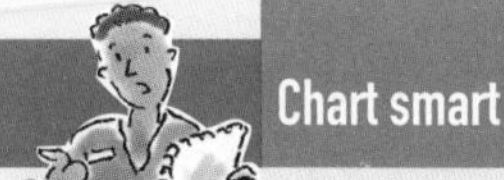

Chart smart

Documenting hypervolemia

For a patient who is hypervolemic, you should document:

- your assessment findings, including vital signs, hemodynamic status, pulmonary status, and edema
- oxygen therapy in use
- intake and output
- interventions, such as administration of a diuretic, and the patient's response
- daily weight and the type of scale used
- pertinent laboratory results
- dietary or fluid restrictions
- safety measures implemented
- patient teaching.

Water intoxication

Water intoxication occurs when excess fluid moves from the extracellular space to the intracellular space. Here's the lowdown on this condition.

How it happens

Excessive low-sodium fluid in the extracellular space is hypotonic to the cells; the cells are hypertonic to the fluid. Because of this imbalance, fluid shifts—by osmosis—into the cells, which have comparatively less fluid and more solutes. That fluid shift, which causes the cells to swell, occurs as a means of balancing the concentration of fluid between the two spaces, a condition called *water intoxication*.

Water, water everywhere

By causing the body to hold on to electrolyte-free water (despite low plasma osmolality [dilute plasma] and high fluid volume), syndrome of inappropriate antidiuretic hormone (SIADH) secretion can cause water intoxication. SIADH can result from central nervous system or pulmonary disorders, head trauma, certain medications, tumors, and some surgeries. (You'll learn more about SIADH when you read the discussion on sodium imbalances in chapter 5.)

Water intoxication can also occur with rapid infusions of hypotonic solutions such as D_5W. Excessive use of tap water as a nasogastric tube irrigant or enema also increases water intake.

Psychogenic polydipsia, a psychological condition, is another cause. It occurs when a person continues to drink water or other fluids in large amounts, even when they aren't needed. The condition is especially dangerous if the person's kidneys don't function well.

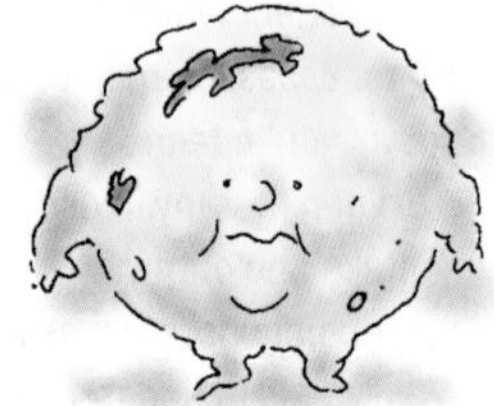
I have *definitely* had too much water to drink . . .

What to look for

Indications of water intoxication include low sodium levels and increased intracranial pressure (ICP), which occurs as brain cells swell. Although headache and personality changes are the first symptoms, suspect any change in behavior or level of consciousness, such as confusion, irritability, or lethargy. The patient may also experience nausea, vomiting, cramping, muscle weakness, twitching, thirst, dyspnea on exertion, and dulled sensorium.

Late signs of increased ICP include pupillary and vital sign changes, such as bradycardia and widened pulse pressure. A patient with water intoxication may develop seizures and coma. Any weight gain reflects additional cellular fluid.

What tests show

Typical laboratory findings for a patient with water intoxication include:

- serum sodium level less than 125 mEq/L
- serum osmolality less than 280 mOsm/kg.

How it's treated

Treatment for water intoxication includes correcting the underlying cause, restricting both oral and parenteral fluid intake, and avoiding the use of hypotonic I.V. solutions, such as D_5W, until serum sodium levels rise. Hypertonic solutions are used only in severe situations to draw fluid out of the cells and require close patient monitoring. The original cause of the intoxication should also be addressed.

How you intervene

The best treatment for water intoxication is prevention. However, if your patient develops water intoxication, you'll want to implement the following nursing actions:

- Closely assess his neurologic status; watch for deterioration, especially changes in personality or level of consciousness.
- Monitor vital signs and intake and output to evaluate the patient's progress.
- Maintain oral and I.V. fluid restrictions as prescribed.
- Alert the dietitian and the patient's family about the restrictions, and post a sign in the patient's room to let staff members know. (See *Teaching about water intoxication*.)
- Insert an I.V. catheter and maintain it as ordered; infuse hypertonic solutions with care using an infusion pump.
- Closely observe the patient's response to therapy.
- Weigh the patient daily to detect retention of excess water.
- Monitor laboratory test results such as serum sodium levels.
- Provide a safe environment for the patient with an altered neurologic status and teach his family to do the same.
- Institute seizure precautions in severe cases.
- Document your assessment findings and interventions. (See *Documenting water intoxication*.)

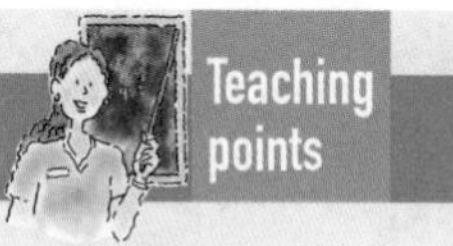

Teaching about water intoxication

When teaching a patient with water intoxication, be sure to cover the following topics and then evaluate the patient's learning:

- nature of the condition and its causes
- need for fluid restriction
- warning signs and symptoms and when they should be reported
- prescribed medications
- importance of being weighed regularly.

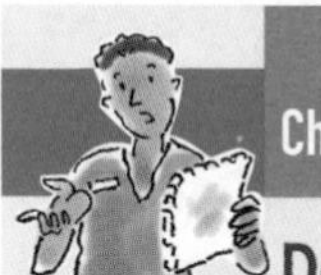

Chart smart

Documenting water intoxication

For a patient with water intoxication, you should document:

- all assessment findings
- intake and output, noting fluid restrictions
- safety measures
- types of seizure activity and treatment
- laboratory results
- daily weight
- nursing interventions and patient's response
- patient teaching.

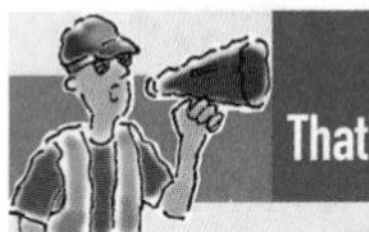

That's a wrap!

Fluid imbalances review

Fluid volume basics

- Blood pressure is related to the amount of blood the heart pumps.
- Fluid volume affects the amount of blood to the heart; therefore, assessing blood pressure also assesses a patient's fluid status.

Measuring blood pressure and fluid volume status

- Sphygmomanometer and stethoscope
  - Provide simple and noninvasive method for measuring blood pressure
  - Require use of proper size cuff
  - Require cuff to be placed over the medial aspect of the arm, over the brachial artery
- Arterial lines
  - Are typically inserted into the radial or the brachial artery
  - Are used to continuously monitor blood pressure
  - Can also be used to sample arterial blood for laboratory tests
- PA catheters
  - Are inserted into the subclavian or the internal jugular vein
  - Measure PAP, PAWP, CVP, and cardiac output
  - Help assess left-sided heart function, including pumping ability, filling pressures, and vascular volume
  - Give clearest picture of fluid volume status

Dehydration

- Lack of water in extracellular spaces that causes fluid to shift out of the cells, which then shrink
- May be caused by any situation that accelerates fluid loss, including diabetes insipidus, prolonged fever, watery diarrhea, renal failure, and hyperglycemia
- Patients who are more prone to dehydration:
  - Comatose, confused, or bedridden patients
  - Infants
  - Elderly patients
  - Patients receiving highly concentrated tube feedings without enough supplemental water
- Assessment findings: irritability, confusion, dizziness, weakness, extreme thirst, fever, dry skin, dry mucous membranes, sunken eyeballs, poor skin turgor, decreased urine output (with diabetes insipidus, urine is pale and plentiful), and increased heart rate with falling blood pressure

Hypovolemia

- Hypotonic fluid loss from extracellular space
- May progress to hypovolemic shock if not detected early and treated properly
- Is caused by excessive fluid loss or third-space fluid shift

Signs and symptoms of fluid loss

- Mild fluid loss
  - Orthostatic hypotension
  - Restlessness
  - Anxiety
  - Weight loss
  - Increased heart rate
- Moderate fluid loss
  - Confusion
  - Dizziness

Fluid imbalances review *(continued)*

- Irritability
- Extreme thirst
- Nausea
- Cool, clammy skin
- Rapid pulse
- Decreased urine output (10 to 30 ml/hour)

• Severe fluid loss
- Decreased cardiac output
- Unconsciousness
- Marked tachycardia
- Hypotension
- Weak or absent peripheral pulses
- Cool, mottled skin
- Decreased urine output (< 10 ml/hour)

Hypervolemia

• Excess isotonic fluid in extracellular spaces
• Can lead to heart failure and pulmonary edema, especially in prolonged or severe hypervolemia or in patients with poor heart function
• Mild to moderate fluid gain equaling a 5% to 10% weight gain
• Severe fluid gain equaling more than a 10% weight gain
• Causes include:
- excessive sodium or fluid intake
- fluid or sodium retention
- shift in fluid from the interstitial space into the intravascular space
- acute or chronic renal failure with low urine output

• Assessment findings: tachypnea; dyspnea; crackles; rapid or bounding pulse; hypertension (unless in heart failure); increased CVP, PAP, and PAWP; distended neck and hand veins; acute weight gain; edema and S_3 gallop

Water intoxication

• Excess fluid in the intracellular space from the extracellular space
• Causes increased ICP
• May lead to seizures and coma
• Causes include:
- SIADH
- rapid infusion of a hypotonic solution
- excessive use of tap water as a nasogastric tube irrigant or an enema
- psychogenic polydipsia

• Test results: low serum sodium levels and low serum osmolality

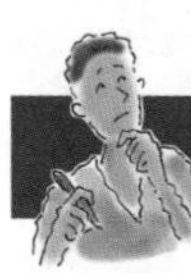

Quick quiz

1. Populations at risk for dehydration include:
   A. infants.
   B. adolescents.
   C. patients with SIADH.
   D. young adults.

Answer: A. Patients at risk for dehydration are those who either have an impaired thirst mechanism or can't respond to the thirst reflex. Infants fall into this category.

2. Checking for orthostatic hypotension allows the nurse to detect early signs of:

A. hypovolemia.
B. low serum osmolality.
C. high serum osmolality.
D. hypervolemia.

Answer: A. Changes in blood pressure—which can result in orthostatic hypotension—and pulse are two initial changes seen with hypovolemia.

3. Of the following options, the first step you should take for a patient with hypovolemic shock is to:

A. assess for dehydration.
B. administer I.V. fluids.
C. insert a urinary catheter.
D. prepare for surgery.

Answer: B. Hypovolemic shock is an emergency that requires rapid infusion of I.V. fluids.

4. One sign of hypervolemia is:

A. increased urine output.
B. clear, watery sputum.
C. severe hypertension.
D. a rapid, bounding pulse.

Answer: D. Excess fluid in the intravascular space causes a rapid, bounding pulse. When hypervolemia progresses, it can fill the lungs with fluid and cause pulmonary edema, as indicated by the presence of pink, frothy sputum.

5. Water intoxication can be caused by:

A. administering too much hypertonic fluid.
B. administering too much hypotonic fluid.
C. encouraging fluid intake.
D. administering too much isotonic fluid.

Answer: B. Administering too much hypotonic fluid can cause water to shift from the blood vessels into the cells, leading to water intoxication and cellular edema.

Scoring

☆☆☆ If you answered all five questions correctly, way to go! Your fluidity leaves us breathless!

☆☆ If you answered four correctly, great going! You certainly know how to go with the flow of understanding fluid imbalances.

☆ If you answered fewer than four correctly, that's okay. Splash a little water on your face and check over the chapter again!

References

Ashford, J. R. (2008). Hydration and dysphagia management: Water: Understanding a necessity of life. *ASHA Leader, 13*(14), 10–12.

Dix, D. (2012). Hypertensive disorders in pregnancy. In D. L. Lowdermilk, S. E. Perry, K. Cashion, & K. R. Alden (Eds.), *Maternity & women's health care* (10th ed., pp. 654–669). St. Louis, MO: Mosby.

Garcia, M. G., Ang, E., Ahmad, M. N., & Lim, C. C. (2012). Correct placement of blood pressure cuff during blood pressure measurement. *International Journal of Evidence-Based Healthcare, 10*(3), 191–196.

Gaspar, L. J., Moreira, N. M., Moutinho, A. A., Pinto, P. J., & Lima, H. B. (2002). Continuous renal replacement therapies. *Journal of Renal Care, 28*(S2), 19–22.

Muralidhar, K. (2002). Central venous pressure and pulmonary capillary wedge pressure monitoring. *Indian Journal of Anaesthesia, 46*(4), 298–303.

Chapter 5

When sodium tips the balance

Just the facts

In this chapter, you'll learn:

- ways that sodium contributes to fluid and electrolyte balance
- the body's mechanisms for regulating sodium balance
- causes, signs and symptoms, and treatments associated with sodium imbalances
- proper care for the patient with a sodium imbalance.

A look at sodium

Sodium is one of the most important elements in the body. It accounts for 90% of extracellular fluid cations (positively charged ions) and is the most abundant solute in extracellular fluid. In the body's normal state, almost all sodium in the body is found in this fluid.

Why it's important

The body needs sodium to maintain proper extracellular fluid osmolality (concentration). Sodium attracts fluid and helps preserve the extracellular fluid volume and fluid distribution in the body. It also helps transmit impulses in nerve and muscle fibers and combines with chloride and bicarbonate to regulate acid-base balance. Because the electrolyte compositions of serum and interstitial fluid are essentially equal, sodium concentration in extracellular fluid is measured in serum levels. The normal range for serum sodium level is 135 to 145 mEq/L. As a comparison, the amount of sodium inside a cell is 10 mEq/L (Deglin, Vallerand, & Sanoski, 2013; Smeltzer, Bare, Hinkle, & Cheever, 2010).

Sodium is vital to life!

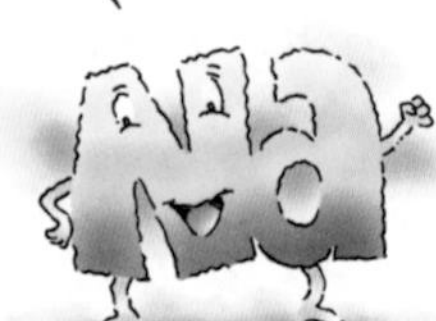

How the body regulates sodium

What a person eats and how the intestines absorb it determine a body's sodium level. Sodium requirements vary according to the individual's size and age. The minimum daily requirement is 0.5 to 2.7 g; however, a salty diet provides at least 6 g/day. The U.S. Department of Agriculture (2013) has released new guidelines suggesting no one should consume more than 2,300 mg of salt per day. They also suggest that people age 51 years and older and those who are African American or have high blood pressure, diabetes, or chronic kidney disease should restrict salt intake to 1,500 mg daily. One teaspoon of table salt has 2,325 mg of sodium (U.S. Department of Agriculture, 2013).

Kidneys naturally balance the amount of sodium stored in the body for optimal health. When sodium levels are low, kidneys essentially hold on to the sodium. When sodium levels are high, kidneys excrete the excess in urine.

If the kidneys can't eliminate enough sodium, the sodium starts to accumulate in the bloodstream. Because sodium attracts and holds water, blood volume increases, which in turn increases workload of the heart and contributes to high blood pressure. (See *Dietary sources of sodium*.)

Sodium is also excreted through the gastrointestinal (GI) tract and through the skin in sweat. When you think *sodium*, you should automatically think *water* as well—the two are that closely related in the body. The normal range of serum sodium levels reflects this close relationship. If sodium intake suddenly increases, extracellular fluid concentration also rises and vice versa (Smeltzer et al., 2010).

Dietary sources of sodium

Major dietary sources of sodium include:

- canned soups and vegetables
- cheese
- ketchup
- processed meats
- table salt
- salty snack foods
- seafood
- pickled foods
- seasonings such as monosodium glutamate, seasoned salt, and soy sauce
- baked goods with baking powder and baking soda.

Not too much!

The body makes adjustments when the sodium level rises. Increased serum sodium levels cause the individual to feel thirsty and the posterior pituitary gland to release antidiuretic hormone (ADH). (For more information about ADH, see chapter 1, Balancing fluids.) ADH causes the kidneys to retain water, which dilutes the blood and normalizes serum osmolality.

When sodium levels decrease and serum osmolality decreases, thirst and ADH secretion are suppressed, and the kidneys excrete more water to restore normal osmolality. (See *Regulating sodium and water*, page 86.)

Aldosterone also regulates extracellular sodium balance via a feedback loop. The adrenal cortex secretes aldosterone, which stimulates the renal tubules to conserve water and sodium when the body's sodium level is low, thus helping to normalize extracellular fluid sodium levels (George, Majeed, Mackenzie, MacDonald, & Wei, 2013; Smeltzer et al., 2010).

The power of the pump

Normally, extracellular sodium levels are very high compared with intracellular sodium levels. The body contains an active transport

Regulating sodium and water

This flowchart shows two of the body's compensatory mechanisms for restoring sodium and water balance.

Serum sodium level decreases (water excess)	Serum sodium level increases (water deficit)
↓	↓
Serum osmolality falls to less than 280 mOsm/kg	Serum osmolality rises to more than 300 mOsm/kg
↓	↓
Thirst diminishes, leading to decreased water intake	Thirst increases, leading to increased water intake
↓	↓
ADH release is suppressed	ADH release increases
↓	↓
Renal water excretion increases	Renal water excretion diminishes
↓	↓
Serum osmolality normalizes	Serum osmolality normalizes

mechanism, called the *sodium-potassium pump*, that helps maintain normal sodium levels. This is how the pump works:

In diffusion (a form of passive transport), a substance moves from an area of higher concentration to one of lower concentration. Sodium ions, normally most abundant outside the cells, tend to diffuse inward, and potassium (K) ions, normally most abundant inside the cells, tend to diffuse outward. To combat this ionic diffusion and maintain normal sodium and potassium levels, the sodium-potassium pump is constantly at work in every cell.

However, moving sodium out of the cell and potassium back in can't happen without some help. Each ion links with a carrier because it can't get through the cell wall alone. This movement requires energy (a form of active transport), which comes from adenosine triphosphate (ATP)—made up of phosphorus, another electrolyte—magnesium, and an enzyme. These substances help move sodium out of the cell and force potassium back into the cell.

Sodium-potassium pump

This illustration shows how the sodium-potassium pump carries ions when their concentrations change.

Normal placement

Normally, more sodium (Na) ions exist outside cells than inside. More potassium (K) ions exist inside cells than outside.

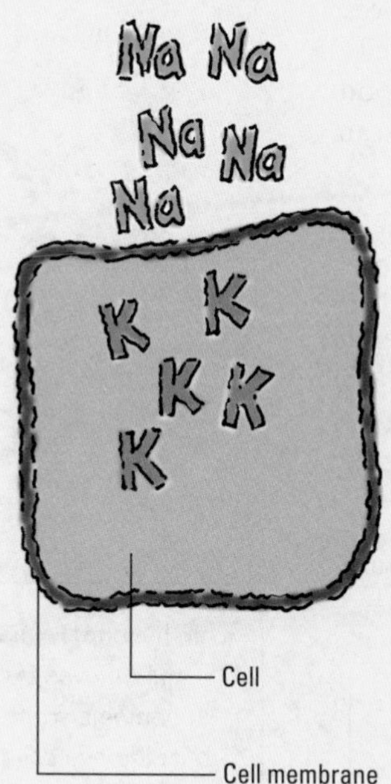

Increased permeability

Certain stimuli increase the membrane's permeability. When this occurs, sodium ions diffuse inward; potassium ions diffuse outward.

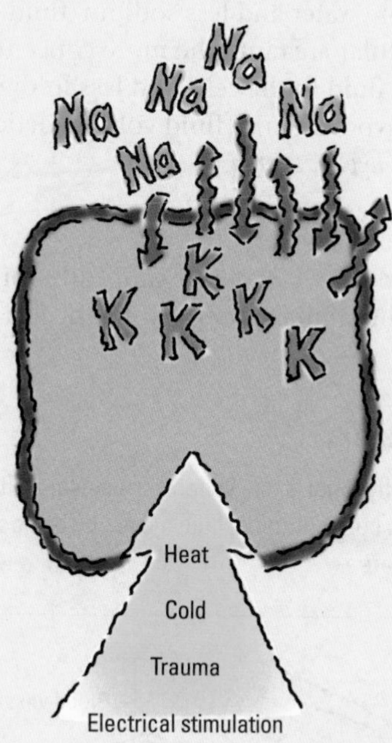

Energy source

The cell links each ion with a carrier molecule that helps the ion return through the cell wall. Energy for the ion's return trip comes from ATP, magnesium (Mg), and an enzyme commonly found in cells.

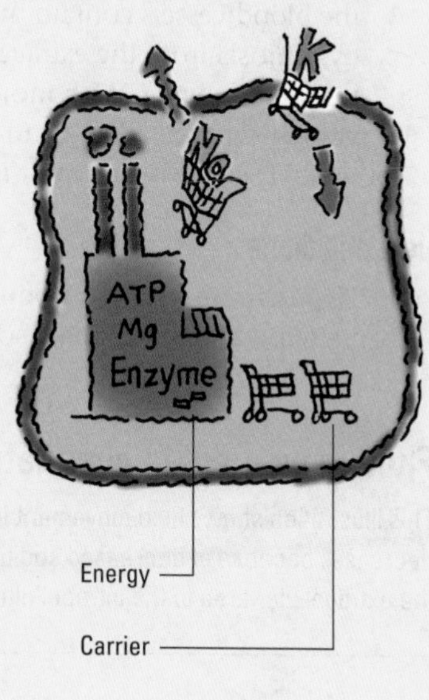

The sodium-potassium pump allows the body to carry out its essential functions and helps prevent cellular swelling caused by too many ions inside the cell attracting excessive amounts of water. The pump also creates an electrical charge in the cell from the movement of ions, permitting transmission of neuromuscular impulses. (See *Sodium-potassium pump*.)

Hyponatremia

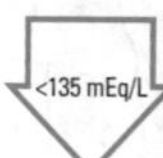

A common electrolyte imbalance, *hyponatremia* is a term that describes a state when sodium concentration in the plasma (outside the cell) is lower than normal. In other words, body fluids are diluted and cells swell from decreased extracellular fluid osmolality. Severe hyponatremia can lead to seizures, coma, and permanent neurologic damage.

How it happens

Normally, the body gets rid of excess water by secreting less ADH; less ADH causes diuresis. For that to happen, the nephrons must be functioning normally, receiving and excreting excess water and reabsorbing sodium.

Hyponatremia develops when this regulatory function goes haywire. Serum sodium levels decrease, and fluid shifts occur. When the blood vessels contain more water and less sodium, fluid moves by osmosis from the extracellular area into the more concentrated intracellular area. With more fluid in the cells and less in the blood vessels, cerebral edema and hypovolemia (fluid volume deficit) can occur. (See *Fluid movement in hyponatremia.*)

Deplete and dilute

Hyponatremia results from sodium loss, water gain (dilutional hyponatremia), or inadequate sodium intake (depletional hyponatremia).

Fluid movement in hyponatremia

This illustration shows fluid movement in hyponatremia. When serum osmolality decreases because of decreased sodium concentration, fluid moves by osmosis from the extracellular area to the intracellular area.

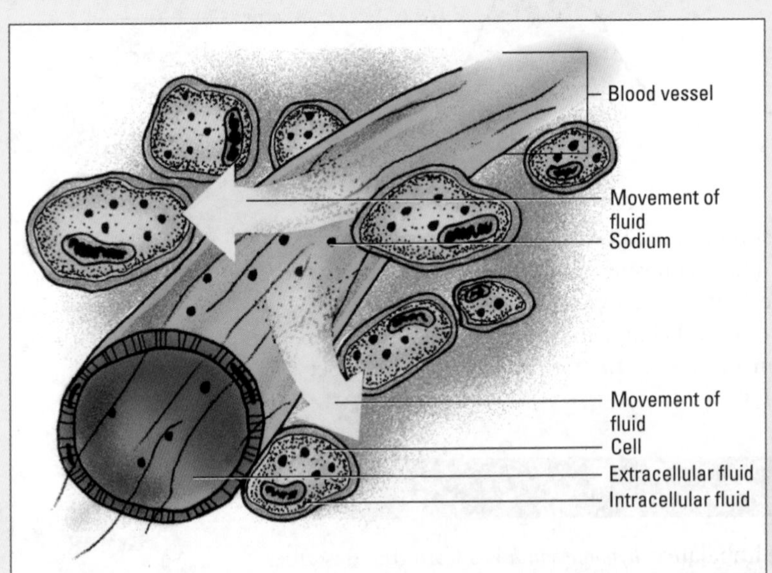

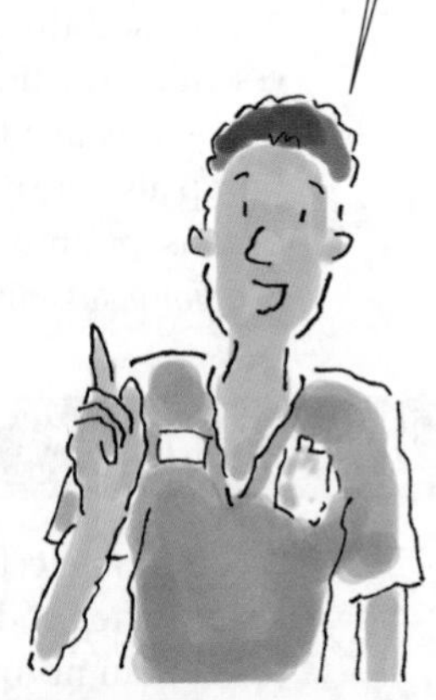
In hyponatremia, fluid moves by osmosis from outside the cell to inside the cell.

It may be classified according to whether extracellular fluid volume is abnormally decreased (hypovolemic hyponatremia), abnormally increased (hypervolemic hyponatremia), or equal to intracellular fluid volume (isovolemic hyponatremia).

Sodium slips lower

In *hypovolemic hyponatremia*, both sodium and water levels decrease in the extracellular area, but sodium loss is greater than water loss. Causes may be nonrenal or renal. Nonrenal causes include vomiting, diarrhea, fistulas, gastric suctioning, excessive sweating, cystic fibrosis, burns, and wound drainage. Renal causes include osmotic diuresis, salt-losing nephritis, adrenal insufficiency, and diuretic use.

Diuretics promote sodium loss and volume depletion from the blood vessels, causing the individual to feel thirsty and his kidneys to retain water. Drinking large quantities of water can worsen hyponatremia. Sodium deficits can also become more pronounced if the patient is on a sodium-restricted diet. Diuretics can cause potassium loss (hypokalemia), which is also linked to hyponatremia. (See *Drugs associated with hyponatremia*.)

Water rises higher

In *hypervolemic hyponatremia*, both water and sodium levels increase in the extracellular area, but the water gain is more impressive. Serum sodium levels are diluted and edema also occurs. Causes include heart failure, liver failure, nephrotic syndrome, excessive administration of hypotonic I.V. fluids, and hyperaldosteronism.

Drugs associated with hyponatremia

Drugs can cause hyponatremia by potentiating the action of ADH or by causing syndrome of inappropriate antidiuretic hormone secretion. Diuretics may also cause hyponatremia by inhibiting sodium reabsorption in the kidneys.

Anticoagulants	Anticonvulsants	Antidiabetics	Antineoplastics	Antipsychotics/ mood altering	Diuretics	Sedatives
• Heparin	• Acetazolamide • Carbamazepine	• Chlorpropamide • Tolbutamide (rarely)	• Cyclophosphamide • Vincristine	• Fluphenazine • Thioridazine • Thiothixene • Amitriptyline • Lithium	• Amiloride • Loop (for example, bumetanide, furosemide, ethacrynic acid) • Thiazides (for example, hydrochlorothiazide)	• Barbiturates • Morphine

(Deglin et al., 2013; Institute for Safe Medicine Practices, 2012)

Water rises alone

In *isovolemic hyponatremia,* also called *dilutional hyponatremia,* sodium levels may appear low because too much fluid is in the body. However, these patients have no physical signs of fluid volume excess, and total body sodium remains stable. Causes include glucocorticoid deficiency (causing inadequate fluid filtration by the kidneys), hypothyroidism (causing limited water excretion), and renal failure (Smeltzer et al., 2010).

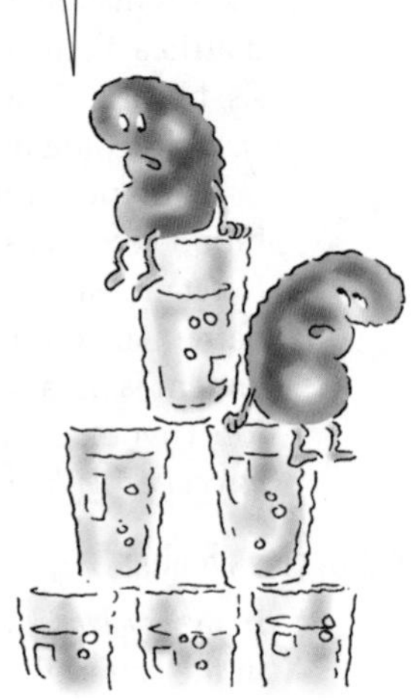
Renal failure can lead to dilutional hyponatremia, which results in water levels that are much higher than we like.

Disturbing the balance

Another cause of isovolemic hyponatremia is syndrome of inappropriate antidiuretic hormone (SIADH) secretion. SIADH causes excessive release of ADH, which causes inappropriate and excessive water retention, thereby disturbing fluid and electrolyte balance. This syndrome is a major cause of low sodium levels. ADH is released when the body doesn't need it, which results in water retention and sodium excretion. (See *What happens in SIADH.*)

SIADH occurs with:

- cancers, especially cancer of the duodenum and pancreas and oat cell carcinoma of the lung
- central nervous system (CNS) disorders, such as trauma, tumors, and stroke
- pulmonary disorders, such as tumors, asthma, and chronic obstructive pulmonary disease
- medications, such as certain oral antidiabetics, chemotherapeutic drugs, psychoactive drugs, diuretics, synthetic hormones, and barbiturates.

What lies beneath

The patient is treated for the underlying cause of SIADH and for hyponatremia. For instance, if a tumor caused the syndrome, the patient would receive cancer treatment; if a medication caused it, the drug would be stopped. The low sodium levels are treated with fluid restriction (about 1 qt [1 L]/day) and diuretics, such as furosemide.

For many patients, initial treatment may be simple. The patient is placed on fluid restriction to lower water intake to match the low volume of urine caused by the increased ADH. Serum osmolality then increases, causing the ADH level to balance it. If this treatment is inadequate, then the patient may receive oral urea or be instructed to follow a high-sodium diet to increase the kidneys' excretion of solutes (water follows). The patient may also receive medications, such as demeclocycline or lithium, to block ADH in the renal tubule. If fluid restriction doesn't raise the patient's sodium levels, he may need a hypertonic saline solution.

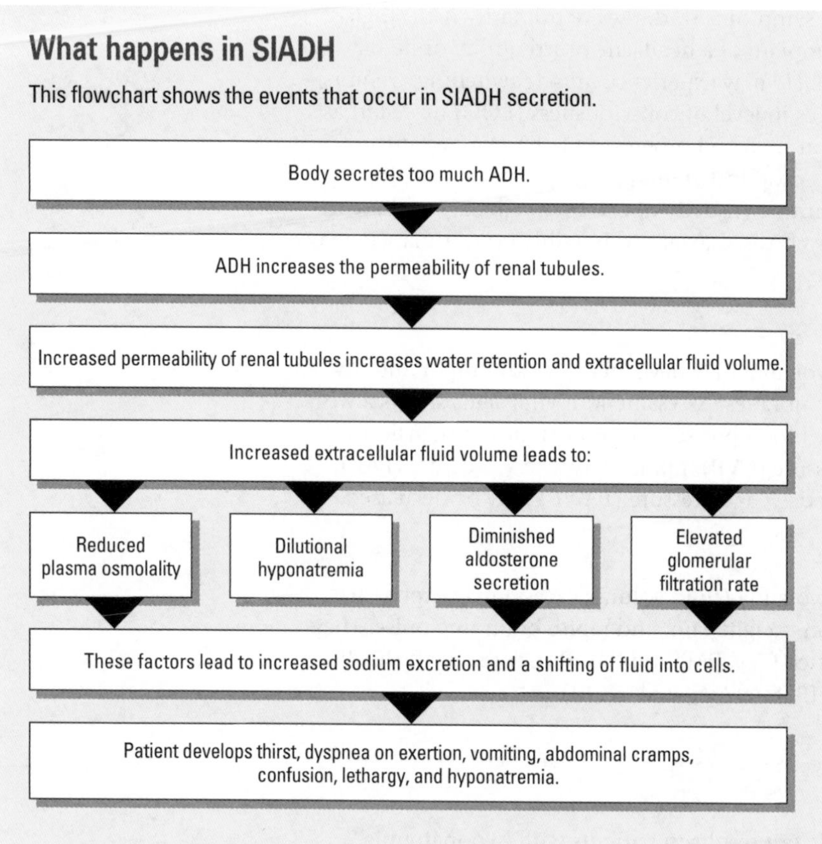

What happens in SIADH

This flowchart shows the events that occur in SIADH secretion.

Body secretes too much ADH.
ADH increases the permeability of renal tubules.
Increased permeability of renal tubules increases water retention and extracellular fluid volume.
Increased extracellular fluid volume leads to:
Reduced plasma osmolality
Dilutional hyponatremia
Diminished aldosterone secretion
Elevated glomerular filtration rate
These factors lead to increased sodium excretion and a shifting of fluid into cells.
Patient develops thirst, dyspnea on exertion, vomiting, abdominal cramps, confusion, lethargy, and hyponatremia.

What to look for

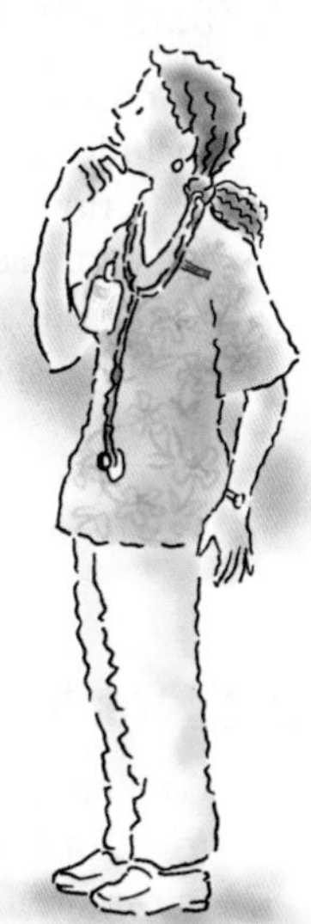

As you look for signs of hyponatremia, remember that they vary from patient to patient. They also vary depending on how quickly the patient's sodium level drops. If the level drops quickly, the patient will be more symptomatic than if the level drops slowly. Patients with sodium levels above 125 mEq/L may not show signs of hyponatremia—but, again, this depends on how quickly sodium levels drop. Usually, acute initial signs and symptoms of nausea, vomiting, and anorexia begin when the serum sodium levels fall between 115 and 120 mEq/L (Smeltzer et al., 2010).

When signs and symptoms start, they're primarily neurologic. The patient may complain of a headache or irritability or he may become disoriented. He may experience muscle twitching, tremors, or weakness. Changes in level of consciousness (LOC) may start as a shortened attention span and progress to lethargy or confusion. When sodium levels drop to 110 mEq/L, the patient's neurologic status deteriorates further (usually due to brain edema), leading to stupor, delirium, psychosis, ataxia, and possibly even coma. He may also develop seizures.

Low show

Patients with hypovolemia may have inelastic skin turgor and dry, cracked mucous membranes. Assessment of vital signs shows a weak, rapid pulse and low blood pressure or orthostatic hypotension. Central venous pressure (CVP), pulmonary artery pressure (PAP), and pulmonary artery wedge pressure (PAWP) may be decreased.

High signs

Patients with hypervolemia (fluid volume excess) may experience edema, hypertension, weight gain, and rapid, bounding pulse. They may also have elevated CVP, PAP, and PAWP (George et al., 2013; Lindner & Funk, 2013; Smeltzer et al., 2010).

What tests show

Common diagnostic test results in patients with hyponatremia include:

- serum osmolality less than 280 mOsm/kg (dilute blood)
- serum sodium level less than 135 mEq/L (low sodium level in blood)
- urine specific gravity less than 1.010
- increased urine specific gravity and elevated urine sodium levels (above 20 mEq/L) in patients with SIADH
- elevated hematocrit and plasma protein levels.

How it's treated

Generally, treatment varies with the cause and severity of hyponatremia. For example, the patient with an underlying endocrine disorder may require hormone therapy.

Milder measures

Therapy for mild hyponatremia associated with hypervolemia or isovolemia usually consists of restricted fluid intake and possibly oral sodium supplements. If hyponatremia is related to hypovolemia, the patient may receive isotonic I.V. fluids such as normal saline solution to restore volume. High-sodium foods may also be offered.

Critical steps

When serum sodium levels fall below 120 mEq/L, treatment in the intensive care unit may include infusion of a hypertonic saline solution (such as 3% or 5% saline) if the patient is symptomatic (seizures, coma). Monitor the patient carefully during the infusion for signs of circulatory overload or worsening neurologic status. A hypertonic saline solution causes water to shift out of cells, which may lead to intravascular volume overload and serious brain damage (osmotic demyelination), especially in the pons.

Fluid volume overload can be fatal if untreated. To prevent fluid overload, a hypertonic sodium chloride solution is infused slowly and in small volumes. Furosemide is usually administered at the same time. Infusions of hypertonic solution (3% to 5%) are only done in the intensive care unit with cardiac monitoring available. Sodium levels should not be raised more than 25 mEq/L in the first 48 hours with the rate not exceeding 1 to 2 mEq/L/hour (Smeltzer et al., 2010).

Hypervolemic patients shouldn't receive hypertonic sodium chloride solutions, except in rare instances of severe symptomatic hyponatremia. During treatment, monitor serum sodium levels and related diagnostic tests to follow the patient's progress (George et al., 2013; Lindner & Funk, 2013; Smeltzer et al., 2010).

How you intervene

Watch patients at risk for hyponatremia, including those with heart failure, cancer, or GI disorders with fluid losses. Review your patient's medications, noting those that are associated with hyponatremia. For patients who develop hyponatremia, you'll want to take the following actions:

- Monitor and record vital signs, especially blood pressure and pulse, and watch for orthostatic hypotension and tachycardia.
- Monitor neurologic status frequently. Report any deterioration in LOC. Assess the patient for lethargy, muscle twitching, seizures, and coma.
- Accurately measure and record intake and output.
- Weigh the patient daily to monitor the success of fluid restriction.
- Assess skin turgor at least every 8 hours for signs of dehydration.
- Watch for and report extreme changes in serum sodium levels and accompanying serum chloride levels. Also monitor other test results, such as urine specific gravity and serum osmolality.

- Restrict fluid intake as ordered. (Fluid restriction is the primary treatment for dilutional hyponatremia.) Post a sign about fluid restriction in the patient's room and make sure the staff, the patient, and his family are aware of the restrictions. (See *Teaching about hyponatremia and hypernatremia*, page 99.)
- Administer oral sodium supplements, if prescribed, to treat mild hyponatremia. If the practitioner has instructed the patient to increase his intake of dietary sodium, teach him about foods high in sodium.
- For severe hyponatremia, make sure a patent I.V. line is in place, then administer prescribed I.V. isotonic or hypertonic saline solutions. Do so cautiously to avoid inducing hypernatremia, brain injury, or fluid volume overload from an excessive or too rapid infusion. Watch closely for signs of hypervolemia (dyspnea, crackles, engorged neck or hand veins), and report them immediately. Use an infusion pump to ensure that the patient receives only the prescribed volume of fluid.
- Keep the patient safe while he undergoes treatment. Provide a safe environment for a patient who has altered thought processes and reorient him as needed. If seizures are likely, pad the bed's side rails and keep suction equipment and an artificial airway handy. (See *Documenting hyponatremia or hypernatremia*, page 99.)

Hypernatremia

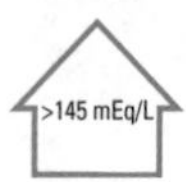

Hypernatremia, a less common problem than hyponatremia, refers to an elevated sodium level in the plasma (blood). Severe hypernatremia can lead to seizures, coma, and permanent neurologic damage.

How it happens

Thirst is the body's main defense against hypernatremia. The hypothalamus (with its osmoreceptors) is the brain's thirst center. High serum osmolality (increased solute concentrations in the blood) stimulates the hypothalamus and initiates the sensation of thirst.

The drive to respond to thirst is so strong that severe, persistent hypernatremia usually occurs only in people who can't drink voluntarily, such as infants, confused elderly patients, and immobile or unconscious patients. Hypothalamic disorders, such as a lesion on the hypothalamus, may cause a disturbance of the thirst mechanism, but this condition is rare. When hypernatremia occurs, it usually has a high mortality rate (> 50%).

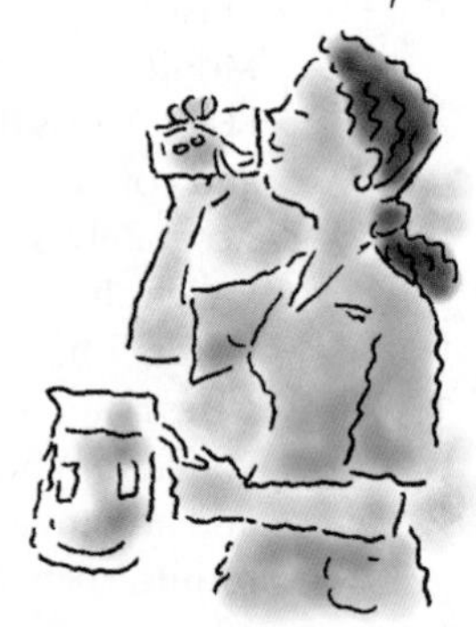
Thirst is the body's main defense against hypernatremia. Drink up!

Striving for balance

The body strives to maintain a normal sodium level by secreting ADH from the posterior pituitary gland. This hormone causes water to be retained, which helps to lower serum sodium levels.

The cells also play a role in maintaining sodium balance. When serum osmolality increases because of hypernatremia, fluid moves by osmosis from inside the cell to outside the cell, to balance the concentrations in the two compartments. (For more information, see chapter 1, Balancing fluids.)

As fluid leaves the cells, they become dehydrated and shrink—especially those of the CNS. When this occurs, patients may show signs of neurologic impairment. They may also show signs of hypervolemia (fluid overload) from increased extracellular fluid volume in the blood vessels. (See *Fluid movement in hypernatremia*.) If the overload is severe enough, subarachnoid hemorrhage may occur.

Increased concentration

A water deficit can cause hypernatremia—that is, more sodium relative to water in the body. Excessive intake of sodium can also cause

Fluid movement in hypernatremia

With hypernatremia, the body tries to maintain balance by shifting fluid from the inside of cells to the outside. This illustration shows fluid movement in hypernatremia.

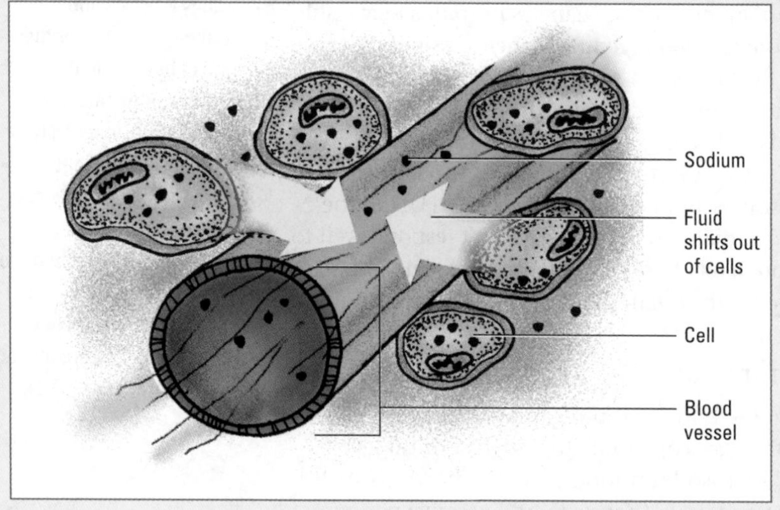

it. Regardless of the cause, body fluids become hypertonic (more concentrated).

Water deficit

A water deficit can occur alone or with a sodium loss (but more water is lost than sodium). In either case, serum sodium levels are elevated. This elevation is more dangerous in debilitated patients and those with deficient water intake.

Insensible water losses of several liters per day can result from fever and heat stroke, with older adults and athletes being equally susceptible. Significant water losses also occur in patients with pulmonary infections, who lose water vapor from the lungs through hyperventilation, and in patients with extensive burns. Vomiting and severe, watery diarrhea are other causes of water loss and subsequent hypernatremia; either can be especially dangerous in children. (See *Infants, children, elderly patients, and critically ill at risk.*)

Patients with **hyperosmolar hyperglycemic nonketotic syndrome** can also develop hypernatremia due to severe water losses from osmotic diuresis. Urea diuresis, another cause of hypernatremia, occurs with administration of high-protein feedings or high-protein diets without adequate water supplementation (George et al., 2013; Lindner & Funk, 2013; Smeltzer et al., 2010).

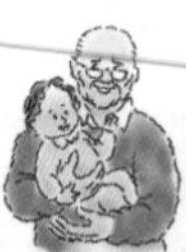

Ages and stages

Infants, children, elderly patients, and critically ill at risk

Hypernatremia is more common in infants and children for two key reasons:

1. They tend to lose more water as a result of diarrhea, vomiting, inadequate fluid intake, and fever.
2. Their intake of water is generally inadequate because they lack access to fluids and can't readily communicate their needs.

Elderly patients are also at increased risk for hypernatremia. They may have an impaired thirst response, or they may have limited access to water because of confusion, immobility, or a debilitating illness.

Critically ill patients who are unconscious, intubated, or sedated are at risk because they cannot express thirst or communicate they are thirsty (Lindner & Funk, 2013).

Thirst to an extreme

Patients with **diabetes insipidus** have extreme thirst and enormous urinary losses, in many cases, more than 4 gal (15 L)/day. Usually, they can drink enough fluids to match the urinary losses; otherwise, severe dehydration and hypernatremia occur. Diabetes insipidus may result from a lack of ADH from the brain (central diabetes insipidus) or a lack of response from the kidneys to ADH (nephrogenic diabetes insipidus) (George et al., 2013; Lindner & Funk, 2013; Smeltzer et al., 2010).

Central diabetes insipidus may be caused by a tumor or head trauma (injury or surgery), or it may be idiopathic (no known cause). It responds well to vasopressin (another name for ADH). On the other hand, nephrogenic diabetes insipidus doesn't respond well to vasopressin and is more likely to occur with an electrolyte imbalance such as hypokalemia or with certain medications such as lithium.

Excessive sodium intake

Like water losses from the body, sodium gains can cause hypernatremia. Several factors can contribute to a high sodium level, including salt tablets, high-sodium foods, and medications such as sodium polystyrene sulfonate (Kayexalate). Excessive parenteral administration of sodium solutions, such as hypertonic saline solutions or sodium bicarbonate preparations, and gastric or enteral

Drugs associated with hypernatremia

The drugs listed below can cause high sodium levels. Ask your patient if any of these medications are part of his drug therapy:

- antacids with sodium bicarbonate
- antibiotics such as ticarcillin disodium-clavulanate potassium (Timentin)
- salt tablets
- sodium bicarbonate injections (such as those given during cardiac arrest)
- I.V. sodium chloride preparations
- sodium polystyrene sulfonate (Kayexalate)
- corticosteroids

(Deglin et al., 2013; Institute for Safe Medicine Practices, 2012)

tube feedings can also cause hypernatremia. (See *Drugs associated with hypernatremia*.)

Other causes of increased sodium levels include inadvertent introduction of hypertonic saline solution into maternal circulation during therapeutic abortion and near drowning in salt water. Excessive amounts of adrenocortical hormones (as in Cushing's syndrome and hyperaldosteronism) also affect water and sodium balance.

What to look for

The most important signs of hypernatremia are neurologic because fluid shifts have a significant effect on brain cells. The hyperosmolarity causes a shift of free water from the intracellular to the extracellular space, leading to brain cell shrinkage. Vascular rupture can occur with permanent neurologic deficits if severe. Remember, the body can tolerate a high sodium level that develops over time better than one that occurs rapidly. Early signs and symptoms of hypernatremia may include restlessness or agitation, anorexia, nausea, and vomiting. These may be followed by weakness, lethargy, confusion, stupor, seizures, and coma. Neuromuscular signs also commonly occur, including twitching, hyperreflexia, ataxia, and tremors.

That flushed, fevered feeling

You may also observe a low-grade fever and flushed skin. The patient may complain of intense thirst from stimulation of the hypothalamus from increased osmolality.

Other signs and symptoms vary depending on the cause of the high sodium levels. If a sodium gain has occurred, fluid may be drawn into the blood vessels and the patient will appear hypervolemic, with an elevated blood pressure, bounding pulse, and dyspnea.

If water loss occurs, fluid leaves the blood vessels and you'll notice signs of hypovolemia, such as dry mucous membranes, oliguria, and orthostatic hypotension (blood pressure drop and heart rate increase with position changes).

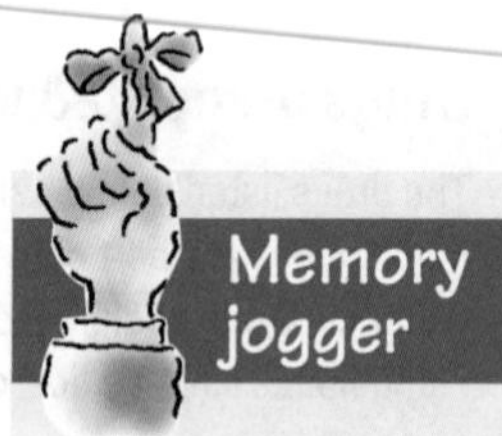

To remember some common signs and symptoms of hypernatremia, think of the word **SALT:**

Skin flushed

Agitation

Low-grade fever

Thirst.

What tests show

Now that you know how hypernatremia progresses, you can better understand how it causes these common diagnostic findings:

- serum sodium level greater than 145 mEq/L
- urine specific gravity greater than 1.030 (except in diabetes insipidus, where urine specific gravity is decreased)
- serum osmolality greater than 300 mOsm/kg.

How it's treated

Treatment for hypernatremia varies with the cause. The underlying disorder must be corrected, and serum sodium levels and related diagnostic tests must be monitored. If too little water in the body is causing the hypernatremia, treatment may include oral fluid replacement. Note that the fluids should be given gradually over 48 hours to avoid shifting water into brain cells.

Brain drain

Remember, as sodium levels in the blood vessels rise, fluid shifts out of the cells—including the brain cells—to dilute the blood and equalize concentrations. If too much water is introduced into the body too quickly, water moves into brain cells and they get bigger, causing cerebral edema.

If the patient can't drink enough fluids, it will be necessary to provide I.V. fluid replacement. A patient may receive salt-free solutions (such as dextrose 5% in water) to return serum sodium levels to normal, followed by infusion of half-normal saline solution to prevent hyponatremia and cerebral edema. Other treatments include restricting sodium intake and administering diuretics along with oral or I.V. fluid replacement to increase sodium loss.

Treatment for diabetes insipidus may include vasopressin, hypotonic I.V. fluids, and thiazide diuretics to decrease free water loss from the kidneys. The underlying cause should also be treated.

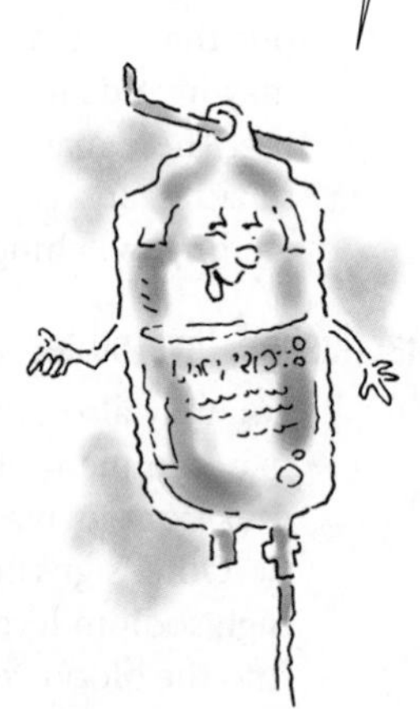
The patient who can't drink enough may need I.V. fluids.

How you intervene

Try to prevent hypernatremia in high-risk patients (such as those recovering from surgery near the pituitary gland) by observing

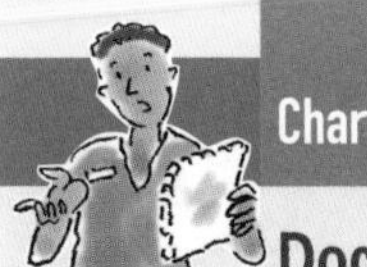

Chart smart

Documenting hyponatremia or hypernatremia

If your patient has hyponatremia or hypernatremia, make sure you document the following information:

- assessment findings (including neurologic status)
- vital signs
- types of seizures, if any
- daily weight
- serum sodium level and other pertinent laboratory test results
- intake and output
- medications given and I.V. therapy implemented
- notification of the practitioner when the patient's condition changes
- nursing interventions and patient response
- patient compliance with fluid restrictions and dietary changes
- patient teaching provided and patient response to the teaching
- safety measures taken to protect the patient (seizure precautions).

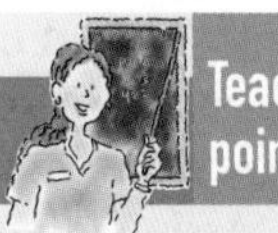

Teaching points

Teaching about hyponatremia and hypernatremia

When teaching a patient with hyponatremia or hypernatremia, be sure to cover the following topics and then evaluate your patient's learning:

- explanation of hyponatremia or hypernatremia, including causes and treatment
- importance of increasing or restricting sodium intake, including both dietary sources and over-the-counter medications that contain sodium
- drug therapy and possible adverse effects
- signs and symptoms and when to report them.

them closely. Also, find out if the patient is taking medications that may cause hypernatremia. If your patient does develop hypernatremia, take the following measures:

- Monitor and record vital signs, especially blood pressure and pulse.
- If the patient needs I.V. fluid replacement, monitor fluid delivery and his response to the therapy. Watch for signs of cerebral edema and check his neurologic status frequently. Report any deterioration in LOC.
- Carefully measure and record intake and output. Weigh the patient daily to check for body fluid loss. (See *Documenting hyponatremia or hypernatremia.*)
- Assess skin and mucous membranes for signs of breakdown and infection as well as water loss from perspiration.
- Monitor the patient's serum sodium level and report any increase. Monitor urine specific gravity and other laboratory test results.
- If the patient can't take oral fluids, recommend the I.V. route to the practitioner. If the patient can drink and is alert and responsible, involve him in his treatment. Give him a target amount of fluid to drink each shift, mark cups with the volume they hold, leave fluids within easy reach, and provide paper and pen to record amounts. If family members want to help the patient drink, give them specific instructions as well. (See *Teaching about hyponatremia and hypernatremia.*)

- Insert and maintain a patent I.V. as ordered. Use an infusion pump to control delivery of I.V. fluids to prevent cerebral edema.
- Assist with oral hygiene. Lubricate the patient's lips frequently with a water-based lubricant and provide mouthwash or gargle if he's alert. Good mouth care helps keep mucous membranes moist and decreases mouth odor.
- Provide a safe environment for confused or agitated patients. If seizures are likely, pad the bed's side rails and keep an artificial airway and suction equipment handy. Reorient the patient as needed, and reduce environmental stimuli (Smeltzer et al., 2010).

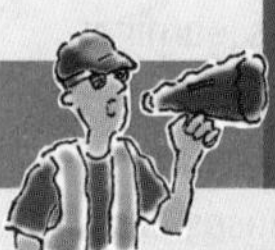

That's a wrap!

Sodium imbalances review

Sodium basics

- Major cation in extracellular fluid (90%)
- Attracts fluids
- Helps transmit impulses in nerve and muscle fibers
- Combines with chloride and bicarbonate to regulate acid-base balance
- Normal serum level: 135 to 145 mEq/L

Sodium balance

- Balance is maintained by ADH, which is secreted from the posterior pituitary gland.
- The balance depends on what's eaten and how sodium is absorbed in the intestines.
- Increased sodium intake results in increased extracellular fluid volume.
- Decreased sodium intake results in decreased extracellular fluid volume.
- Increased sodium levels result in increased thirst, release of ADH, retention of water by the kidneys, and dilution of blood.
- Decreased sodium levels results in suppressed thirst, suppressed ADH secretion, excretion of water by the kidneys, and secretion of aldosterone to conserve sodium.
- Balance is maintained by diffusion, which moves sodium ions into cells and potassium out.
- Sodium-potassium pump uses energy to move sodium ions back out of cells and return potassium to cells; it also creates an electrical charge within the cell from the movement of ions, allowing transmission of nerve impulses.

Hyponatremia

- Common electrolyte imbalance
- Caused by an inadequate sodium intake, excessive water loss, or water gain
- Serum sodium level less than 135 mEq/L
- Varied signs and symptoms, depending on the individual
- Results from decreased serum osmolality

Sodium imbalances review *(continued)*

- Fluid shifts into intracellular areas: neurologic symptoms are related to cerebral edema
- May cause stupor and coma if serum sodium level drops to 110 mEq/L

Types

- *Hypovolemic*—both sodium and water are decreased in extracellular area, but sodium loss is greater than water loss
- *Hypervolemic*—both sodium and water are increased in extracellular area, but water gain is more than sodium gain
- *Isovolemic*—water increases, but total sodium levels remain stable; may also be caused by SIADH

Signs and symptoms

- Abdominal cramps
- Lethargy and confusion (altered LOC)
- Headache
- Muscle twitching
- Nausea and vomiting
- Anorexia

Signs and symptoms with depletional hyponatremia

- Dry mucous membranes
- Orthostatic hypotension
- Poor skin turgor
- Tachycardia

Signs and symptoms with dilutional hyponatremia

- Hypertension
- Rapid, bounding pulse
- Weight gain

Hypernatremia

- Caused by water loss, inadequate water intake (rarely from failure of the thirst mechanism), excessive sodium intake, or diabetes insipidus
- Patients at increased risk: infants, elderly, immobile and comatose patients
- Always results in increased serum osmolality
- Fluid shifts out of the cells, causing cells to shrink
- Must be corrected slowly to prevent a rapid shift of water back into the cells, which could cause cerebral edema

Signs and symptoms

- Agitation
- Confusion
- Flushed skin
- Lethargy
- Low-grade fever
- Thirst
- Restlessness
- Muscle twitching
- Weakness

Signs and symptoms of hypervolemia with sodium gain

- Bounding pulse
- Dyspnea
- Hypertension

Signs and symptoms of hypervolemia with water loss

- Dry mucous membranes
- Oliguria
- Orthostatic hypotension

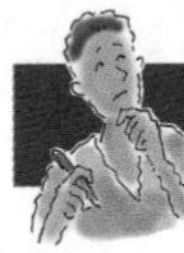

Quick quiz

1. In addition to its responsibility for fluid balance, sodium is also responsible for:
   A. good eyesight and vitamin balance.
   B. bone structure.
   C. impulse transmission.
   D. muscle mass.

Answer: C. Besides its role as the main extracellular cation responsible for regulating fluid balance in the body, sodium is also involved in impulse transmission in nerve and muscle fibers.

2. Signs and symptoms of hyponatremia include:
   A. change in LOC, abdominal cramps, and muscle twitching.
   B. headache, rapid breathing, and high energy level.
   C. chest pain, fever, and pericardial rub.
   D. weight loss, slow pulse, and vision changes.

Answer: A. The signs and symptoms of hyponatremia include change in LOC, abdominal cramps, and muscle twitching. A patient with hyponatremia may also exhibit headache, nausea, coma, blood pressure changes, and tachycardia.

3. The minimum daily requirement of sodium for an average adult is:
   A. 2 g.
   B. 4 g.
   C. 5 g.
   D. 8 g.

Answer: A. Although the minimum daily requirement is 2 g, most people consume more than 6 g/day.

4. Increased serum sodium levels cause thirst and the release of:
   A. potassium into the cells.
   B. fluid into the interstitium.
   C. ADH into the bloodstream.
   D. aldosterone into the kidneys.

Answer: C. Higher blood sodium levels prompt the release of ADH from the posterior pituitary gland.

5. The sodium-potassium pump transports sodium ions:
   A. into cells.
   B. out of cells.
   C. into and out of cells in equal amounts.
   D. into skeletal muscles.

Answer: B. Normally most abundant outside of cells, sodium tends to diffuse inward. The sodium-potassium pump returns sodium to the extracellular area. Potassium ions tend to diffuse out of the cells and require transport back into cells.

6. You're teaching a patient with hypernatremia that he needs to restrict daily intake of sodium. Which foods high in sodium should you tell him to avoid?
   A. Bananas, peaches, and broccoli
   B. Red meat, chicken, and pork
   C. Milk, nuts, and liver
   D. Canned soups, ketchup, and cheese

Answer: D. Major dietary sources of sodium include canned soups and vegetables, cheese, ketchup, processed meats, table salt, salty snack foods, and seafood.

7. Which of the following disorders causes isovolemic hyponatremia?
   A. Hyperthyroidism
   B. SIADH
   C. Heart failure
   D. Dementia

Answer: B. Causes of isovolemic hyponatremia include glucocorticoid deficiency, hypothyroidism, renal failure, and SIADH.

8. Drugs that may cause high sodium levels include:
   A. antacids.
   B. diuretics.
   C. antipsychotics.
   D. antidepressants.

Answer: A. If taken on a regular basis, antacids with sodium bicarbonate may cause high sodium levels.

Scoring

☆☆☆ If you answered all eight questions correctly, congratulations! You're a Sodium Somebody!

☆☆ If you answered six or seven correctly, good job. You're a pillar of strength and intelligence (and not salt)!

☆ If you answered fewer than six correctly, don't fret. You'll strike the proper balance in the following chapters!

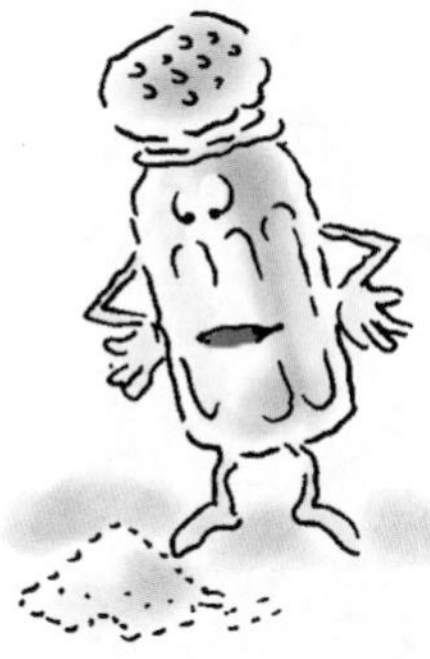

References

Deglin, J. H., Vallerand, A. H., & Sanoski, C. A. (2013). *Davis's drug guide for nurses* (13th ed.). Philadelphia, PA: F. A. Davis.

George, J., Majeed, W., Mackenzie, I. S., MacDonald, T. M., & Wei, L. (2013). Association between cardiovascular events and sodium-containing effervescent, dispersible, and soluble drugs: Nested case-control study. *British Medical Journal*, 347. doi:10.1136/bmj.f6954

Institute for Safe Medicine Practices. (2012). *ISMP's list of high alert medications. Institute for Safe Medicine Practices Tools*. Retrieved from https://www.ismp.org/tools/highalertmedicationLists.asp

Lindner, G., & Funk, G. C. (2013). Hypernatremia in critically ill patients. *Journal of Critical Care, 28*, 216.e11–216.e20.

Smeltzer, S., Bare, B., Hinkle, J., & Cheever, K. (2010). *Textbook of medical-surgical nursing* (12th ed.). Philadelphia, PA: Lippincott Williams & Wilkins.

U.S. Department of Agriculture. (2013). *Dietary guidelines*. Retrieved from http://www.cnpp.usda.gov/Dietary Guidelines.htm

Chapter 6

When potassium tips the balance

Just the facts

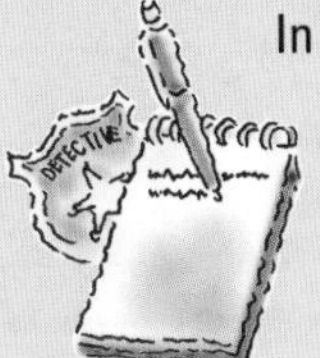

In this chapter, you'll learn:

- ways that potassium contributes to fluid and electrolyte balance
- the body's mechanisms for regulating serum potassium levels
- treatments for potassium imbalances
- care for patients with potassium imbalances
- documentation tips for patients with potassium imbalances.

A look at potassium

A major cation (ion with a positive charge) in intracellular fluid, potassium plays a critical role in many metabolic cell functions. Only 2% of the body's potassium is found in extracellular fluid; 98% is in intracellular fluid. That significant difference in location affects nerve impulse transmission.

Diseases, injuries, medications, and therapies can all disturb potassium levels. Small, untreated alterations in serum potassium levels can seriously affect neuromuscular and cardiac functioning.

Potassium plays a critical role in many metabolic cell functions.

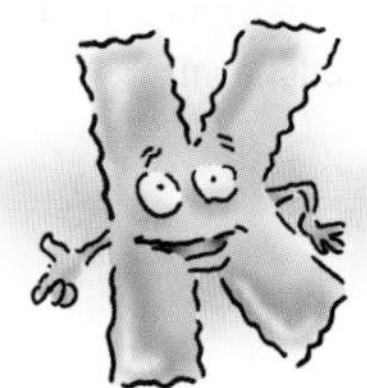

Why it's important

Potassium directly affects how well the body's cells, nerves, and muscles function by:

- maintaining cells' electrical neutrality and osmolality
- aiding neuromuscular transmission of nerve impulses
- assisting skeletal and cardiac muscle contraction and electrical conductivity
- affecting acid-base balance in relationship to the hydrogen (H) ion (another cation). (See *Potassium's role in acid-base balance,* page 106.)

Potassium's role in acid-base balance

The illustrations below show the movement of potassium ions in response to changes in extracellular hydrogen ion concentration. Hydrogen ion concentration changes with acidosis and alkalosis.

Normal balance

Under normal conditions, the potassium ion (K) content in intracellular fluid is much greater than the content in extracellular fluid. Hydrogen ion (H) concentration is low in both compartments.

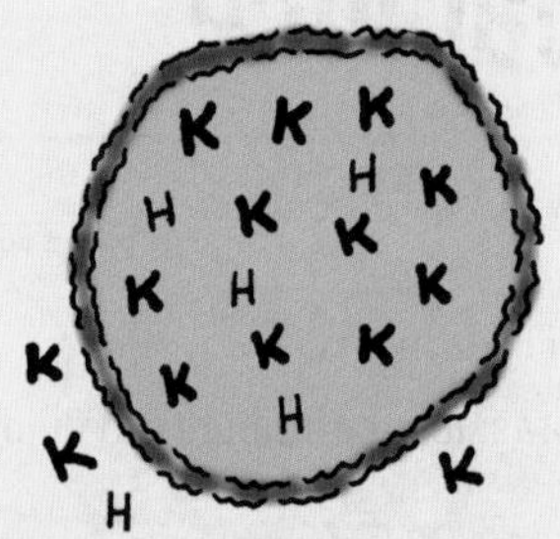

Acidosis

In acidosis, hydrogen ion content in extracellular fluid increases and the ions move into the intracellular fluid. To keep the intracellular fluid electrically neutral, an equal number of potassium ions leave the cell, which causes hyperkalemia (excessive potassium in the bloodstream).

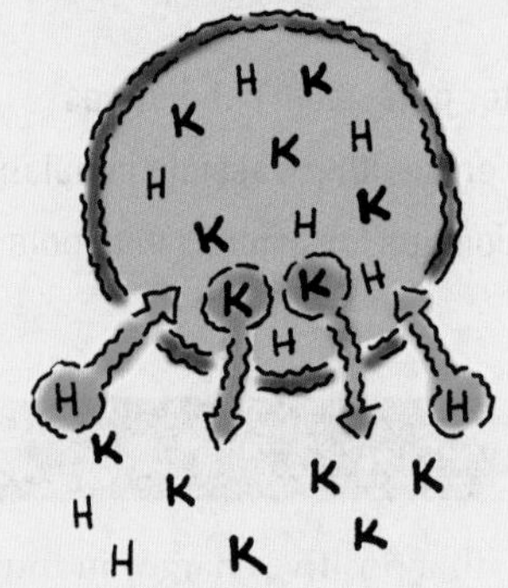

Alkalosis

In alkalosis, more hydrogen ions are present in intracellular fluid than in extracellular fluid. Therefore, hydrogen ions move from the intracellular fluid into the extracellular fluid. To keep the intracellular fluid electrically neutral, potassium ions move from the extracellular fluid into the intracellular fluid, which causes hypokalemia (too little potassium in the bloodstream).

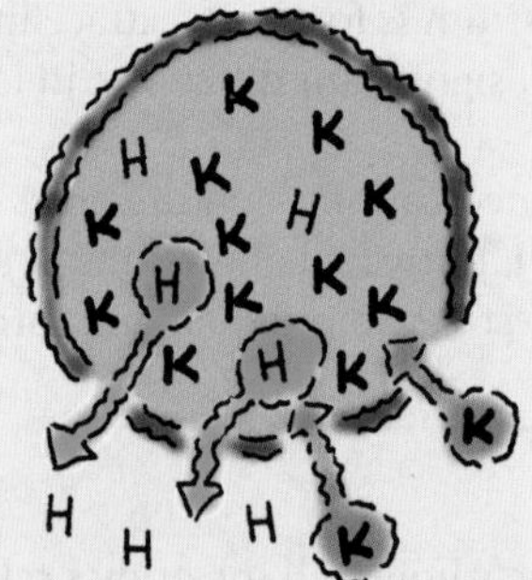

How the body regulates potassium

Normal serum potassium levels range from 3.5 to 5 mEq/L. In the cell, the potassium level (usually not measured) is much higher at 140 mEq/L. Potassium must be ingested daily because the body can't conserve it. The recommended daily requirement for adults is about 40 mEq; the average daily intake in the United States is 60 to 100 mEq. (See *Dietary sources of potassium*.)

Extracellular fluid also gains potassium when cells are destroyed (thus, releasing intracellular potassium) and when potassium shifts out of the intracellular fluid into the extracellular fluid.

Just passing through

About 80% of the potassium taken in is excreted in urine, with each liter of urine containing 20 to 40 mEq of the electrolyte. Any remaining potassium is excreted in feces and sweat.

Extracellular potassium loss also occurs when potassium moves from the extracellular fluid to the intracellular fluid and when cells undergo anabolism. Three more factors that affect potassium levels include the sodium-potassium pump, renal regulation, and pH level.

Pumping action

The sodium-potassium pump is an active transport mechanism that moves ions across the cell membrane against a concentration gradient. Specifically, the pump moves sodium from the cell into the extracellular fluid and maintains high intracellular potassium levels by pumping potassium into the cell.

The body also rids itself of excess potassium through the kidneys. As serum potassium levels rise, the renal tubules excrete more potassium, leading to increased potassium loss in the urine.

Sodium and potassium have a reciprocal relationship. The kidneys reabsorb sodium and excrete potassium when the hormone aldosterone is secreted. The kidneys, however, have no effective mechanism to combat loss of potassium and may excrete it even when the serum potassium level is low. Even when potassium intake is zero, the kidneys will excrete 10 to 15 mEq/day.

Free trade

A change in pH may affect serum potassium levels because hydrogen ions and potassium ions freely exchange across plasma cell membranes. For example, in acidosis, excess hydrogen ions move into cells and push potassium into the extracellular fluid. Thus, acidosis can cause hyperkalemia as potassium moves out of the cell to maintain balance. Likewise, alkalosis can cause hypokalemia by increasing potassium movement into the cell to maintain balance.

Dietary sources of potassium

Here are some main dietary sources of potassium:

- chocolate
- dried fruit, nuts, and seeds
- fruits, such as oranges, bananas, avocados, apricots, and cantaloupe
- meats
- vegetables, especially beans, potatoes, mushrooms, tomatoes, and celery
- yogurt (Tufts University, 2012).

Hypokalemia

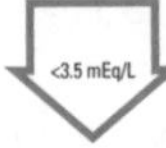

In hypokalemia, the serum potassium level drops below 3.5 mEq/L. In moderate hypokalemia, the serum potassium level ranges from 2.5 to 3 mEq/L. In severe hypokalemia, it's less than 2.5 mEq/L. Because the normal range for serum potassium is narrow (3.5 to 5 mEq/L), a slight decrease has profound effects.

How it happens

Remember, the body can't conserve potassium. Inadequate intake and excessive output of potassium can cause a moderate drop in its level, upsetting the balance and causing a potassium deficiency.

Conditions such as prolonged intestinal suction, recent ileostomy, and villous adenoma can cause a decrease in the body's overall potassium level. In certain situations, potassium shifts from the extracellular space to the intracellular space and hides in the cells. Because the cells contain more potassium than usual, less can be measured in the blood.

Not enough in . . .

Inadequate potassium intake causes a drop in the body's overall potassium level. That could mean a person isn't eating enough potassium-rich foods, is receiving potassium-deficient I.V. fluids, or is getting total parenteral nutrition that lacks potassium supplementation. Also, large intake of natural black licorice produces an aldosterone effect, which can lead to sodium retention and potassium loss.

. . . Too much out

Intestinal fluids contain large amounts of potassium. Severe gastrointestinal (GI) fluid losses from suction, lavage, or prolonged vomiting can deplete the body's potassium supply. As a result, potassium levels drop. Diarrhea, fistulas, laxative abuse, and severe diaphoresis also contribute to potassium loss. (See *Common causes of hypokalemia in the old and young*.)

Potassium can also be depleted through the kidneys. Diuresis that occurs with a newly functioning transplanted kidney can lead to hypokalemia. High urine glucose levels cause osmotic diuresis, and potassium is lost through the urine. Other potassium losses are seen in renal tubular acidosis, magnesium depletion, Cushing's syndrome, and periods of high stress.

Depleting drugs

Drugs, such as diuretics (especially thiazides and furosemide), corticosteroids, insulin, cisplatin, and certain antibiotics (gentamicin,

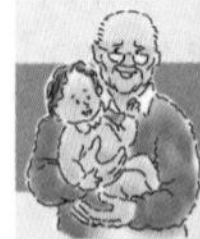

Ages and stages

Common causes of hypokalemia in the old and young

In elderly patients, the most common causes of hypokalemia are diuretic therapy, diarrhea, and chronic laxative abuse. Individuals who can't cook for themselves or have difficultly chewing and swallowing may have poor potassium intake.

In pediatric patients, gastroenteritis that produces vomiting and diarrhea is more likely to lead to dehydration and hypokalemia.

Drugs associated with hypokalemia

These drugs can deplete potassium and cause hypokalemia:

- adrenergics, such as albuterol and epinephrine
- antibiotics, such as amphotericin B, carbenicillin, and gentamicin
- cisplatin
- corticosteroids
- diuretics, such as furosemide and thiazides
- insulin
- laxatives (when used excessively).

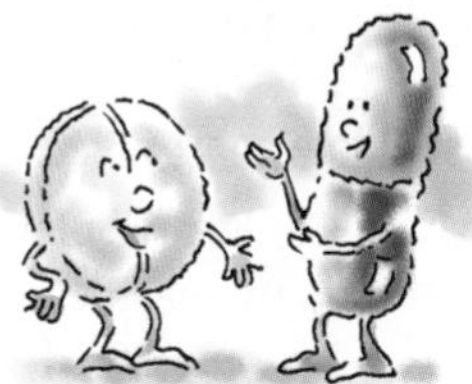
Drugs can
also cause
potassium
loss.

carbenicillin, and amphotericin B, for instance), also cause potassium loss. (See *Drugs associated with hypokalemia.*)

Excessive secretion of insulin, whether endogenous or exogenous, may shift potassium into the cells. Insulin can be released from the body and cause hypokalemia in patients receiving large amounts of dextrose solutions. Potassium levels also drop when adrenergics, such as epinephrine or albuterol, are used to treat asthma as they cause potassium to move into the cell (Lehnhardt & Kemper, 2011).

Damaging diseases

Conditions (such as vomiting or diarrhea) that lead to the loss of GI fluids can cause alkalosis and hypokalemia. Alkalosis moves potassium ions into the cells as hydrogen ions move out.

Other disorders associated with hypokalemia are hepatic disease, hyperaldosteronism, acute alcoholism, heart failure, malabsorption syndrome, nephritis, Bartter's syndrome, and acute leukemias.

What to look for

The signs and symptoms of a low potassium level reflect how important the electrolyte is to normal body functions.

Feeling weak in the knees

Skeletal muscle weakness, especially in the legs, is a sign of a moderate loss of potassium. Weakness progresses and paresthesia develops. Leg cramps occur. Deep tendon reflexes may be decreased or absent. Rarely, paralysis occurs and may involve the respiratory muscles. If respiratory muscles become weak, the patient may also become tachycardic and tachypneic.

Because potassium affects cell function, severe hypokalemia can lead to rhabdomyolysis, a breakdown of muscle fibers leading to myoglobin in the urine. As hypokalemia affects smooth muscle, the patient may develop anorexia, nausea, and vomiting.

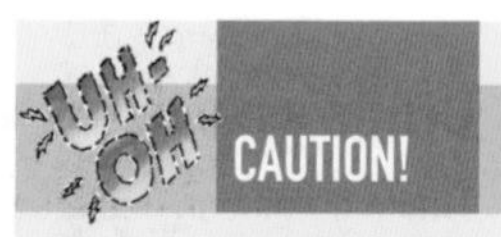

Danger signs of hypokalemia

- Dysrhythmias
- Cardiac arrest
- Digoxin toxicity
- Muscle paralysis
- Paralytic ileus
- Respiratory arrest

GI trouble

The patient may experience intestinal problems, such as decreased bowel sounds, constipation, and paralytic ileus. The patient may also have difficulty concentrating urine (when hypokalemia is prolonged) and therefore pass large volumes of dilute urine.

The telltale heart

Cardiac problems can also result from a low potassium level. The pulse may be weak and irregular. The patient may have orthostatic hypotension or experience palpitations. The electrocardiogram (ECG) may show a flattened or inverted T wave, a depressed ST segment, and a characteristic U wave. In moderate to severe hypokalemia, ventricular dysrhythmias, ectopic beats, bradycardia, tachycardia, and full cardiac arrest may occur.

A patient taking digoxin, especially if he's also taking a diuretic, should be watched closely for hypokalemia, which can potentiate the action of the digoxin and cause a toxic reaction. (See *Danger signs of hypokalemia*.)

What tests show

The following test results may help confirm the diagnosis of hypokalemia:

- serum potassium level less than 3.5 mEq/L
- increased 24-hour urine level
- elevated pH and bicarbonate levels
- slightly elevated serum glucose level
- decreased serum magnesium level
- characteristic ECG changes
- increased digoxin level (if the patient is taking this drug).

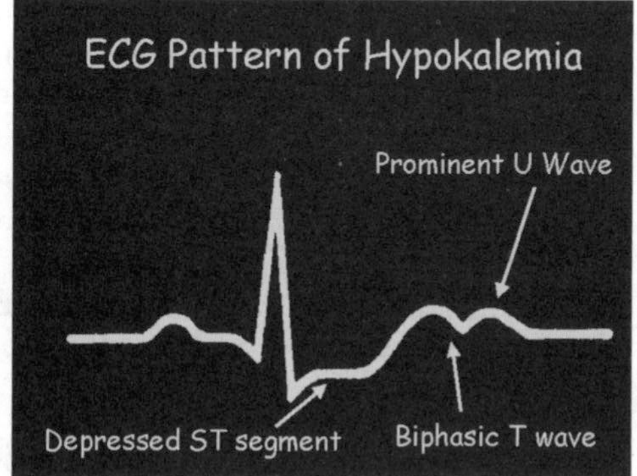

How it's treated

Treatment for hypokalemia focuses on restoring a normal potassium balance, preventing serious complications, and removing or treating the underlying causes. Treatment varies depending on the severity of the imbalance and the underlying cause.

The patient should be placed on a high-potassium, low-sodium diet. However, increasing the intake of dietary potassium may be insufficient to treat more acute hypokalemia. The patient may need oral potassium supplements using potassium salts, in which case potassium chloride is preferred.

Patients who have severe hypokalemia or who can't take oral supplements may need I.V. potassium replacement therapy. Oral and parenteral potassium can be safely given at the same time. Whether through a peripheral or central catheter, I.V. potassium must be administered with care to prevent serious complications.

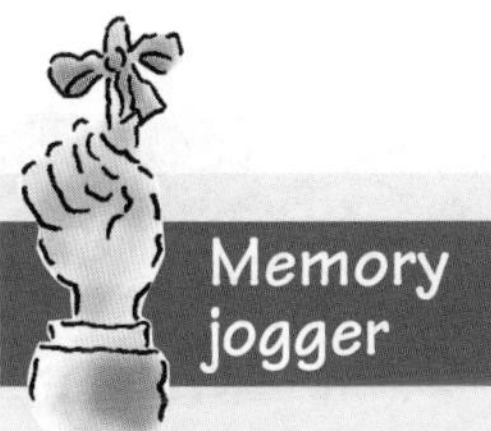

Memory jogger

To remember some of the signs and symptoms of hypokalemia, think of the word **SUCTION** (keep in mind that hypokalemia can be caused by a loss of stomach contents from nasogastric suctioning):

Skeletal muscle weakness

U wave (ECG changes)

Constipation

Toxic effects of digoxin (from hypokalemia)

Irregular, weak pulse

Orthostatic hypotension

Numbness (paresthesia).

Bouncing back to balanced

After the serum potassium level is back to normal, the patient may receive a sustained-release oral potassium supplement and may need to increase the dietary intake of potassium. Also, after the underlying cause of the hypokalemia has been determined and treated, make sure the treatment plan is adequate and implemented. A patient taking a diuretic may be switched to a potassium-sparing diuretic to prevent excessive loss of potassium in the urine. The patient may need his serum potassium levels monitored to determine if there is a need to adjust the potassium supplement.

Careful monitoring and skilled interventions

Careful monitoring and skilled interventions can help prevent hypokalemia and spare your patient from its associated complications. For patients who are at risk for developing hypokalemia or who already have hypokalemia, you'll want to perform these actions:

- Monitor vital signs, especially pulse and blood pressure. Hypokalemia is commonly associated with hypovolemia, which can cause orthostatic hypotension.
- Check heart rate and rhythm and ECG tracings in patients with serum potassium levels less than 3 mEq/L (severe hypokalemia) because hypokalemia is commonly associated with hypovolemia, and hypovolemia can cause tachyarrhythmias.
- Assess the patient's respiratory rate, depth, and pattern. Hypokalemia may weaken or paralyze respiratory muscles. Notify the practitioner immediately if respirations become shallow and rapid or if oxygen saturation values fall. Keep a manual resuscitation bag at the bedside of a patient with severe hypokalemia. (See *When treatment doesn't work,* page 112.)
- Monitor serum potassium levels. Changes in serum potassium levels can lead to serious cardiac complications.
- Assess the patient for clinical evidence of hypokalemia, especially if he's receiving a diuretic or digoxin.

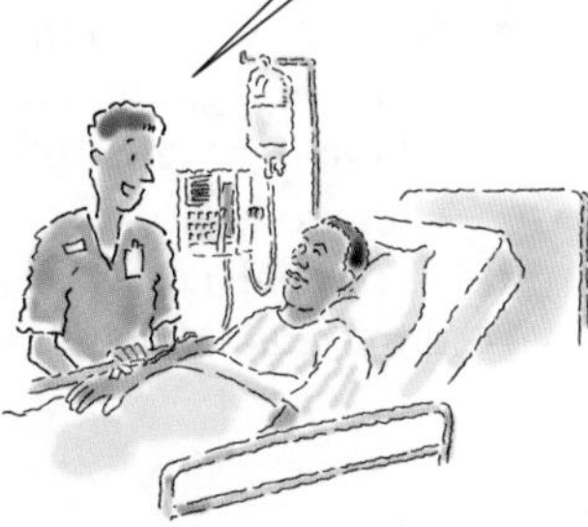
Prevent hypokalemia with careful monitoring and skilled interventions.

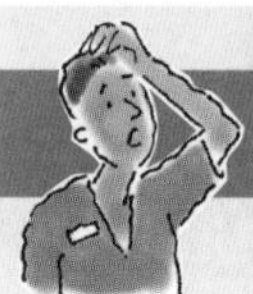

It's not working

When treatment doesn't work

If you're having trouble raising a patient's potassium level, step back and take a look at the entire fluid and electrolyte picture. Ask yourself these questions to guide your assessment of the problem:

- Is the patient still experiencing diuresis or suffering losses from the GI tract or the skin? (If so, he's losing fluid and potassium.)
- Is the patient's magnesium level normal, or does he need supplementation? (Keep in mind that low magnesium levels make it hard for the kidneys to conserve potassium.)

A patient who has hypokalemia and takes digoxin is at increased risk for digoxin toxicity because the body has less potassium with which to work. (Potassium is needed to balance the level of the digoxin in the blood.)

- Monitor and document fluid intake and output. About 40 mEq of potassium is lost in each liter of urine. Diuresis can put the patient at risk for potassium loss.
- Check for signs of hypokalemia-related metabolic alkalosis, including irritability and paresthesia.
- Insert and maintain patent I.V. access as ordered. When choosing a vein, remember that I.V. potassium preparations can irritate peripheral veins and cause discomfort.
- Administer I.V. potassium replacement solutions as prescribed. (See *Guidelines for I.V. potassium administration*.)
- Monitor heart rate and rhythm and ECG tracings of patients receiving potassium infusions of more than 5 mEq/hour or a concentration of more than 40 mEq/L of fluid.
- Administer I.V. potassium infusions cautiously. Make sure infusions are diluted and mixed thoroughly in adequate amounts of fluid. Use premixed potassium solutions when possible.
- Watch the I.V. infusion site for infiltration.
- Never give potassium by I.V. push or as a bolus. It could be fatal.
- To prevent gastric irritation from oral potassium supplements, administer the supplements in at least 4 oz (118 ml) of fluid or with food.
- To prevent a quick load of potassium from entering the body, don't crush slow-release tablets.

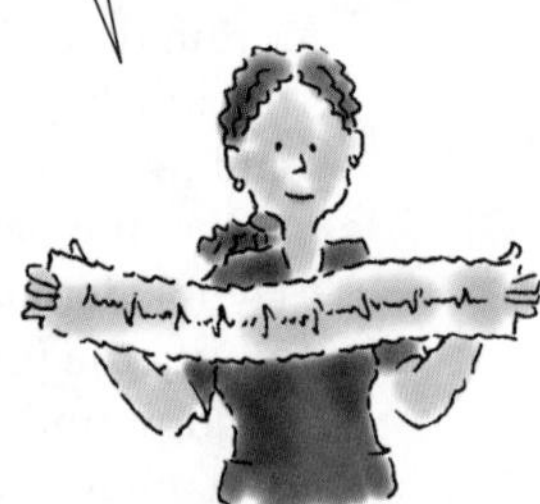
Monitor ECG tracings of patients receiving potassium infusions of more than 5 mEq/hour.

Guidelines for I.V. potassium administration

Below are some guidelines for administering I.V. potassium and for monitoring patients receiving it. Remember, potassium only needs to be replaced intravenously if hypokalemia is severe or if the patient can't take oral potassium supplements.

Administration

- To prevent or reduce toxic effects, I.V. infusion concentrations shouldn't exceed 40 mEq/L. Rates are usually 10 mEq/hour. More rapid infusions may be used in severe cases; however, rapid infusion requires closer monitoring of cardiac status. A rapid rise in serum potassium levels can lead to hyperkalemia, resulting in cardiac complications. The maximum adult dose generally shouldn't exceed 200 mEq/24 hours unless prescribed.
- Use infusion devices when administering potassium solutions to control flow rate.
- Never administer potassium by I.V. push or bolus; doing so can cause cardiac arrhythmias and cardiac arrest, which could be fatal.

Patient monitoring

- Monitor the patient's cardiac rhythm during rapid I.V. potassium administration to prevent toxic effects from hyperkalemia. Immediately report any irregularities.
- Evaluate the results of treatment by checking serum potassium levels and assessing the patient for signs of toxic reaction, such as muscle weakness and paralysis.
- Watch the I.V. site for signs of infiltration, phlebitis, or tissue necrosis.
- Monitor the patient's urine output and notify the practitioner if volume is inadequate. Urine output should exceed 30 ml/hour to avoid hyperkalemia.
- Repeat potassium level measurements every 1 to 3 hours.

When treating a patient with diabetic ketoacidosis (DKA), the following guidelines are recommended:

- Typical deficits of potassium in DKA are between 3 and 5 mEq/kg.
  - If potassium levels are lower than 3.5 mmol/L, replacement should start immediately before insulin therapy is initiated.
  - If potassium levels are between 3.5 and 5.5 mmol/L, replacement is indicated.
  - If potassium levels are greater than 5.5 mmol/L, replacement should not commence (Garcia-Pascual & Kidby, 2012).

- Use the same care when giving an oral supplement as you would when administering an I.V. supplement.
- Provide a safe environment for the patient who is weak from hypokalemia. Explain any imposed activity restrictions. (See *Teaching about hypokalemia and hyperkalemia,* page 120.)
- Check for signs of constipation, such as abdominal distention and decreased bowel sounds. Although medication may be prescribed to combat constipation, don't use laxatives that promote potassium loss. (See *Documenting hypokalemia or hyperkalemia,* page 120.)

- Emphasize the importance of taking potassium supplements as prescribed, especially when the patient is also taking digoxin or a diuretic. If appropriate, teach the patient to recognize and report signs and symptoms of digoxin toxicity, such as pulse irregularities, anorexia, nausea, and vomiting.
- Make sure the patient can identify the signs and symptoms of hypokalemia.

Hyperkalemia

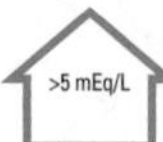

Hyperkalemia occurs when the serum potassium level rises above 5 mEq/L. Moderate hyperkalemia is characterized by potassium levels of 6.1 to 7.0 mEq/L. Severe hyperkalemia is characterized by levels greater than 7.0 mEq/L. Because the normal serum potassium range is so narrow (3.5 to 5 mEq/L), a slight increase can have profound effects. Although it occurs less commonly than hypokalemia, hyperkalemia is more serious. Treatments and underlying conditions are common causes of hyperkalemia. (See *Hyperkalemia in premature infants and elderly patients*.)

How it happens

Remember, potassium is gained through intake and lost by excretion. If either is altered, hyperkalemia can result.

The kidneys, which excrete potassium, are vital in preventing a toxic buildup of this electrolyte. Acid-base imbalances can alter potassium balance as well. Acidosis moves potassium outside the cells as hydrogen ions shift into the cells and inhibit potassium movement into the cells. Cell injury results in release, or spilling, of potassium into the serum, which is reflected in the patient's laboratory test results.

Too much intake

Increased dietary intake of potassium (especially with decreased urine output) can cause potassium level to rise. Excessive use of salt substitutes (most of which use potassium as a substitute for sodium) further compounds the situation. Potassium supplements, whether oral or I.V., also raise the potassium level. Excessive doses can lead to hyperkalemia.

Dangerous donations

The serum potassium level of donated blood increases the longer the blood is stored. Therefore, a patient's potassium level may rise if he's given a large volume of donated blood that's nearing its expiration date.

Certain medications are associated with high potassium levels, such as beta-adrenergic blockers (which inhibit potassium shifts into cells),

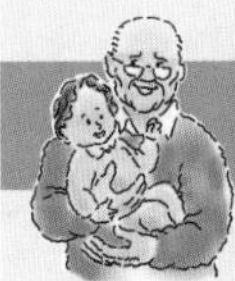

Ages and stages

Hyperkalemia in premature infants and elderly patients

Premature infants and elderly patients are at greatest risk for hyperkalemia. Premature infants are at high risk because of their immature renal function. They commonly experience hyperkalemia within the first 48 hours of life, depending on gestational age.

Individuals age 60 years and older are also at high risk because renal function deteriorates with age, renal blood flow decreases, and oral fluid intake decreases (thereby decreasing urine flow rates). Their plasma renin activity and aldosterone levels also decrease with age, thus decreasing the ability to secrete potassium. Elderly people are more likely to take medications that interfere with potassium excretion, such as nonsteroidal anti-inflammatory drugs, angiotensin-converting enzyme inhibitors, and potassium-sparing diuretics. Patients who are bedridden may be placed on subcutaneous heparin, which also decreases aldosterone production, thereby decreasing potassium excretion.

Drugs associated with hyperkalemia

These drugs are associated with increased potassium levels:

- ACEs (angiotensin-converting enzyme inhibitors) and ARBs (angiotensin receptor blockers) (Lehnhardt & Kemper, 2011)
- antibiotics
- beta-adrenergic blockers
- chemotherapeutic drugs
- digoxin
- heparin
- nonsteroidal anti-inflammatory drugs
- potassium (in excessive amounts)
- potassium-sparing diuretics (such as spironolactone).

potassium-sparing diuretics such as spironolactone, and some antibiotics such as penicillin G potassium. Chemotherapy, which causes cell death (and sometimes renal injury), can also lead to hyperkalemia.

Angiotensin-converting enzyme inhibitors and angiotensin receptor blockers, nonsteroidal anti-inflammatory drugs, and heparin are thought to cause hyperkalemia by suppressing aldosterone secretion, which decreases potassium excretion in the kidneys. When administering any medication that can cause renal injury (such as an aminoglycoside), monitor the patient for hyperkalemia. (See *Drugs associated with hyperkalemia*).

Too little output

Potassium excretion is diminished in patients with acute or chronic renal failure, especially patients who are on dialysis. Any disease that can cause kidney damage (for example, diabetes, sickle cell disease, or systemic lupus erythematosus) can lead to hyperkalemia. Addison's disease and hypoaldosteronism can also decrease potassium excretion from the body.

Keep in mind that the potassium level of donated blood increases the longer blood is stored.

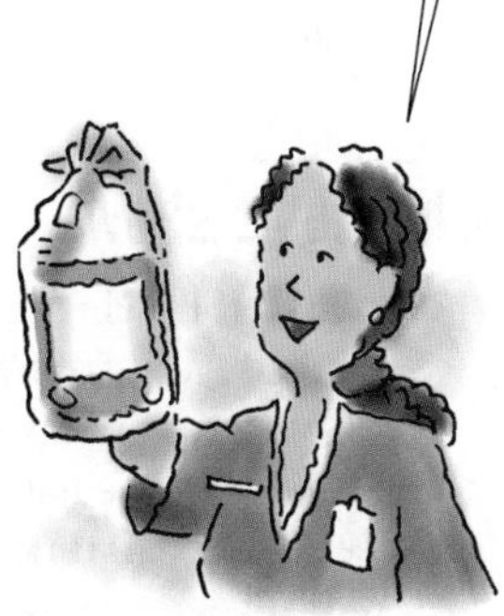

An insult from injury

When a burn, severe infection, trauma, crush injury (rhabdomyolysis), or intravascular hemolysis has injured a cell, potassium may leave the cell. This is also called *relative hyperkalemia*.

Chemotherapy causes cell lysis and the release of potassium. Metabolic acidosis and insulin deficiency decrease the movement of potassium into cells. (See *Make sure the results are true.*)

What to look for

Signs and symptoms of hyperkalemia reflect its effects on neuromuscular and cardiac functioning in the body. Paresthesia, an early symptom, and irritability signal hyperkalemia.

Muscle messages

Hyperkalemia may cause skeletal muscle weakness that, in turn, may lead to flaccid paralysis. Deep tendon reflexes may be decreased. Muscle weakness tends to spread from the legs to the trunk and involves respiratory muscles. Hyperkalemia also causes smooth muscle hyperactivity, particularly in the GI tract, which can result in nausea, abdominal cramping, and diarrhea (an early sign).

Heart signs

Other possible complications of hyperkalemia include a decreased heart rate, irregular pulse, decreased cardiac output, hypotension and, possibly, cardiac arrest.

A tall, tented T wave is a prominent ECG characteristic of a patient with hyperkalemia. Other ECG changes include a flattened P wave, a prolonged PR interval, bundle-branch blocks causing a widened QRS complex, and a depressed ST segment. In the late phase, seen in prolonged hyperkalemic states, the QRS complex and T wave may combine to form a biphasic or "sine" wave, which precedes ventricular standstill. The condition can also lead to heart block, ventricular arrhythmias, and asystole. The more serious arrhythmias become especially dangerous when serum potassium levels reach 7 mEq/L or more.

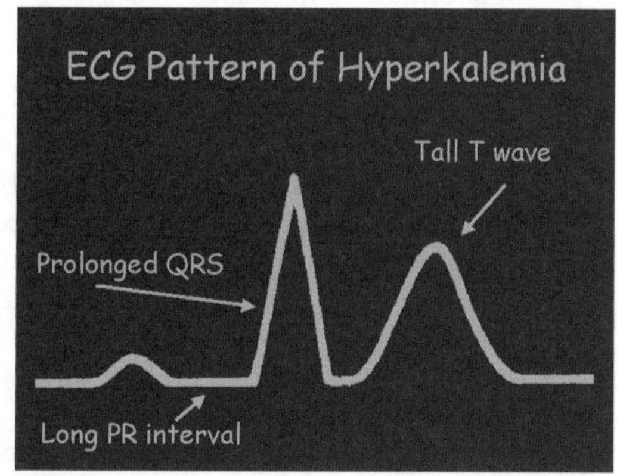

What tests show

The following test results help confirm the diagnosis and determine the severity of hyperkalemia:

- serum potassium level greater than 5 mEq/L
- decreased arterial pH, indicating acidosis
- ECG abnormalities.

Make sure the results are true

When a laboratory test result indicates that your patient has a high serum potassium level and the result just doesn't seem to make sense, make sure it's a true result. If the sample was drawn using poor technique, the results may be falsely high. Some causes of high potassium levels that don't truly reflect the patient's serum potassium level include:

- drawing the sample above an I.V. infusion containing potassium
- using a recently exercised extremity for the venipuncture site
- causing hemolysis (cell damage) by rough handling of the specimen as it's obtained or transported.

How it's treated

Treatment for hyperkalemia aims to lower the potassium level, treat its cause, stabilize the myocardium, and promote renal and GI excretion of potassium. The severity of hyperkalemia dictates how it should be treated.

Mild measures

The patient with mild hyperkalemia may receive a loop diuretic to increase potassium loss from the body or to resolve any acidosis present. Patients will be put on a potassium-restricted diet and have any medications associated with high potassium level readjusted or stopped. Underlying disorders leading to the high potassium level should also be treated.

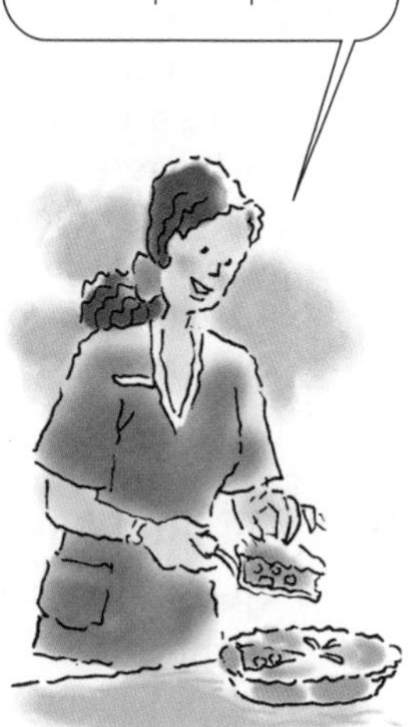

A patient with mild hyperkalemia will have to modify his diet to restrict potassium. That may mean saying no to pecan pie!

Stronger steps

A patient with moderate to severe hyperkalemia may require further measures or treatment. If the patient has renal failure, a diuretic may not be effective. If the patient has acute symptomatic hyperkalemia, he may need hemodialysis.

Sodium polystyrene sulfonate (Kayexalate), a cation-exchange resin, is a common treatment for hyperkalemia. Sorbitol or another osmotic substance should be given with this medication to promote its excretion. Kayexalate can be given orally, through a nasogastric tube, or as a retention enema (may require repeated treatments). The onset of action may take several hours; the duration of action is 4 to 6 hours. As the medication sits in the intestines, sodium moves across the bowel wall into the blood and potassium moves out of the blood into the intestines. Loose stools remove potassium from the body.

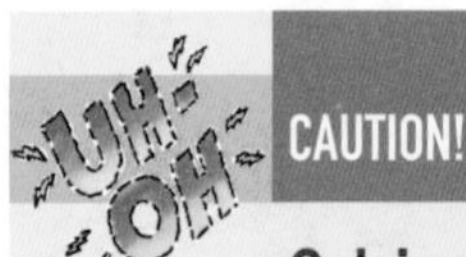

CAUTION!

Calcium alert!

Either calcium chloride or calcium gluconate may be ordered. But there is a difference between the two: One ampule of calcium chloride has three times more calcium than calcium gluconate. Therefore, when preparing a dose for administration, check the order and read the label carefully. If bradycardia develops during administration, stop either type of infusion.

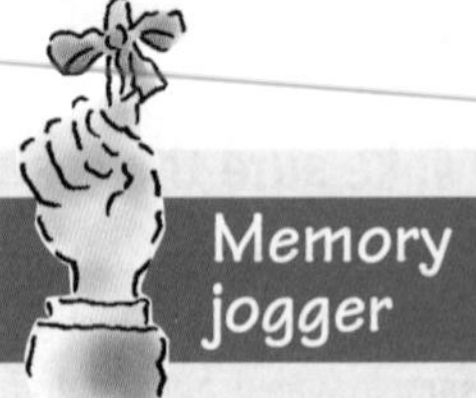

Memory jogger

To help you remember how to treat hyperkalemia, think "see big kid" **(CBIGKD):**

Calcium gluconate

Bicarbonate

Insulin

Glucose

Kayexalate

Dialysis.

The perils of potassium

More severe hyperkalemia is treated as an emergency. Closely monitor the patient's cardiac status. ECGs are obtained to follow progress.

To counteract the myocardial effects of hyperkalemia, administer 10% calcium gluconate (usually 10 ml) or 10% calcium chloride (usually 5 ml) I.V. over 2 minutes as ordered. The patient must be connected to a cardiac monitor. However, calcium gluconate isn't a treatment for hyperkalemia itself, and the hyperkalemia must still be treated because the effects of calcium last only a short time. (See *Calcium alert!*)

A patient with acidosis may receive I.V. sodium bicarbonate (usually 50 mEq), which helps decrease serum potassium by temporarily shifting potassium into the cells. It also raises blood pH. The drug becomes effective within 15 to 30 minutes and lasts 1 to 3 hours. This alkalinizing agent may be given with insulin to enhance its effects.

Another way to move potassium into the cells and lower the serum level is to administer 10 units of regular insulin I.V. The drug becomes active within 15 to 60 minutes and lasts 4 to 6 hours. It's given with I.V. hypertonic dextrose (10% to 50% dextrose solution). Closely watch the cardiac status of a patient with severe hyperkalemia. And lastly, an aerosolized beta-2 agonist, such as albuterol, will drive potassium into the cells.

Closely watch the cardiac status of a patient with severe hyperkalemia.

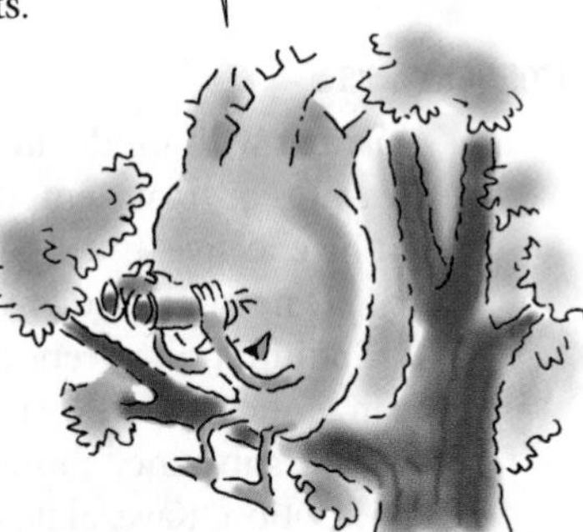

How you intervene

Patients at risk for hyperkalemia require frequent monitoring of serum potassium and other electrolyte levels. Those at risk include patients with acidosis or renal failure and those receiving a potassium-sparing diuretic, an oral potassium supplement, or an

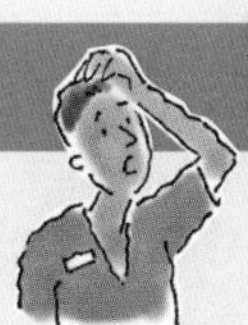

It's not working!

The next step

If you can't lower your patient's potassium level as expected, consider the following questions:

- Is the patient taking an antacid? (Antacids containing magnesium or calcium can interfere with ion exchange resins.)
- Is the patient's renal status worsening?
- Is the patient taking a medication that could raise the potassium level?
- Is the patient receiving old donated blood during transfusions?

I.V. potassium preparation. If a patient develops hyperkalemia, take these actions:

- Assess vital signs. Anticipate cardiac monitoring if the patient's serum potassium level exceeds 6 mEq/L. A patient with ECG changes may need aggressive treatment to prevent cardiac arrest.
- Monitor the patient's intake and output. Report an output of less than 30 ml/hour. An inability to excrete potassium adequately may lead to dangerously high potassium levels. (See *The next step*.)
- Prepare to administer a slow calcium chloride or gluconate I.V. infusion in acute cases to counteract the myocardial depressant effects of hyperkalemia.
- For a patient receiving repeated insulin and glucose treatment, check for clinical signs and symptoms of hypoglycemia, including muscle weakness, syncope, hunger, and diaphoresis.
- Keep in mind when giving Kayexalate that serum sodium levels may rise. Watch for signs of heart failure.
- Monitor bowel sounds and the number and character of bowel movements. Hyperactive bowel sounds result from the body's attempt to maintain homeostasis by causing significant potassium excretion through the bowels.
- Monitor the patient's serum potassium level and related laboratory test results. Keep in mind that patients with serum potassium levels exceeding 6 mEq/L require cardiac monitoring because asystole may occur as hyperkalemia makes depolarization of cardiac muscle easier and shortens repolarization times.
- Monitor the patient's digoxin level if he is taking this medication. He may be at risk for digoxin toxicity.
- Administer prescribed medications and monitor the patient for their effectiveness and for adverse effects.

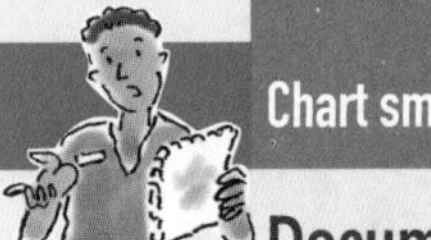

Chart smart

Documenting hypokalemia or hyperkalemia

If your patient has hypokalemia or hyperkalemia, make sure you document the following information:

- assessment findings
- vital signs (including arrhythmias)
- serum potassium level and other pertinent laboratory test results
- intake and output
- practitioner notification
- medications administered
- nursing interventions and patient's response
- safety measures implemented
- patient teaching provided and patient response to the teaching.

- Encourage the patient to retain Kayexalate enemas for 30 to 60 minutes. Monitor the patient for hypokalemia when administering this drug on 2 or more consecutive days.
- If the patient has acute hyperkalemia that doesn't respond to other treatments, prepare him for dialysis.
- If the patient has muscle weakness, implement safety measures. Advise him to ask for help before attempting to get out of bed and walk. Continue to evaluate muscle strength.
- Administer prescribed antidiarrheals and monitor the patient's response.

Diet details

- Help the patient select foods low in potassium (such as apples, pears, berries, carrots, corn, asparagus, rice, noodles, and bread). (See *Teaching about hypokalemia and hyperkalemia.*)
- If the patient with hyperkalemia needs a transfusion, obtain fresh blood.
- Watch for signs of hypokalemia after treatment.
- Document all care given and the patient's response. (See *Documenting hypokalemia or hyperkalemia.*)
- Explain the signs and symptoms of hyperkalemia, including muscle weakness, diarrhea, and pulse irregularities. Urge the patient to report such signs and symptoms to the practitioner.
- Describe the signs and symptoms of hypokalemia to patients taking medications to lower serum potassium levels.

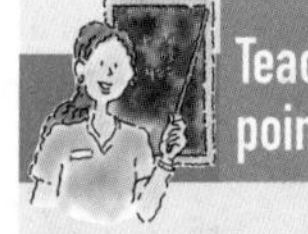

Teaching points

Teaching about hypokalemia and hyperkalemia

When teaching a patient with hypokalemia or hyperkalemia, be sure to cover the following topics and then evaluate your patient's learning:

- explanation of hypokalemia or hyperkalemia, including its signs and symptoms and its complications
- medication, including dosage and potential for hypokalemia or hypokalemia
- need for a potassium-restricted diet and importance of avoiding salt substitutes
- prevention of future episodes of hypokalemia or hyperkalemia
- warning signs and symptoms to report to the practitioner.

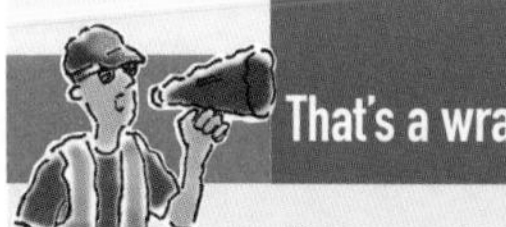

Potassium imbalances review

Potassium basics

- Major cation in intracellular fluid (98%)
- Affects nerve impulse transmission
- Can be disturbed by diseases, injuries, medications, and therapies
- Normal range in blood: 3.5 to 5 mEq/L

Potassium balance

- Potassium must be ingested daily (40 mEq); the body can't conserve it.
- The sodium-potassium pump, renal regulation, and pH level help to maintain balance.

Hypokalemia

- Serum potassium levels less than 3.5 mEq/L (moderate hypokalemia: 2.5 to 3 mEq/L; severe hypokalemia: < 2.5 mEq/L)
- Underlying mechanisms: medications or inadequate intake or excessive output of potassium
- Caused by prolonged intestinal suction, prolonged vomiting or diarrhea, laxative abuse, severe diaphoresis, recent ileostomy, and villous adenoma

Signs and symptoms

- **S**keletal muscle weakness, **U** wave (ECG changes), **C**onstipation, **T**oxicity (digoxin), **I**rregular and weak pulse, **O**rthostatic hypotension, **N**umbness (**SUCTION** is the acronym to remember.)
- Other signs and symptoms
  - Anorexia
  - Cramps
  - Decreased bowel sounds
  - ECG changes
  - Hyporeflexia
  - Nausea
  - Paresthesia
  - Polyuria
  - Vomiting
  - Leg cramps
  - Decreased or absent deep tendon reflexes
  - Paralysis

Treatment

- High-potassium diet
- Oral potassium supplements
- I.V. potassium therapy
- Potassium-sparing diuretic, if needed

Hyperkalemia

- Most dangerous electrolyte disorder
- Commonly accompanies metabolic acidosis
- Underlying mechanisms: increased intake of potassium, decreased urine excretion of potassium, shift of potassium out of the cells to extracellular fluid, medications
- Best clinical indicators: serum potassium levels and ECG tracings
- Serum potassium levels exceeding 7 mEq/L: possible serious cardiac arrhythmias leading to cardiac arrest (could be fatal)

Signs and symptoms

- Abdominal cramping
- Diarrhea
- ECG changes (classic sign: tall, tented T wave with early stages and sine wave with late stages)
- Hypotension
- Irregular pulse rate
- Irritability

(continued)

Potassium imbalances review *(continued)*

- Muscle weakness, especially in the lower extremities, which may lead to flaccid paralysis
- Nausea
- Paresthesia
- Bradycardia

Treatment

For mild to moderate cases

- Loop diuretics

For severe cases

- **C**alcium chloride or gluconate
- **B**icarbonate
- **I**nsulin
- **G**lucose
- **K**ayexalate
- **D**ialysis

(**CBIGKD** ["see big kid"] is the acronym to remember.)

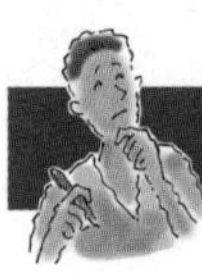

Quick quiz

1. Potassium is responsible for:
   A. building muscle mass.
   B. building bone structure and strength.
   C. maintaining the heartbeat.
   D. maintaining weight.

Answer: C. Potassium is vital for proper cardiac function because it plays a key role in cardiac muscle contraction and electrical conductivity. Changes in serum potassium level call for early recognition and treatment.

2. When the hormone aldosterone is secreted, the kidneys reabsorb:
   A. sodium.
   B. potassium.
   C. magnesium.
   D. calcium.

Answer: A. The kidneys reabsorb sodium and excrete potassium when aldosterone is secreted.

3. Neuromuscular signs and symptoms of hypokalemia include:
   A. Tourette's syndrome.
   B. confusion and irritability.
   C. diminished deep tendon reflexes.
   D. Parkinsonian-type tremors.

Answer: C. Deep tendon reflexes may be decreased or absent in hypokalemia. Also, leg cramps may occur and respiratory muscles may be paralyzed.

4. Medications to help treat severe hyperkalemia include:
   A. methylprednisolone and mannitol.
   B. mannitol and regular insulin.
   C. digoxin and diuretics.
   D. 10% calcium gluconate and regular insulin.

Answer: D. Calcium gluconate helps to stabilize cardiac cell membranes, although it doesn't lower a high potassium level itself. Regular insulin, given with hypertonic dextrose, causes potassium to move into the cells, thus lowering the serum potassium level.

5. A hallmark ECG characteristic of hyperkalemia is the presence of:
   A. irregular PR intervals.
   B. narrowed QRS complexes.
   C. tall, tented T waves.
   D. peaked P waves.

Answer: C. Tall, tented T waves are a hallmark of hyperkalemia, a condition that can also lead to heart block, ventricular arrhythmias, and asystole.

6. An 83-year-old patient with heart failure develops hypokalemia as a result of her diuretic therapy. You suggest that she increase her dietary intake of potassium. Which foods should she consume?
   A. Chocolate, orange juice, and bananas
   B. Canned soups, peas, and milk
   C. Apples, whole wheat bread, and oatmeal
   D. Dairy products and whole grains

Answer: A. Major dietary sources of potassium include chocolate, dried fruit, nuts and seeds, oranges, bananas, apricots, cantaloupes, potatoes, mushrooms, tomatoes, and celery.

7. When administering I.V. potassium for severe hypokalemia, you should:
   A. avoid infusing the potassium with all other I.V. solutions.
   B. infuse through a small I.V. catheter.
   C. verify that the concentration of the solution doesn't exceed 40 mEq/L.
   D. use the drip method to infuse the potassium.

Answer: C. To prevent or reduce toxic effects, the I.V. infusion concentration shouldn't exceed 40 mEq/L.

Scoring

☆☆☆ If you answered all seven questions correctly, wow! You're Top Banana!

☆☆ If you answered five or six correctly, super! You've great potassium power!

☆ If you answered fewer than five correctly, hang in there. Rereading the chapter may help you raise your potassium understanding level.

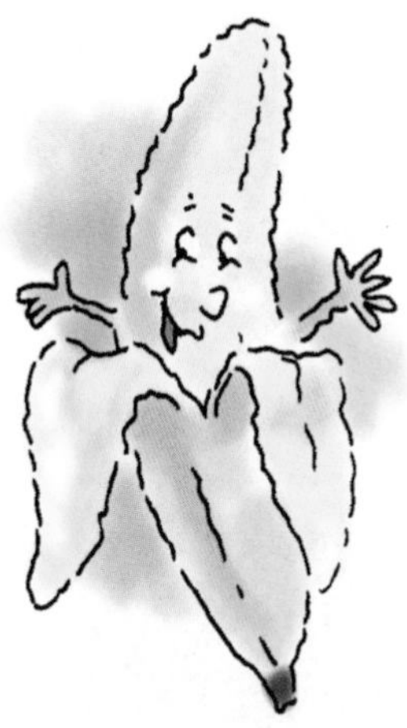

References

Garcia-Pascual, M., & Kidby, J. (2012). Procedures and medications to help patients control their diabetes. *Emergency Nurse, 20*(8), 30–35.

Lehnhardt, A., & Kemper, M. J. (2011). Pathogenesis, diagnosis, and management of hyperkalemia. *Pediatric Nephrology, 26*, 377–384.

Tufts University. (2012). Potassium power: Increased potassium associated with decreased hypertension. *Tufts University Health and Nutrition Letter, 30*(1), 4–5.

Chapter 7

When magnesium tips the balance

Just the facts

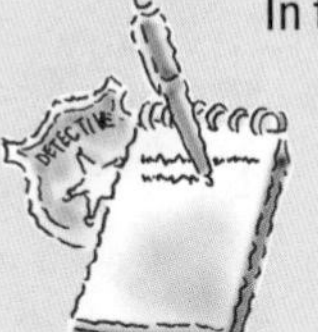

In this chapter, you'll learn:

- the importance of magnesium
- the challenges of interpreting your patient's serum magnesium level
- causes and steps to take when your patient's serum magnesium level is above or below normal.

A look at magnesium

After potassium, magnesium is the most abundant cation (positively charged ion) in intracellular fluid. The bones contain about 60% of the body's magnesium; extracellular fluid contains less than 1%. Intracellular fluid holds the rest.

Why it's important

Magnesium performs many important functions in the body. For example, it:

- promotes enzyme reactions within the cell during carbohydrate metabolism
- helps the body produce and use adenosine triphosphate (ATP) for energy
- takes part in DNA and protein synthesis
- influences vasodilation and irritability and contractility of the cardiac muscles, thereby helping the cardiovascular system function normally
- aids in neurotransmission and hormone-receptor binding
- makes the production of parathyroid hormone (PTH) possible

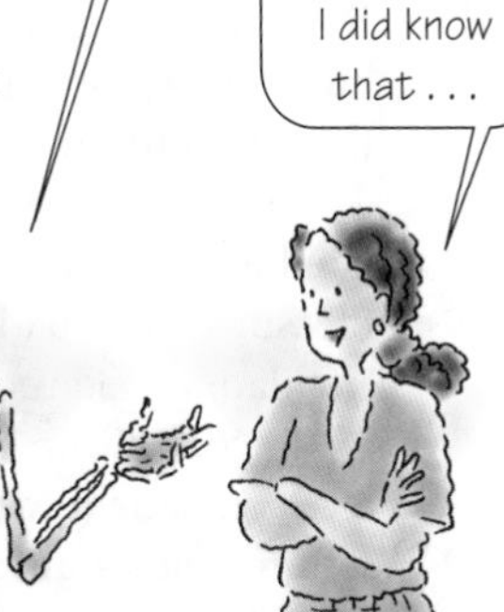
Did you know bones contain 60% of the body's magnesium?
Actually, I did know that . . .

- helps sodium and potassium ions cross the cell membrane (this explains why magnesium affects sodium, calcium, and potassium ion levels both inside and outside the cell).

Managing those muscles

Magnesium also regulates muscle contractions, making it especially vital to the neuromuscular system. By acting on the myoneural junctions—the sites where nerve and muscle fibers meet—magnesium affects the irritability and contractility of cardiac and skeletal muscle. Magnesium is important in maintaining cardiac rhythm (Del Gobo et al., 2013). One study concluded that patients with vascular disease and low magnesium levels were at greater risk for neuromuscular events (most notably, strokes).

What's calcium got to do with it?

Magnesium has another function that's worth remembering: It influences the body's calcium level through its effect on PTH. You might recall that PTH maintains a constant calcium level in extracellular fluid.

Interpreting magnesium levels

You'll need to keep the magnesium-calcium connection in mind when assessing a patient's laboratory values. However, that isn't the only thing you'll need to remember for adults.

Your patient's serum magnesium level *itself* may be misleading. Normally, the body's total serum magnesium level is 1.5 to 2.5 mEq/L. (See *At different levels*.) But the level may not accurately reflect your patient's *actual* magnesium stores. That's because most magnesium is found within cells, where it measures about 40 mEq/L. In serum, magnesium levels are relatively low.

Ties that bind

Here's another reason why interpreting a patient's serum magnesium level can pose a challenge. More than half of circulating magnesium moves in a free, ionized form. Another 30% binds with a protein—mostly albumin—and the remainder binds with other substances.

Ionized magnesium is physiologically active and must be regulated to maintain homeostasis. However, this form alone can't be measured, so a patient's measured levels reflect the total amount of circulating magnesium.

To complicate matters, magnesium levels are linked to albumin levels. A patient with a low serum albumin level also has a low total serum magnesium level—even if the level of ionized magnesium remains unchanged. That's why serum albumin levels need to be measured with serum magnesium levels.

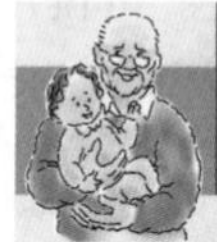

Ages and stages

At different levels

Don't forget that normal magnesium levels in neonates and children are different from adult levels. In neonates, magnesium levels range from 1.4 to 2.9 mEq/L; in children, 1.6 to 2.6 mEq/L.

Serum calcium and certain other laboratory values also come into play when assessing and treating magnesium imbalances. Because magnesium is mainly an intracellular electrolyte, changes in the levels of other intracellular electrolytes, such as potassium and phosphorus, can affect serum magnesium levels, too.

How the body regulates magnesium

The gastrointestinal (GI) and urinary systems regulate magnesium through absorption, excretion, and retention—that is, through dietary intake and output in urine and feces. A well-balanced diet should provide roughly 25 mEq (or 300 to 350 mg) of magnesium daily. (See *Dietary sources of magnesium.*) The Dietary Reference Intakes (DRIs) vary with a person's age and sex. Of this amount, about 40% is absorbed in the small intestine (U.S. Department of Agriculture, 2014).

I know what I have to do to keep things in balance!

A balancing act

The body tries to adjust to any change in the magnesium level. For instance, if the serum magnesium level drops, the GI tract may absorb more magnesium and, if the magnesium level rises, the GI tract excretes more in the feces.

The kidneys, for their part, balance magnesium by altering its reabsorption at the proximal tubule and loop of Henle. So, if serum magnesium levels climb, the kidneys excrete the excess in the urine. Diuretics heighten this effect. The reverse occurs, too: If serum magnesium levels fall, the kidneys conserve magnesium. That conservation is so efficient that the daily loss of circulating ionized magnesium can be restricted to just 1 mEq.

Dietary sources of magnesium

Most healthy people can get all the magnesium they need by eating a well-balanced diet that includes foods rich in magnesium. Here are the "lucky 7" foods high in magnesium:

- chocolate (especially dark chocolate)
- dry beans and peas
- green, leafy vegetables
- meats
- nuts
- seafood
- whole grains.

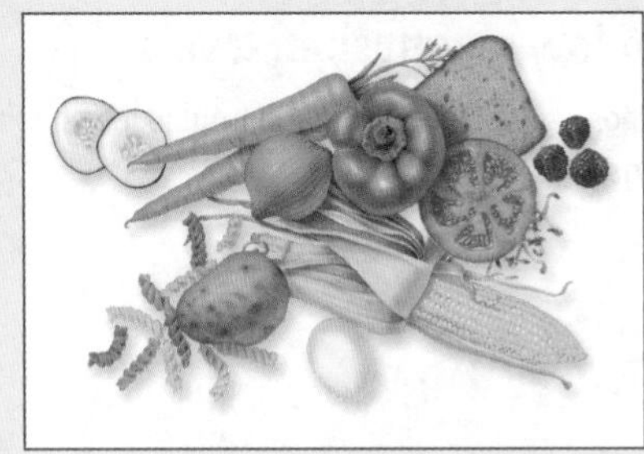

Hypomagnesemia

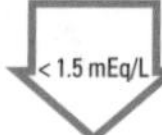

Hypomagnesemia occurs when the body's serum magnesium level falls below 1.5 mEq/L. This imbalance is relatively common, affecting about 10% of all hospitalized patients. The condition is most common among critically ill patients. (See *Danger signs of low magnesium levels*.) Patients with a history of alcoholism, diabetes mellitus, GI disorders, and renal disease along with the elderly are at higher risk for developing hypomagnesemia.

Most symptoms of hypomagnesemia occur when the magnesium level drops below 1 mEq/L. Signs and symptoms of hypomagnesemia tend to be nonspecific but may include hyperactive deep tendon reflexes (DTRs), weakness, muscle cramping, restless leg syndrome, rapid heartbeat, tremor, vertigo, insomnia, ataxia, anxiety, agitation, and depression. At its worst, hypomagnesemia can lead to:

- respiratory muscle paralysis
- complete heart block
- altered mental status or coma.

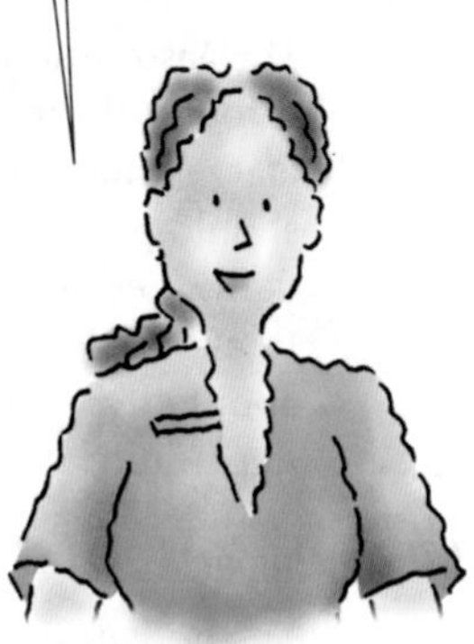
Any condition that impairs either of the body's magnesium regulators can lead to a magnesium shortage.

How it happens

Any condition that impairs either of the body's magnesium regulators—the GI system or the urinary system—can lead to a magnesium shortage. These conditions fall into four main categories:

- poor dietary intake of magnesium
- poor magnesium absorption by the GI tract
- excessive magnesium loss from the GI tract
- excessive magnesium loss from the urinary tract.

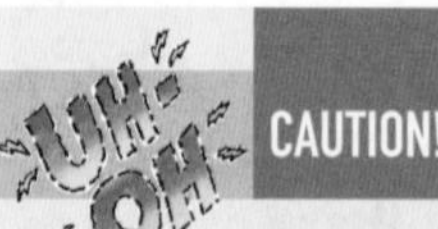

CAUTION!

Danger signs of low magnesium levels

Suspect that your patient with hypomagnesemia is *really* in trouble if he has any of these late-developing danger signs or symptoms:

- cardiac arrhythmias
- digoxin toxicity
- laryngeal stridor
- respiratory muscle weakness
- seizures.

The price of alcohol

Chronic alcoholics are at risk for hypomagnesemia because they tend to eat a poor diet. What's worse, alcohol overuse causes the urinary system to excrete more magnesium than normal. Alcoholics can also lose magnesium through poor intestinal absorption or from frequent or prolonged vomiting.

At risk!

Patients who can't take magnesium orally are at high risk for developing a magnesium deficiency unless they get adequate supplementation. These include patients receiving prolonged I.V. fluid therapy, total parenteral nutrition (TPN), or enteral feeding formulas that contain insufficient magnesium.

Patients who have diabetes mellitus are also at risk for magnesium loss due to osmotic diuresis.

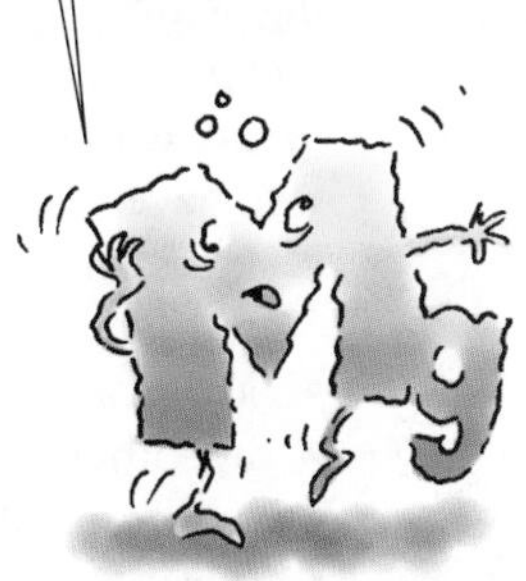

There seem to be so many ways my levels can be low that it makes me dizzy!

Absorption problems

If a patient's dietary intake seems adequate but his serum magnesium level remains low, poor GI absorption may be the culprit. For instance, malabsorption syndromes, steatorrhea, ulcerative colitis, celiac disease, and Crohn's disease can diminish magnesium absorption. Surgery to treat these disorders can also reduce absorption. Bowel resection or bypass, for example, reduces potential absorption sites by decreasing the surface area within the GI tract.

Other conditions that can cause hypomagnesemia from poor GI absorption include cancer, pancreatic insufficiency, and excessive calcium or phosphorus in the GI tract.

GI problems

Fluids in the GI tract (especially the lower part) contain magnesium. That's why a person who loses a great deal of these fluids—from prolonged diarrhea or fistula drainage, for example—can have a magnesium deficiency. A patient who abuses laxatives or who has a nasogastric tube connected to suction is also at risk. In the latter case, the magnesium is lost from the upper, not the lower, GI tract.

In acute pancreatitis, magnesium forms soaps with fatty acids (steatorrhea). This process takes some of the magnesium out of circulation, causing serum levels to drop.

Urinary problems

Greater excretion of magnesium in urine can also lead to a low serum magnesium level. Conditions that boost such excretion include the following:

- primary aldosteronism (overproduction of aldosterone, an adrenal hormone)

- hyperparathyroidism (hyperfunction of the parathyroid glands) or hypoparathyroidism (hypofunction of the parathyroid glands)
- diabetic ketoacidosis (DKA)
- use of amphotericin B, cisplatin, cyclosporine, pentamidine isethionate, or aminoglycoside antibiotics, such as tobramycin or gentamicin
- prolonged administration of loop or thiazide diuretics (See *Drugs associated with hypomagnesemia.*)
- impaired renal absorption of magnesium resulting from diseases such as glomerulonephritis, pyelonephritis, and renal tubular acidosis.

Other causes

Magnesium levels may also drop dramatically in patients undergoing hemodialysis; pregnant patients (second and third trimester); and patients receiving magnesium-free, sodium-rich I.V. fluids to induce extracellular fluid expansion. Others at risk include those who have:

- excessive loss of body fluids (for example, from sweating, breast-feeding, diuretic abuse, or chronic diarrhea)
- hypercalcemia or excessive intake of calcium
- hypothermia
- syndrome of inappropriate antidiuretic hormone secretion
- sepsis
- serious burns
- wounds requiring debridement
- any condition that predisposes them to excessive calcium or sodium in the urine.

Drugs associated with hypomagnesemia

Because certain drugs can cause or contribute to hypomagnesemia, you should monitor your patient's serum magnesium levels if he's receiving:

- an aminoglycoside antibiotic, such as amikacin, gentamicin, streptomycin, or tobramycin
- amphotericin B
- cisplatin
- cyclosporine
- insulin
- a laxative
- loop (such as bumetanide, furosemide, or torsemide) or thiazide diuretics (such as chlorothiazide or hydrochlorothiazide)
- pentamidine isethionate.

What to look for

Signs and symptoms of hypomagnesemia can range from mild to life-threatening and can involve the:

- central nervous system (CNS)
- neuromuscular system
- cardiovascular system
- GI system.

Generally speaking, your patient's signs and symptoms may resemble those you would see with a potassium or calcium imbalance. However, you can't always count on detecting hypomagnesemia from clinical findings alone. Occasionally, a patient remains symptom-free even though his serum magnesium level measures less than 1.8 mEq/L. (See *Identifying hypomagnesemia.*)

So irritating!

A low serum magnesium level irritates the CNS. Such irritation can lead to:

- altered level of consciousness (LOC)
- ataxia
- confusion
- delusions
- depression
- emotional lability
- hallucinations
- insomnia
- psychosis
- seizures
- vertigo.

When magnesium moves out

The body compensates for a low serum magnesium level by moving magnesium out of the cells. Such movement can take an especially high toll on the neuromuscular system. As cells become magnesium starved, skeletal muscles grow weak and nerves and muscles become hyperirritable.

The three Ts and hyperactive DTRs

Watch your patient for neuromuscular signs of hypomagnesemia, such as:

- tremors
- twitching
- tetany
- hyperactive DTRs. (See *Grading DTRs,* page 132.)

Respiratory muscles may be affected, too, resulting in breathing difficulties. Some patients also experience laryngeal stridor, foot or leg cramps, and paresthesia.

Sign language

If you suspect hypomagnesemia, you'll also want to test your patient for hypocalcemia by checking for these signs:

- Chvostek's sign—facial twitching when the facial nerve is tapped
- Trousseau's sign—carpal spasm when the upper arm is compressed. (For more information about these signs, see chapter 8, When calcium tips the balance.)

Hard on the heart

You'll recall that magnesium promotes cardiovascular function. So if you're thinking that hypomagnesemia must affect the heart and blood vessels, you're right. A drop in the magnesium level can irritate the myocardium—with potentially disastrous consequences.

Identifying hypomagnesemia

Consult the list of signs and symptoms below whenever you need to assess your patient for hypomagnesemia.

- *CNS*: altered LOC, confusion, hallucinations, nystagmus
- *Neuromuscular*: muscle weakness, leg and foot cramps, hyperactive DTRs, tetany, Chvostek's and Trousseau's signs (Garrison, Allan, Sekhon, Musini, & Khan, 2012)
- *Cardiovascular*: tachycardia, hypertension, characteristic electrocardiogram changes (Del Gobo et al., 2013)
- *GI*: dysphagia, anorexia, nausea, vomiting

Grading DTRs

If you suspect your patient has hypomagnesemia, you'll want to test his DTRs to determine whether his neuromuscular system is irritable—a clue that his magnesium level is too low. When grading your patient's DTRs, use the following scale:

0	Absent
+	Present but diminished
++	Normal
+++	Increased but not necessarily abnormal
++++	Hyperactive, clonic

To record the patient's reflex activity, draw a stick figure and mark the strength of the response at the proper locations. This figure indicates normal DTR activity.

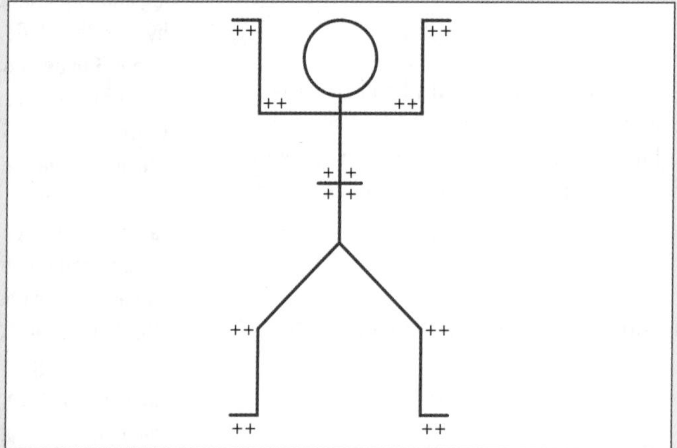
++
++
++
++
++
++
++
++
++
++
++

Wrongful rhythms

Myocardial irritability can lead to cardiac arrhythmias, which can cause a drop in cardiac output. Arrhythmias are likely to develop in patients with coexisting potassium and calcium imbalances, especially after a myocardial infarction (MI) or cardiac surgery. Arrhythmias triggered by a low serum magnesium level include:

- atrial fibrillation
- heart block
- paroxysmal atrial tachycardia
- premature ventricular contractions
- supraventricular tachycardia
- torsades de pointes
- ventricular fibrillation
- ventricular tachycardia.

Because of the risk of arrhythmia, patients with severe hypomagnesemia (serum levels below 1 mEq/L) should undergo continuous

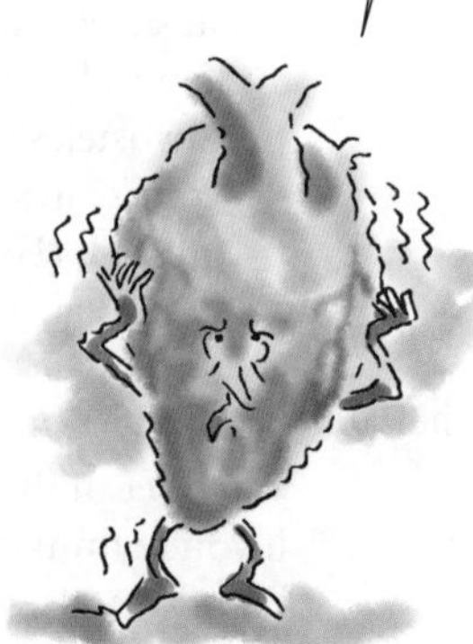
A drop in magnesium irritates me so much!

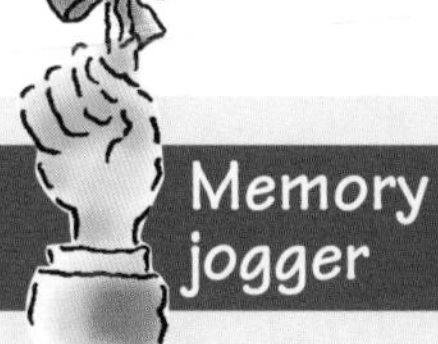

Memory jogger

You'll recall that starvation may cause a below-normal serum magnesium level. The word **STARVED** can help you remember some signs and symptoms of hypomagnesemia. Each of its letters stands for a typical clinical finding:

Seizures

Tetany

Anorexia and arrhythmias

Rapid heart rate

Vomiting

Emotional lability

DTRs increased.

cardiac monitoring. Patients who have had an MI or cardiac surgery may be given oral magnesium supplements to prevent arrhythmias.

General electrocardiogram (ECG) changes that can occur with a low serum magnesium level include:

- prolonged PR interval
- widened QRS complex
- prolonged QT interval
- depressed ST segment
- broad, flattened T wave
- prominent U wave.

The plot may turn toxic

If your patient with hypomagnesemia is receiving digoxin, watch him closely for signs and symptoms of digoxin toxicity—another condition that can trigger arrhythmias. A low magnesium level may increase the body's retention of digoxin. Digoxin may also cause more magnesium to be lost in the urine. Suspect digoxin toxicity if your patient has:

- anorexia
- arrhythmias
- nausea
- vomiting
- yellow-tinged vision.

Tough times for the GI tract

A patient who doesn't have a sufficient amount of magnesium in the bloodstream may suffer such GI problems as:

- anorexia
- dysphagia
- nausea and vomiting.

These conditions can lead to poor dietary magnesium intake or loss of magnesium through the GI tract, which in turn worsen the patient's condition.

What tests show

Diagnostic test results that point to hypomagnesemia include:

- a serum magnesium level below 1.5 mEq/L (possibly with a below-normal serum albumin level)
- other electrolyte abnormalities, such as a below-normal serum potassium or calcium level
- characteristic ECG changes
- elevated serum levels of digoxin in a patient receiving the drug.

How it's treated

Treatment for hypomagnesemia depends on the underlying cause of the condition and the patient's clinical findings. For patients with mild magnesium shortages, a change in diet and teaching may be enough to correct the imbalance. Some doctors also prescribe an oral supplement, such as magnesium gluconate, magnesium oxide, or magnesium hydroxide. Because it may take a few days to replenish magnesium stores inside the cell, magnesium replacement may be necessary for several days after the serum magnesium level returns to normal.

Patients with more severe hypomagnesemia may need I.V. or deep I.M. injections of magnesium sulfate. Before magnesium administration, renal function should be assessed. If renal function is impaired, magnesium levels should be monitored closely. (See *Check the label.*)

Check the label

When you prepare a magnesium sulfate injection, keep in mind that the drug comes in various concentrations, such as 10%, 12.5%, and 50%. Check the label (such as the one shown here) to make sure you're using the correct concentration. The label shows other dosage information as well.

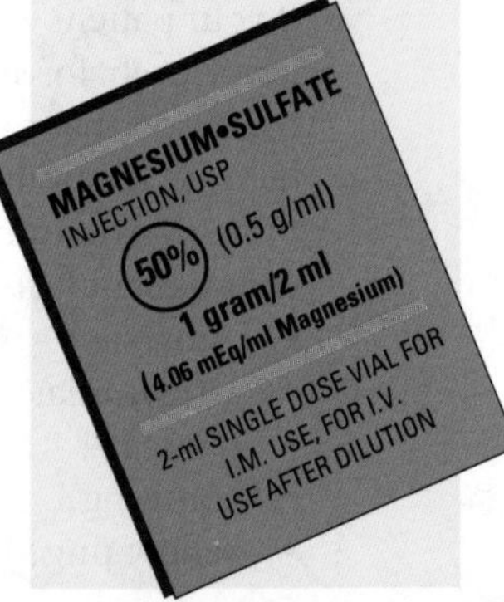

MAGNESIUM•SULFATE
INJECTION, USP
50% (0.5 g/ml)
1 gram/2 ml
(4.06 mEq/ml Magnesium)
2-ml SINGLE DOSE VIAL FOR
I.M. USE, FOR I.V.
USE AFTER DILUTION

How you intervene

The best treatment for hypomagnesemia is prevention, so keep a watchful eye on patients at risk for this imbalance such as those who can't tolerate oral intake. For patients who have already been diagnosed with hypomagnesemia, take the following actions:

- Assess the patient's mental status and report changes.
- Evaluate the patient's neuromuscular status regularly by checking for hyperactive DTRs, tremors, and tetany. Check for

Chvostek's and Trousseau's signs if hypocalcemia is also suspected.
- Check the patient for dysphagia before he's given food, oral fluids, or oral medications. Hypomagnesemia may impair his ability to swallow.
- Monitor and record your patient's vital signs. Report findings that indicate hemodynamic instability.
- Monitor the patient's respiratory status. A magnesium deficiency can cause laryngeal stridor and compromise the airway.
- Connect your patient to a cardiac monitor if his magnesium level is below 1 mEq/L. Watch the rhythm strip closely for arrhythmias. Be sure to follow your facility's policy regarding magnesium levels and when cardiac monitoring is required.
- Monitor patients who have lost an excessive amount of fluid (for example, due to prolonged diarrhea or fistula drainage or nasogastric suction). Patients who have experienced excessive fluid loss are at risk for magnesium deficiency.
- Monitor urine output at least every 4 hours. Magnesium generally isn't administered if urine output is less than 100 ml in 4 hours.
- Assess vital signs every 15 minutes. If patient is experiencing respiratory distress, assess him for a sharp decrease in blood pressure.
- If the patient is receiving digoxin, monitor him closely for signs and symptoms of digoxin toxicity (such as nausea, vomiting, and bradycardia). Magnesium deficiency enhances the pharmacologic action of digoxin.
- If the patient is receiving a medication that can affect magnesium levels, such as an aminoglycoside antibiotic, amphotericin B, cisplatin, cyclosporine, insulin, a laxative, a loop or thiazide diuretic, or pentamidine isethionate, monitor his serum magnesium levels closely.
- Monitor the patient's serum electrolyte levels, and notify the practitioner if the serum potassium level or calcium level is low. Both hypocalcemia and hypokalemia can cause hypomagnesemia.
- Monitor patients who have received nothing by mouth and who have been receiving I.V. fluids without magnesium salts. Prolonged administration of magnesium-free fluids can result in low serum magnesium levels.
- Institute seizure precautions.
- If a seizure occurs, report the type of seizure, its length, and the patient's behavior during the seizure. Reorient him as needed.
- Keep emergency equipment nearby for airway protection.
- Ensure your patient's safety at all times.
- To ease your patient's anxiety, tell him what to expect before each procedure. (See *Teaching about hypomagnesemia*, page 136.)
- Establish I.V. access and maintain a patent I.V. line in case your patient needs I.V. magnesium replacement or I.V. fluids.

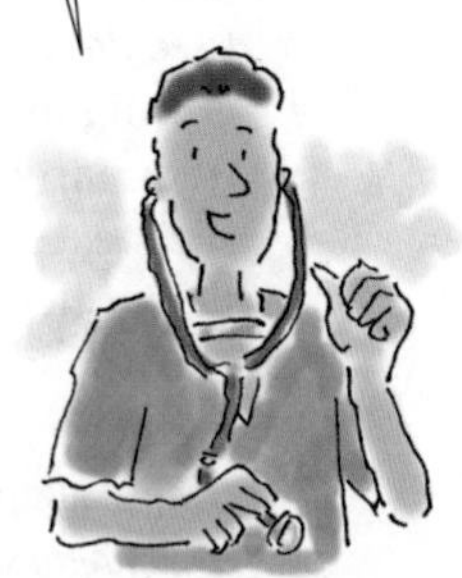
Assess vital signs
every 15 minutes in
a patient with
hypomagnesemia.

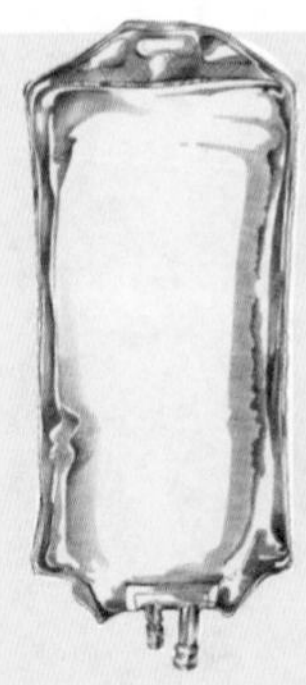

Infusing magnesium sulfate

If the practitioner prescribes magnesium sulfate to boost your patient's serum magnesium level, you'll need to take some special precautions. Read on for details.

- Using an infusion pump, administer magnesium sulfate *slowly*—no faster than 150 mg/minute. Injecting a bolus dose too rapidly can trigger cardiac arrest.
- Monitor your patient's vital signs and DTRs during magnesium sulfate therapy. Every 15 minutes, check for signs and symptoms of magnesium excess, such as hypotension and respiratory distress.
- Check the patient's serum magnesium level after each bolus dose or at least every 6 hours if he has a continuous I.V. drip.
- Stay especially alert for an above-normal serum magnesium level if your patient's renal function is impaired.
- Place the patient on continuous cardiac monitoring. Observe him closely, especially if he's also receiving digoxin.
- Monitor urine output before, during, and after magnesium sulfate infusion. Notify the doctor if output measures less than 100 ml over 4 hours.
- Keep calcium gluconate on hand to counteract adverse reactions. Have resuscitation equipment nearby, and be prepared to use it if the patient goes into cardiac or respiratory arrest.

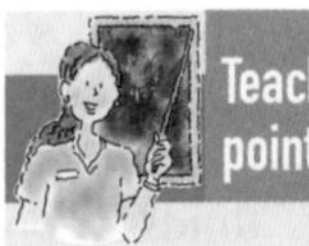

Teaching about hypomagnesemia

When teaching a patient with hypomagnesemia, be sure to cover the following topics and then evaluate your patient's learning:

- explanations about hypomagnesemia, its risk factors, and its treatment
- prescribed medications
- avoidance of drugs that deplete magnesium in the body, such as diuretics and laxatives
- consumption of high-magnesium diet
- danger signs and symptoms and when to report them
- referral to appropriate support groups such as Alcoholics Anonymous.

- When preparing an infusion of magnesium sulfate, keep in mind that I.V. magnesium sulfate comes in various concentrations (such as 10%, 12.5%, and 50%). Clarify a practitioner's order that specifies only the number of ampules or vials to give. A proper order states how many grams or milliliters of a particular concentration to administer, the volume of desired solution for dilution, and the length of time for infusion. (See *Infusing magnesium sulfate.*)
- When administering I.M. magnesium, inject the dose into the deep gluteal muscle. I.M. injections of magnesium can be painful. If giving more than one injection, alternate injection sites.
- Administer magnesium supplements as needed and ordered. (See *Preventing med errors.*)
- During magnesium replacement, check the cardiac monitor frequently and assess the patient closely for signs of magnesium excess, such as hypotension and respiratory distress. Keep calcium gluconate at the bedside in case such signs occur.
- Maintain an accurate record of your patient's fluid intake and output. Report any decrease in urine output. (See *Documenting hypomagnesemia.*)

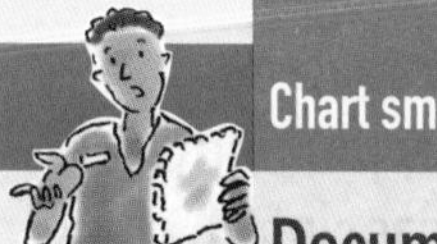

Chart smart

Documenting hypomagnesemia

If your patient has hypomagnesemia, make sure you document the following information:

- vital signs
- heart rhythm
- neurologic, neuromuscular, and cardiac assessment findings
- magnesium sulfate or other drugs administered and the patient's response
- fluid intake and output
- seizures and safety measures used
- your interventions and patient's response
- pertinent laboratory values, including serum electrolyte, albumin and, if appropriate, digoxin levels
- practitioner notification
- patient teaching.

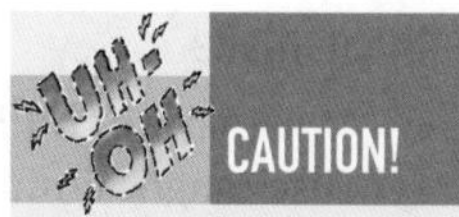

CAUTION!

Preventing med errors

When documenting magnesium sulfate administration, always write out magnesium sulfate to prevent serious medication errors. The abbreviation for magnesium sulfate, $MgSO_4$, is easily confused with that for morphine sulfate, MSO_4.

Hypermagnesemia

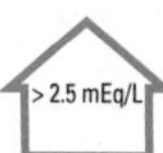

Having too much magnesium can be just as bad as having too little. Hypermagnesemia occurs when the body's serum magnesium level rises above 2.5 mEq/L. However, hypermagnesemia is uncommon; typically, the kidneys can rapidly reduce the amount of excess magnesium in the body, especially if the excess is from food sources.

How it happens

Hypermagnesemia results from the conditions opposite those that bring on a magnesium shortage. Its main causes are impaired magnesium excretion (for example, from renal dysfunction) and excessive magnesium intake.

Keeping it in

Renal dysfunction is the most common cause of hypermagnesemia. Just as some renal conditions boost magnesium excretion to cause *hypo*magnesemia, others can make the body retain too much magnesium, causing *hyper*magnesemia. Causes of poor renal excretion of magnesium include:

- advancing age, which tends to reduce renal function
- renal failure
- Addison's disease
- adrenocortical insufficiency
- untreated DKA.

Too much intake

Magnesium buildup is common in patients with renal failure who use magnesium-containing antacids or laxatives. (See *Drugs and supplements associated with hypermagnesemia.*)

Other causes of excessive magnesium intake include the following:

- hemodialysis with a magnesium-rich dialysate
- TPN solutions that contain too much magnesium
- continuous infusion of magnesium sulfate to treat such conditions as seizures, pregnancy-induced hypertension, and preterm labor. (The fetus of a woman receiving magnesium sulfate may develop a higher serum magnesium level, too.)

Drugs and supplements associated with hypermagnesemia

Monitor your patient's serum magnesium level closely if he's receiving or taking any of these medications:

- antacids (Di-Gel, Gaviscon, Maalox)
- laxatives (Milk of Magnesia, Haley's M-O, magnesium citrate)
- magnesium supplements (magnesium oxide, magnesium sulfate)
- rectal enemas
- potassium-sparing diuretics.

What to look for

Just as an abnormally low serum magnesium level overstimulates the neuromuscular system, an abnormally high one depresses it. Specifically, hypermagnesemia blocks neuromuscular transmission, so expect neuromuscular signs and symptoms opposite those of hypomagnesemia, such as:

- decreased muscle and nerve activity
- hypotension, bradycardia, and respiratory paralysis
- hypoactive DTRs
- facial paresthesia (usually with moderately elevated serum levels)
- generalized weakness (for instance, a patient who has a weak hand grasp or difficulty repositioning himself in bed); in severe cases, weakness progresses to flaccid paralysis
- occasional nausea and vomiting. (See *Signs and symptoms of hypermagnesemia.*)

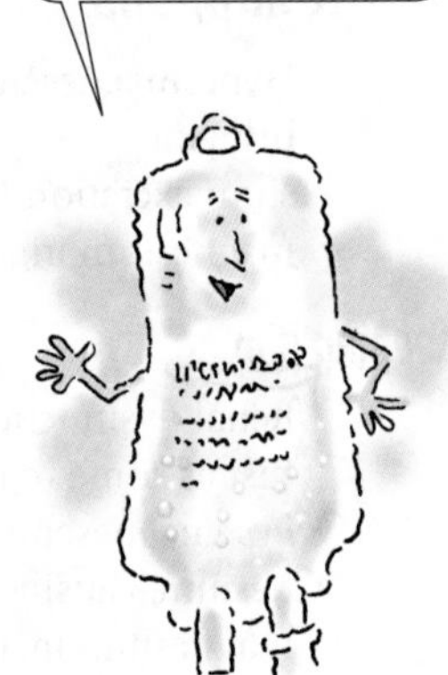

Continuous magnesium sulfate infusions can result in hypermagnesemia.

You're feeling very sleepy . . .

Because excess magnesium depresses the CNS, the patient may appear drowsy and lethargic. His LOC may even diminish to the point of coma.

Hypermagnesemia can pose a danger to the respiratory system—and to life itself—if it weakens the respiratory muscles. Typically, slow, shallow, depressed respirations are indicators of such muscle weakness. Eventually, the patient may suffer respiratory arrest and require mechanical ventilation.

A high serum magnesium level also may trigger serious heart problems—among them a weak pulse, bradycardia, heart block, and cardiac arrest. Arrhythmias may lead to diminished cardiac output.

A high serum magnesium level also causes vasodilation, which lowers the blood pressure and may make your patient feel flushed and warm all over.

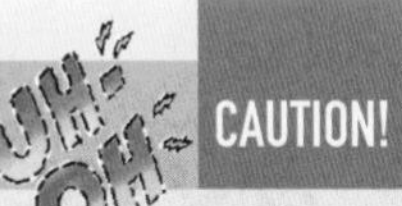

CAUTION!

Signs and symptoms of hypermagnesemia

Use this chart to compare total serum magnesium levels with the typical signs and symptoms that may appear.

Total serum magnesium level	Signs and symptoms
3 mEq/L	• Feelings of warmth • Flushed appearance • Mild hypotension • Nausea and vomiting
4 mEq/L	• Facial paresthesia • Diminished DTRs • Muscle weakness
5 mEq/L	• Drowsiness • ECG changes • Bradycardia • Worsening hypotension
7 mEq/L	• Loss of DTRs
8 mEq/L	• Respiratory compromise
12 mEq/L	• Heart block • Flaccid paralysis • Coma
15 mEq/L	• Respiratory arrest
20 mEq/L	• Cardiac arrest

What tests show

To help confirm the diagnosis of hypermagnesemia, look for a serum magnesium level above 2.5 mEq/L and these telltale ECG changes: prolonged PR intervals, widened QRS complexes, and tall T waves.

How it's treated

After hypermagnesemia is confirmed, the practitioner works to correct both the magnesium imbalance and its underlying cause.

Fluid up, magnesium down

If the patient has normal renal function, expect the practitioner to order oral or I.V. fluids. Increased fluid intake raises the patient's urine output, ridding his body of excess magnesium. If the patient doesn't respond to increased fluid intake, the practitioner may order a loop diuretic to promote magnesium excretion.

Worst-case scenarios

In an emergency, expect to give calcium gluconate, a magnesium antagonist. (You'll probably give 10 to 20 ml of a 10% solution.) Some patients with toxic levels of magnesium in the blood also need mechanical ventilation to relieve respiratory depression.

Patients who have severe renal dysfunction may need hemodialysis with magnesium-free dialysate to lower the serum magnesium level. (See *If treatment doesn't work.*)

How you intervene

Whenever possible, take steps to prevent hypermagnesemia by identifying high-risk patients. Those at risk include:

- elderly people
- patients with renal insufficiency or failure
- pregnant women in preterm labor or with gestational hypertension
- neonates whose mothers received magnesium sulfate during labor
- patients receiving magnesium sulfate to control seizures
- those with a high intake of magnesium or magnesium-containing products, such as antacids or laxatives
- those with adrenal insufficiency
- those with severe DKA
- dehydrated patients
- those with hypothyroidism.

If your patient already has hypermagnesemia, you may need to take the following actions:

- Monitor your patient's vital signs frequently. Stay especially alert for hypotension, bradycardia, and respiratory depression—indicators of hypermagnesemia. Notify the practitioner immediately if the patient's respiratory status deteriorates. (See *Teaching about hypermagnesemia.*)
- Check for flushed skin and diaphoresis.
- Assess the patient's neuromuscular system, including DTRs and muscle strength. (See *Testing the patellar reflex.*)
- Monitor laboratory tests and report abnormal results. Monitor serum electrolyte levels and other laboratory test results that reflect renal function, such as blood urea nitrogen and creatinine levels. Monitor the patient for hypocalcemia, which may accompany hypermagnesemia, because a low serum calcium level suppresses PTH secretion.
- Monitor urine output. The kidneys excrete most of the body's magnesium.

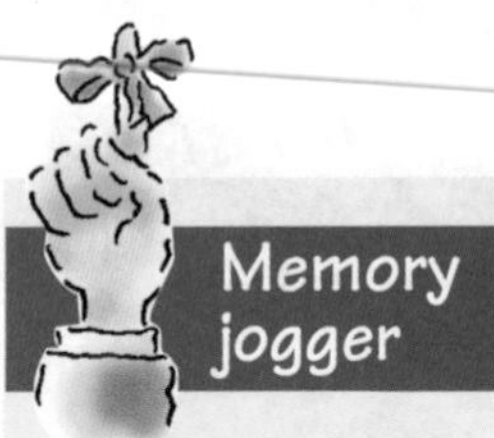

Memory jogger

To remember the signs and symptoms of hypermagnesemia, think **RENAL** because poor renal excretion is a major cause of this electrolyte imbalance. Here's a letter-by-letter rundown:

Reflexes decreased (plus weakness and paralysis)

ECG changes (bradycardia) and hypotension

Nausea and vomiting

Appearance flushed

Lethargy (plus drowsiness and coma).

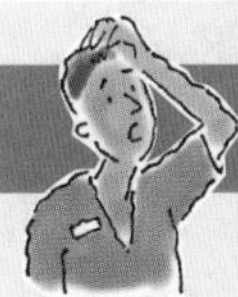

It's not working!

If treatment doesn't work

What should you do if your patient's laboratory test results continue to show that his serum magnesium level is above normal, despite treatment?

Your first step is to notify the practitioner. Expect to prepare the patient for peritoneal dialysis or hemodialysis using magnesium-free dialysate. The patient needs to get rid of the excess magnesium fast—especially if his renal function is failing.

Testing the patellar reflex

One way to gauge your patient's magnesium status is to test the patellar reflex, one of the DTRs that the serum magnesium level affects. To test the reflex, strike the patellar tendon just below the patella with the patient sitting or lying in a supine position, as shown below. Look for leg extension or contraction of the quadriceps muscle in the front of the thigh.

If the patellar reflex is absent, notify the doctor immediately. This finding may mean your patient's serum magnesium level is 7 mEq/L or higher.

Sitting	Supine position
Have the patient sit on the side of the bed with the legs dangling freely (as shown here). Then test the reflex.	Flex the patient's knee at a 45-degree angle, and place your nondominant hand behind it for support (as shown here). Then test the reflex.

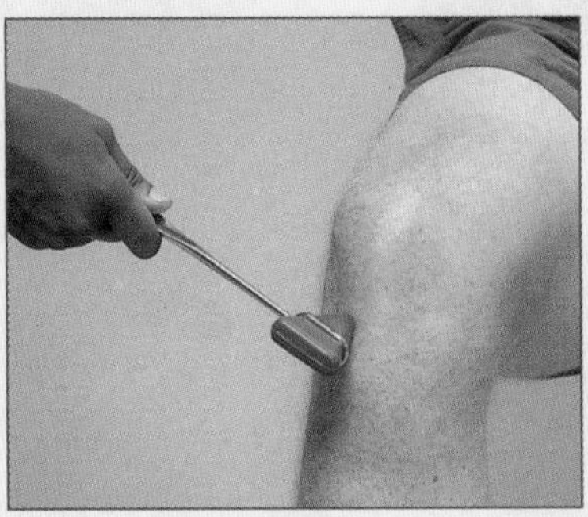

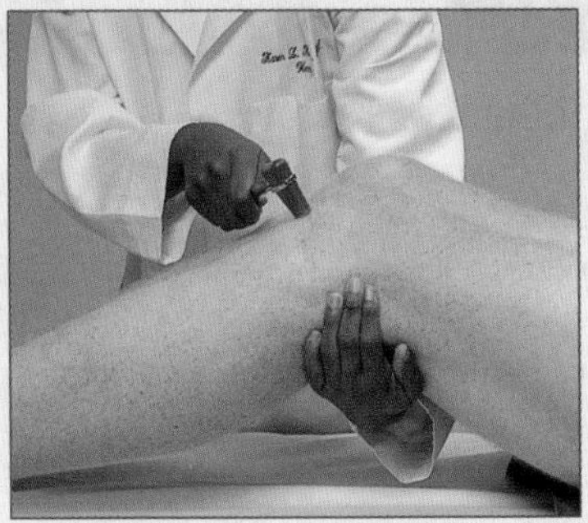

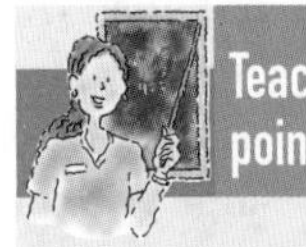

Teaching points

Teaching about hypermagnesemia

When teaching a patient with hypermagnesemia, be sure to cover the following topics and then evaluate your patient's learning:

- explanation of hypermagnesemia
- risk factors
- hydration requirements
- dietary modifications, if needed
- prescribed medications
- warning signs and symptoms
- need to avoid medications that contain magnesium
- dialysis, if needed.

- Evaluate the patient for changes in mental status. If the patient's LOC decreases, institute safety measures. Reorient the patient if he's confused.
- Prepare the patient for continuous cardiac monitoring. Assess ECG tracings for pertinent changes.
- Be prepared to administer resuscitation drugs, maintain a patent airway, and provide calcium gluconate, as ordered, in case of a hypermagnesemia emergency.
- If the patient's magnesium level becomes dangerously high, prepare him for dialysis as ordered.
- Be prepared to provide mechanical ventilation as ordered for the patient with compromised respiratory function.
- Be prepared to apply a transcutaneous external pacemaker or to assist with the insertion of a transvenous pacemaker for patients with bradyarrhythmias.
- Establish I.V. access and maintain a patent I.V. line.
- Provide adequate fluids, both I.V. and oral if prescribed, to help your patient's kidneys excrete excess magnesium. When giving large volumes of fluids, remember to keep accurate intake and output records and to watch closely for signs of fluid overload and kidney failure. Both conditions can arise quickly. (See *Documenting hypermagnesemia*.)
- Avoid giving your patient medications that contain magnesium. To make sure no other staff members give them, flag the patient's chart and medication administration record with a note that says, "No magnesium products."
- Restrict the patient's dietary magnesium intake as needed.

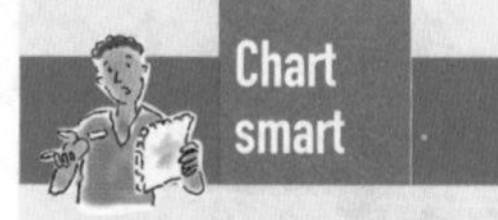

Chart smart

Documenting hypermagnesemia

If your patient has hypermagnesemia, make sure you document the following information:

- LOC
- vital signs
- ECG changes
- signs and symptoms of hemodynamic instability
- DTR assessment
- I.V. fluid therapy
- drugs administered
- safety measures
- your interventions and the patient's responses
- pertinent laboratory values, including serum electrolyte and albumin levels
- intake and output
- practitioner notification
- patient teaching.

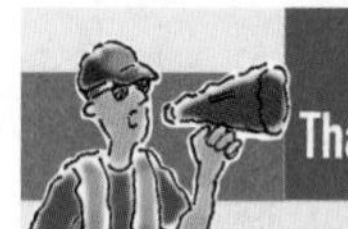

That's a wrap!

Magnesium imbalances review

Magnesium basics

- Second most abundant cation in intracellular fluid
- Performs many functions
  - Promotes enzyme reactions within the cells during carbohydrate metabolism
  - Helps the body produce and use ATP for energy
  - Takes part in DNA and protein synthesis
  - Influences vasodilation and cardiac muscle contractility
  - Aids in neurotransmission
  - Plays an essential role in the production of parathyroid hormone
  - Helps sodium and potassium cross cell membranes

Magnesium imbalances review *(continued)*

- Normal serum levels: 1.5 to 2.5 mEq/L; ranges differ for neonates and children

Magnesium balance

- More than half of magnesium ions are free, circulating ions; others bind to albumin and other substances.
- Magnesium levels relate to albumin levels; low magnesium equals low albumin; high magnesium equals high albumin.
- GI and urinary systems regulate magnesium levels to maintain balance.

Hypomagnesemia

- Occurs when serum magnesium levels are less than 1.5 mEq/L
- Results from poor dietary intake of magnesium, poor GI absorption, and increased loss from GI tract or urinary tract
- Occurs in patients who are pregnant; those with chronic diarrhea, hemodialysis, hypercalcemia, hypothermia, sepsis, burns, and wound debridement; and patients taking certain medications

Signs and symptoms

- Altered LOC
- Ataxia
- Confusion
- Depression
- Hallucinations and/or delusions
- Seizures
- Vertigo
- Skeletal muscle weakness
- Hyperactive DTRs
- Tetany
- Chvostek's and Trousseau's signs
- Arrhythmias
- Rapid heart rate
- Vomiting
- Insomnia (Crawford & Harris, 2011)

Treatment

- Change in diet
- Oral or I.V. magnesium replacement

Hypermagnesemia

- Occurs when serum magnesium levels are greater than 2.5 mEq/L
- Is usually uncommon except in patients with renal failure (especially patients taking antacids or laxatives or the elderly with decreased renal function)
- Caused by Addison's disease, adrenocortical insufficiency, and untreated DKA
- May result from increased intake of magnesium, usually from hemodialysis using magnesium-rich dialysate, TPN with excess magnesium, or continuous magnesium sulfate infusion to treat certain conditions

Signs and symptoms

- Decreased muscle and nerve activity
- Hypoactive DTRs
- Generalized weakness, drowsiness, and lethargy
- Facial paresthesias
- Nausea and vomiting
- Slow, shallow, depressed respirations or respiratory paralysis
- Respiratory arrest
- ECG changes
- Vasodilation and hypotension
- Arrhythmias and bradycardia

Treatment

- Oral or I.V. fluids
- Avoidance of magnesium products
- Calcium gluconate, in emergent situations
- Hemodialysis with magnesium-free dialysate (for dialysis patients)
- Mechanical ventilation (for severe cases in which respiration depression is present)

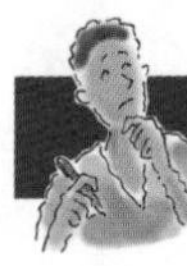

Quick quiz

1. Magnesium is an important electrolyte because it:
   A. helps control urine volume.
   B. promotes the production of growth hormone.
   C. promotes bone growth and strength.
   D. assists in neuromuscular transmission.

Answer: D. Magnesium acts at the myoneural junction and is vital to nerve and muscle activity.

2. Your patient with Crohn's disease develops tremors while receiving TPN. Suspecting she might have hypomagnesemia, you assess her neuromuscular system. You should expect to see:
   A. Homans' sign.
   B. elevated serum potassium.
   C. hyperactive DTRs.
   D. slowed heart rate.

Answer: C. In a patient with hypomagnesemia, expect to see hyperactive DTRs because hypomagnesemia increases neuromuscular excitability.

3. When teaching your patient with hypomagnesemia about a proper diet, you should recommend that he consume plenty of:
   A. seafood.
   B. fruits.
   C. corn products.
   D. dairy products.

Answer: A. Magnesium is found in seafood as well as in chocolate; dry beans and peas; meats; nuts; whole grains; and green, leafy vegetables.

4. The doctor prescribes I.V. magnesium sulfate for your patient with hypomagnesemia. Before giving the magnesium preparation, you review the practitioner's order to make sure it specifies the:
   A. number of grams or milliliters to give.
   B. number of ampules to give.
   C. number of vials to give.
   D. number of uses per vial.

Answer: A. Magnesium sulfate comes in several different concentrations. The practitioner's order should specify the number of grams or milliliters of a particular concentration, plus either the amount of solution to use for dilution or the duration of the infusion.

5. Your patient is diagnosed with hypermagnesemia. To treat this imbalance, the practitioner is likely to order:

A. magnesium citrate.
B. magnesium sulfate diluted in fluids.
C. potassium-sparing diuretics.
D. oral and I.V. fluids.

Answer: D. Both oral and I.V. fluids may be used to treat hypermagnesemia. By causing diuresis, the fluids promote excretion of excess magnesium by the kidneys.

6. Your hemodialysis patient needs a laxative. When you see that the practitioner has ordered magnesium citrate, you decide to question the order because:

A. this magnesium salt would be too strong for the patient.
B. magnesium administration could worsen the patient's condition.
C. magnesium citrate must be given orally.
D. magnesium citrate can cause nausea and vomiting.

Answer: B. Magnesium citrate is a poor laxative choice for a patient with a renal impairment whose kidneys can't excrete magnesium properly. The patient could develop hypermagnesemia.

Scoring

☆☆☆ If you answered all six questions correctly, you should be twitching with pride. You're a magnesium magician!

☆☆ If you answered four or five correctly, excellent! You're ready to become a magnesium magician's assistant!

☆ If you answered fewer than four correctly, try not to worry. You're now enrolled as a first-year learner in the Magical Magnesium College of Fine Electrolytes.

References

Crawford, A., & Harris, H. (2011). Balancing act: Hypomagnesemia & hypermagnesemia. *Nursing, 41*(10), 52–55. doi:10.1097/01.NURSE.0000403378.71042.f0.

Davidson, K., & Kaplan, B. J. (2011).Vitamin and mineral intakes in adults with mood disorders: Comparisons to nutrition standards and associations with sociodemographic and clinical variables. *Journal of the American College of Nutrition, 30*(6), 547–558.

Del Gobo, L., Imamura, F., Wu, J., de Oliveira Otto, M., Chiuve, S., & Mozaffarian, D. (2013). Circulating and dietary magnesium and risk of cardiovascular disease: A systematic review and meta-analysis of prospective studies. *American Journal of Clinical Nutrition, 98*(1), 160–173. doi:10.3945/ajcn.112.053132

Ellam, S., & Williamson, G. (2013). Cocoa and human health. *Annual Review of Nutrition, 33*, 105–128. doi:10.1146/annurev-nutr-071811-150642

Garrison, S., Allan, G. M., Sekhon, R. K., Musini, V. M., & Khan, K. M. (2012). Magnesium for skeletal muscle cramps. *Cochrane Database of Systemic Reviews, 9*, CD009402. doi:10.1002/14651858.CD009402.pub2

Harris, R., Chavarro, J. E., Malspeis, S., Willett, W. C., & Missmer, S. A. (2013). Dairy-food, calcium, magnesium, and vitamin D intake and endometriosis: A prospective cohort study. *American Journal of Epidemiology, 177*(5), 420–430. doi:10.1093/aje/kws247

Islam, M. R., Ahmed, M. U., Mitu, S. A., Islam, M. S., Rahman, G. K., Qusar, M. M., & Hasnat, A. (2013). Comparative analysis of serum zinc, copper, manganese, iron, calcium, and magnesium level and complexity of interelement relations in generalized anxiety disorder patients. *Biological Trace Element Research, 154*(1), 21–27. doi:10.1007/s12011-013-9723-7

Joosten, M., Gansevoort, R. T., Mukamal, M. J., Kootstra-Ros, J. E., Feskens, E. J., Geleijnse, J. M., . . . Bakker, S. J. (2013). Urinary magnesium excretion and risk of hypertension: The prevention of renal and vascular end-stage disease study. *Hypertension, 61*(6), 1161–1167. doi:10.1161/HYPERTENSIONAHA.113.01333

Kanbay, M. Yilmaz, M. I., Apetrii, M., Saglam, M., Yaman, H., Unal, H. U., . . . Covic, A. (2012). Relationship between serum magnesium levels and cardiovascular events in chronic kidney disease patients. *American Journal of Nephrology, 36*(3), 228–237.

Kim, Y., Jung, K. I., & Song, C. H. (2012). Effects of serum calcium and magnesium on heart rate variability in adult women. *Biological Trace Element Research, 150*(1–3), 116–122. doi:10.1007/s12011-012-9518-2

Kisters, K., & Gröber, U. (2013). Lowered magnesium in hypertension. *Hypertension, 62*(4), e19. doi:10.1161/HYPERTENSIONAHA.113.02060

Lopes, P. J., Mei, M. F., Guardia, A. C., Stucchi, R. S., Udo, E. Y., Warwar, M. I., & Boin, I. F. (2013). Correlation between serum magnesium levels and hepatic encephalopathy in immediate post liver transplantation period. *Transplantation Proceedings, 45*(3), 1122–1125. doi:10.1016/j.transproceed.2013.02.011

Merrill, L. (2013). Magnesium sulfate during anticipated preterm birth for infant neuroprotection. *Nursing for Women's Health, 17*(1), 42–51. doi:10.1111/1751-486X.12005

Oka, R., & Alley, H. F. (2012). Differences in nutrition status by body mass index in patients with peripheral artery disease. *Journal of Vascular Nursing, 30*(3), 77–87. doi:10.1016/j.jvn.2012.04.003

Rude, R. (2014). Magnesium. In A.C. Ross, B. Caballero, R. J. Cousins, K. L. Tucker & T. R. Zeigler (Eds.), *Modern nutrition in health and disease* (11th ed., pp. 159–175). Baltimore, MD: Lippincott Williams & Wilkins.

U.S. Department of Agriculture. (2014). *Dietary reference intakes (DRI) and recommended dietary allowances (RDA) resources*. Retrieved from http://www.nutrition.gov/smart-nutrition-101/dietary-reference-intakes-rdas

Van Laecke, S., Nagler, E. V., Verbeke, F., Van Biesen, W., & Vanholder, R. (2013). Hypomagnesemia and the risk of death and GFR decline in chronic kidney disease. *American Journal of Medicine, 126*(9), 825–831. doi:10.1016/j.amjmed.2013.02.036

Volpe, S. (2013). Magnesium in disease prevention and overall health. *Advances in Niutrition, 4*(3), 378S–383S. doi:10.3945/an.112.003483

Wyskida, K., Witkowicz, J., Chudek, J., & Więcek, A. (2012). Daily magnesium intake and hypermagnesemia in hemodialysis patients with chronic kidney disease. *Journal of Renal Nutrition, 22*(1), 19–26. doi:10.1053/j.jrn.2011.03.001

Chapter 8

When calcium tips the balance

Just the facts

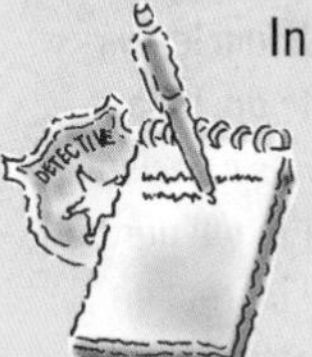

In this chapter, you'll learn:

- ways that calcium works in the body
- the relationship between calcium and albumin
- parathyroid hormone's role in calcium regulation
- ways to assess a patient for signs of calcium imbalance
- proper care for a patient with hypocalcemia or hypercalcemia.

A look at calcium

Calcium is a positively charged ion, or cation, found in both extracellular fluid and intracellular fluid. About 99% of the body's calcium is found in the bones and the teeth. Only 1% is found in serum and in soft tissue. However, that 1% is what matters when measuring calcium levels in the blood.

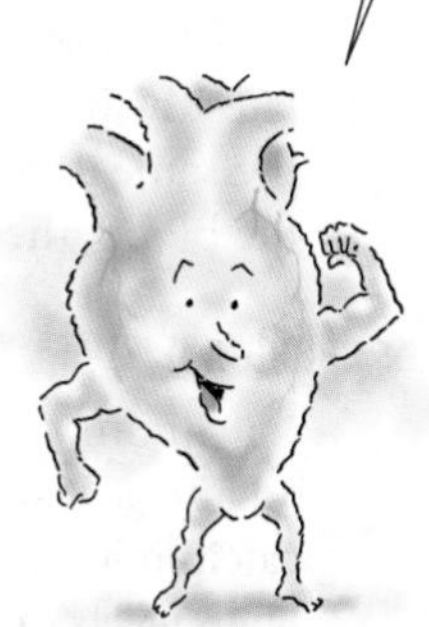

Calcium affects how cardiac muscle contracts. I think my muscles are contracting quite well!

Why it's important

Calcium is involved in numerous body functions. Together with phosphorus, calcium is responsible for the formation and structure of bones and teeth. It helps maintain cell structure and function and plays a role in cell membrane permeability and impulse transmission.

Calcium affects the contraction of cardiac muscle, smooth muscle, and skeletal muscle. It also plays a role in the blood clotting process and in the release of certain hormones.

Measuring up

Calcium can be measured in two ways. The most commonly ordered laboratory test is a total serum calcium level, which measures the total amount of calcium in blood. The normal range for total serum calcium is 8.9 to 10.1 mg/dl. (See *Calcium levels by age,* page 148.)

The second test measures the various forms of calcium in extracellular fluid. About 41% of all extracellular calcium is bound to protein; 9% is bound to citrate or other organic ions. The other half is ionized (or free) calcium, the only biologically active form of calcium. Ionized calcium carries out most of the ion's physiologic functions. In adults, the normal range for ionized calcium is 4.4 to 5.3 mg/dl; in children, it's 4.4 to 6.0 mg/dl. Normal values may vary slightly from laboratory to laboratory.

Because nearly half of all calcium is bound to the protein albumin or immunoglobulins, serum protein abnormalities can influence total serum calcium levels. For example, in hypoalbuminemia, the total serum calcium level decreases. However, ionized calcium levels—the more important of the two levels—remain unchanged. So when considering total serum calcium levels, you should also consider serum albumin levels. (See *Calculating calcium and albumin levels*.)

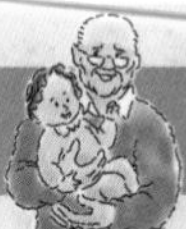

Ages and stages

Calcium levels by age

Children have higher serum calcium levels than adults do. In fact, serum levels can rise as high as 11 mg/dl during periods of increased bone growth.

The normal range for ionized calcium levels is narrower for elderly people. For elderly men, the range is 2.3 to 3.7 mg/dl; for elderly women, the range is 2.8 to 4.1 mg/dl. These values may vary slightly from laboratory to laboratory.

How the body regulates calcium

Both intake of dietary calcium and existing stores of calcium affect calcium levels in the body. For adults, the range for the recommended daily requirement of calcium is 800 to 1,200 mg/day. Requirements vary for children, pregnant patients, and patients with osteoporosis.

Dairy products are the most common calcium-rich foods, but calcium can also be found in large quantities in green, leafy vegetables. (See *Dietary sources of calcium*.) Calcium is absorbed by the small intestine and is excreted in urine and feces.

PTH is on the scene

Several factors influence calcium levels in the body. The first is parathyroid hormone (PTH). When serum calcium levels are low, the parathyroid glands release PTH, which draws calcium from the bones and promotes the transfer of calcium (along with phosphorus) into plasma. That transfer increases serum calcium levels.

PTH also promotes kidney reabsorption of calcium and stimulates the intestines to absorb the mineral. Phosphorus is excreted at the same time. In hypercalcemia, where too much calcium exists in the blood, the body suppresses the release of PTH.

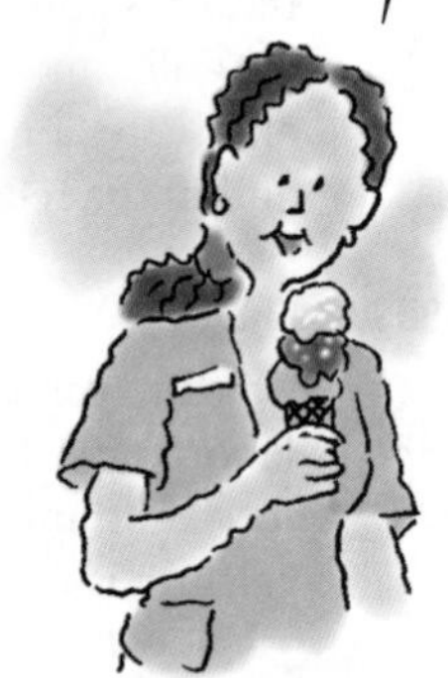
Dairy products have loads of calcium.

Enter calcitonin

Calcitonin, a hormone produced in the thyroid gland that acts as an antagonist to PTH, also helps to regulate calcium levels. When calcium levels are too high, the thyroid gland releases calcitonin. High levels of this hormone inhibit bone resorption, which causes a decrease in the amount of calcium available from bone. This causes a

Calculating calcium and albumin levels

For every 1 g/dl that a patient's serum albumin level drops, his total calcium level decreases by 0.8 mg/dl. To determine what your patient's calcium level would be if his serum albumin level were normal—and to help find out if treatment is necessary—just do a little math.

Correcting a level

A normal albumin level is 4 g/dl. The formula for correcting calcium level is:

$$\text{Total serum calcium level} + 0.8\,(4 - \text{albumin level}) = \text{corrected calcium level}$$

Sample problem

For example, if a patient's serum calcium level is 8.2 mg/dl and his albumin level is 3 g/dl, what would his corrected calcium be?

$$8.2 + 0.8\,(4 - 3) = 9\ \text{mg/dl}$$

The corrected calcium level is within the normal range, and therefore, the patient probably wouldn't require treatment.

Dietary sources of calcium

Here's a list of the most common dietary sources of calcium:

- canned sardines and salmon
- dairy products, such as milk, buttermilk, cheese, and yogurt
- green, leafy vegetables
- legumes
- molasses
- nuts
- whole grains.

decrease in serum calcium level. Calcitonin also decreases absorption of calcium and enhances its excretion by the kidneys.

Vitamin D delivers

Another factor that influences calcium levels is vitamin D. Vitamin D is ingested with foods, particularly dairy products. Also, when the skin is exposed to ultraviolet light, it synthesizes vitamin D.

The active form of vitamin D promotes calcium absorption through the intestines, calcium resorption from bone, and kidney reabsorption of calcium, all of which raise the serum calcium level. (See *Calcium in balance*, page 150.)

Phosphorus follows

Phosphorus also affects serum calcium levels. Phosphorus inhibits calcium absorption in the intestines, the opposite effect of vitamin D. When calcium levels are low and the kidneys retain calcium, phosphorus is excreted.

An inverse relationship between calcium and phosphorus exists in the body. When calcium levels rise, phosphorus levels drop. The opposite is also true: When calcium levels drop, phosphorus levels rise.

Serum pH's part

Serum pH also has an inverse relationship with ionized calcium. If the serum pH level rises (blood becomes alkaline), more calcium binds with protein and the ionized calcium level drops. Thus, a patient with alkalosis typically has hypocalcemia as well.

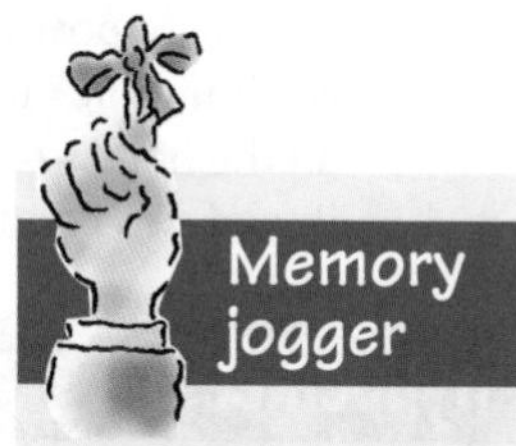

To recall the roles of calcitonin and PTH, think "**Parathyroid pulls, calcitonin keeps.**" PTH pulls calcium out of the bone. Calcitonin keeps it there.

Calcium in balance

Extracellular calcium levels are normally kept constant by several interrelated processes that move calcium ions into and out of extracellular fluid. Calcium enters the extracellular space through resorption of calcium ions from bone, through the absorption of dietary calcium in the gastrointestinal (GI) tract, and through reabsorption of calcium from the kidneys. Calcium leaves extracellular fluid as it's excreted in feces and urine and deposited in bone tissues. This illustration shows how calcium moves throughout the body.

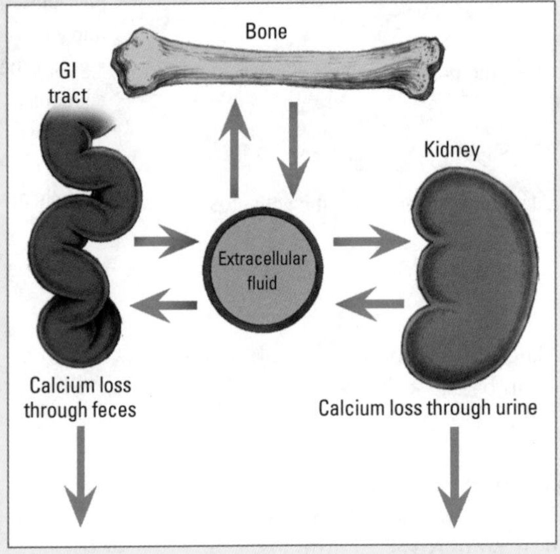

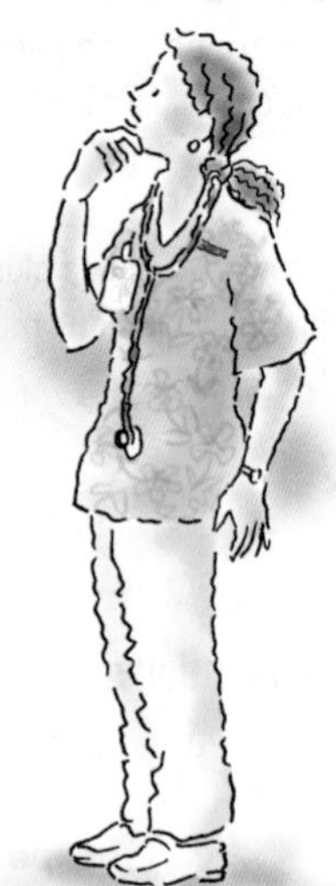

The opposite is true for acidosis. When the pH level drops, less calcium binds to protein and the ionized calcium level rises. When all the body's regulatory efforts fail to control the level of calcium, one of two conditions may result: hypocalcemia or hypercalcemia.

Hypocalcemia

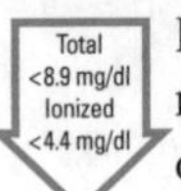

Hypocalcemia occurs when calcium levels fall below the normal range—that is, when total serum calcium levels fall below 8.9 mg/dl or ionized calcium levels fall below 4.4 mg/dl.

How it happens

Hypocalcemia occurs when a person doesn't take in enough calcium, when the body doesn't absorb the mineral properly, or when excessive amounts of calcium are lost from the body. A decreased level of ionized calcium can also cause hypocalcemia. (See *Hypocalcemia in elderly patients.*)

Intake issues

Inadequate intake of calcium can put a patient at risk for hypocalcemia. Alcoholics—who typically have poor nutritional intake, poor calcium absorption, and low magnesium levels (magnesium affects PTH secretion)—are especially prone.

A breast-fed infant can have low calcium and vitamin D levels if his mother's intake of those nutrients is inadequate. Also, anyone who doesn't receive sufficient exposure to sunlight may suffer from vitamin D deficiency and, subsequently, lower calcium levels.

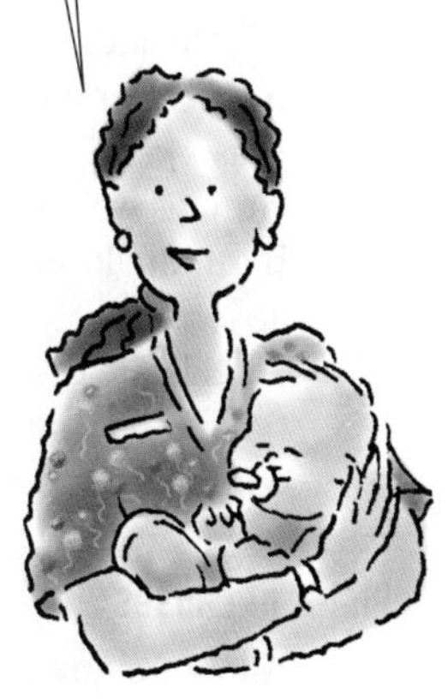
A breast-fed infant can suffer from low calcium and vitamin D levels if his mother's intake is inadequate.

Malabsorption maladies

Hypocalcemia can result when calcium isn't absorbed properly from the GI tract, a condition commonly caused by malabsorption. Malabsorption can result from increased intestinal motility from severe diarrhea, laxative abuse, or chronic malabsorption syndrome.

Absorption is also affected by a lack of vitamin D in the diet. Anticonvulsants, such as phenobarbital and phenytoin (Dilantin), can interfere with vitamin D metabolism and calcium absorption.

A high phosphorus level in the intestines can also interfere with absorption, as can a reduction in gastric acidity, which decreases the solubility of calcium salts.

Too much in the loss column

Pancreatic insufficiency can cause malabsorption of calcium and a subsequent loss of calcium in the feces. Acute pancreatitis can cause hypocalcemia as well, although the mechanism isn't well understood. PTH or possibly the combining of free fatty acids and calcium in pancreatic tissue may be involved.

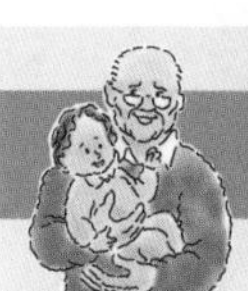

Ages and stages

Hypocalcemia in elderly patients

Several factors contribute to hypocalcemia in elderly patients. Such factors include:

- inadequate dietary intake of calcium
- poor calcium absorption (especially in postmenopausal women lacking estrogen)
- reduced activity or inactivity (inactivity causes a loss of calcium from the bones and osteoporosis, in which serum levels may be normal but bone stores of the mineral are depleted)
- medications. (See *Drugs associated with hypocalcemia,* page 152.)

Hypocalcemia can also occur when PTH secretion is reduced or eliminated. Thyroid surgery, surgical removal of the parathyroid gland, removal of a parathyroid tumor, or injury or disease of the parathyroid gland (such as hypoparathyroidism) can all reduce or prevent PTH secretion.

Hypocalcemia can also result from medications such as calcitonin and mithramycin because these drugs decrease calcium resorption from bone.

The kidneys may also excrete too much excess calcium and cause hypocalcemia. Diuretics, especially loop diuretics such as furosemide (Lasix) and ethacrynic acid (Edecrin), increase renal excretion of calcium as well as water and other electrolytes. Renal failure may also harm the kidneys' ability to activate vitamin D, which affects calcium absorption.

Edetate disodium (disodium EDTA), which is used to treat lead poisoning, can combine with calcium and carry it out of the body when excreted.

A cluster of causes

A low magnesium level (hypomagnesemia) can affect the function of the parathyroid gland and cause a decrease in calcium reabsorption in the GI tract and kidneys. Drugs that lower serum magnesium levels, such as cisplatin and gentamicin, may decrease calcium absorption from bone. (See *Drugs associated with hypocalcemia.*)

Low serum albumin (hypoalbuminemia) is the most common cause of hypocalcemia. Hypoalbuminemia may result from cirrhosis, nephrosis, malnutrition, burns, chronic illness, and sepsis.

Hyperphosphatemia (a high level of phosphorus in the blood) can cause calcium levels to fall as phosphorus levels rise. Excess phosphorus combines with calcium to form salts, which are then deposited in tissues.

When phosphates are administered orally, I.V., or rectally, the phosphorus binds with calcium and serum calcium levels drop. Infants receiving cow's milk are predisposed to hypocalcemic tetany because of the high levels of phosphorus in the milk.

Alkalosis can cause calcium to bind to albumin, thereby decreasing ionized calcium levels. Citrate, added to stored blood to prevent clotting, binds with calcium and renders it unavailable for use. Therefore, patients receiving massive blood transfusions are at risk for hypocalcemia. That risk can also apply to pediatric patients.

Other causes of hypocalcemia include increased caffeine intake, severe burns, and infections. Burned or diseased tissues trap calcium ions from extracellular fluid, thereby reducing serum calcium levels.

Drugs associated with hypocalcemia

Drugs that can cause hypocalcemia include:

- antibiotics such as rifampin
- aluminum-containing antacids
- aminoglycosides
- anticonvulsants, especially phenytoin and phenobarbital
- beta-adrenergic blockers
- caffeine
- calcitonin
- corticosteroids
- drugs that lower serum magnesium levels (such as cisplatin and gentamicin)
- edetate disodium (disodium EDTA)
- heparin
- loop diuretics
- mithramycin
- phosphates (oral, I.V., rectal).

What to look for

Signs and symptoms of hypocalcemia reflect calcium's effects on nerve transmission and muscle and heart function. Because of that, you're most likely to observe neuromuscular and cardiovascular findings. The neurologic effects of a low calcium level include anxiety, confusion, and irritability. These symptoms can progress to seizures or dementia in adults and mental retardation in children.

Neuromuscular symptoms may also develop. The patient may experience paresthesia of the toes, fingers, or face, especially around the mouth. Patients may also experience twitching, muscle cramps, or tremors. Laryngeal and abdominal muscles are particularly prone to spasm, leading to laryngospasm and bronchospasm. An increase in nerve excitability can lead to the classic manifestation of tetany, which may be evidenced by positive Trousseau's or Chvostek's signs. (See *Checking for Trousseau's and Chvostek's signs*, page 154.)

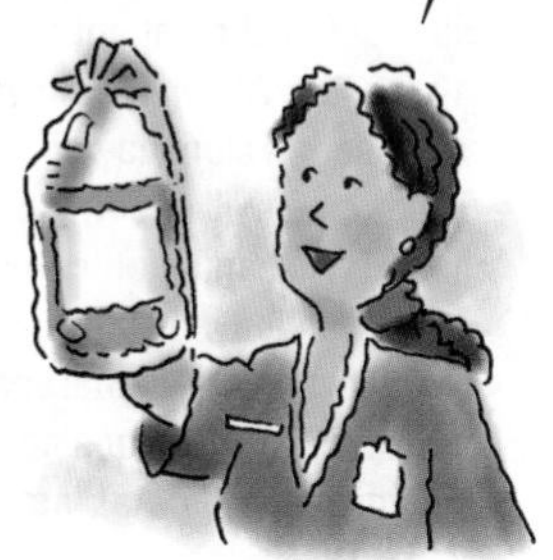
Patients receiving massive blood transfusions are at risk for hypocalcemia.

More signs

Fractures may occur more easily in a patient who's hypocalcemic for an extended period. A patient may also have brittle nails and dry skin or hair.

Other signs of hypocalcemia include:

- diarrhea
- hyperactive deep tendon reflexes
- hypotension
- diminished response to digoxin, dopamine, and norepinephrine
- decreased cardiac output and subsequent arrhythmias
- prolonged ST segment on electrocardiogram (ECG)
- lengthened QT interval on ECG, which puts the patient at risk for torsades de pointes (a form of ventricular tachycardia)
- decreased myocardial contractility, leading to angina, bradycardia, hypotension, and heart failure.

What tests show

These test results can help diagnose hypocalcemia and determine the severity of the deficiency:

- total serum calcium level less than 8.9 mg/dl
- ionized calcium level below 4.4 mg/dl (ionized calcium measurement is the definitive method to diagnose hypocalcemia)
- low albumin level
- characteristic ECG changes.

Note that falsely decreased levels may be seen with hyperbilirubinemia or administration of heparin, oxalate, or citrate or excessive I.V. fluids.

Checking for Trousseau's and Chvostek's signs

Testing for Trousseau's and Chvostek's signs can help diagnose tetany and hypocalcemia. Here's how to check for these important signs.

Trousseau's sign	Chvostek's sign
To check for Trousseau's sign, apply a blood pressure cuff to the patient's upper arm and inflate it to a pressure 20 mm Hg above the systolic pressure. Trousseau's sign may appear after 1 to 4 minutes. The patient will experience an adducted thumb, flexed wrist and metacarpophalangeal joints, and extended interphalangeal joints (with fingers together)—carpopedal spasm—indicating tetany, a major sign of hypocalcemia. Note: Trousseau's sign usually indicates late tetany.	You can induce Chvostek's sign by tapping the patient's facial nerve adjacent to the ear. A brief contraction of the upper lip, nose, or ipsilateral side of the face indicates Chvostek's sign. Note: Chvostek's sign may be present in healthy infants and, therefore, may not indicate tetany.

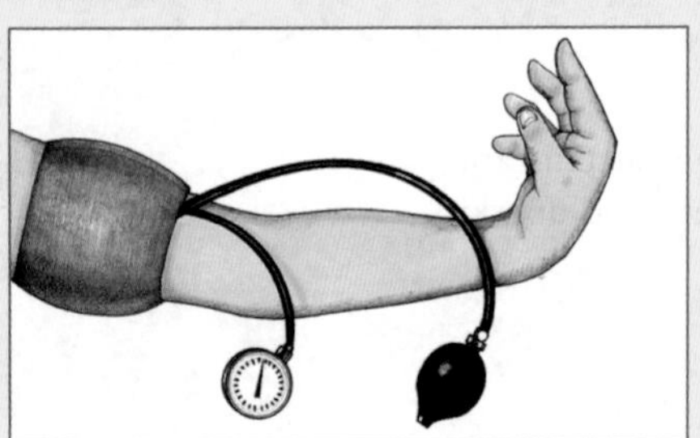

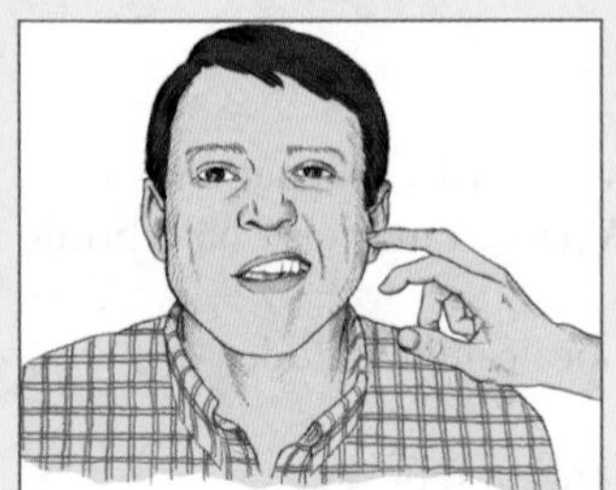

How it's treated

Treatment for hypocalcemia focuses on correcting the imbalance as quickly and safely as possible. The underlying cause should be addressed to prevent recurrence.

Acute hypocalcemia requires immediate correction by administering either I.V. calcium gluconate or I.V. calcium chloride. Although calcium chloride contains three times as much available calcium as calcium gluconate, the latter is more commonly used. Calcium chloride is advised for patients in cardiac arrest. Magnesium replacement may also be needed because hypocalcemia doesn't always respond to calcium therapy alone. (See *Administering I.V. calcium safely,* page 156.)

Chronic hypocalcemia requires vitamin D supplements to promote GI absorption of calcium. Oral calcium supplements also help increase calcium levels.

Diet differences

The patient's diet should also be adjusted to allow for adequate intake of calcium, vitamin D, and protein. In cases where the patient also has a high phosphorus level, aluminum hydroxide antacids may be given to bind with excess phosphorus. (See *When treatment doesn't work.*)

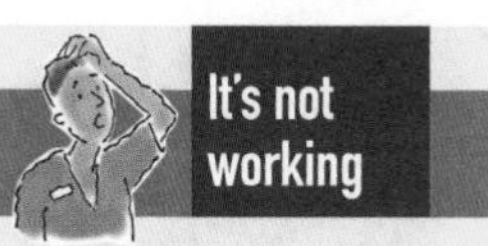

When treatment doesn't work

If treatment for hypocalcemia doesn't seem to be working, consider these interventions:

- Check the magnesium level. A low magnesium level must be corrected before I.V. calcium can increase serum calcium levels.
- Check the phosphate level. If the phosphate level is too high, calcium won't be absorbed. Reduce the phosphate level first.
- Mix I.V. calcium in dextrose solutions only because normal saline may cause calcium to be excreted. Whenever possible, use premixed solutions.

How you intervene

If your patient is at increased risk for hypocalcemia, assess carefully, especially if the patient has had parathyroid or thyroid surgery or has received massive blood transfusions. If your patient is a breast-feeding mother, assess her for adequate vitamin D intake and exposure to sunlight.

When assessing a patient you suspect has hypocalcemia, obtain a complete medical history. Note if the patient has ever had neck surgery. Hypoparathyroidism may develop immediately or several years after neck surgery. Ask a patient who has chronic hypocalcemia if he has a history of fractures. Obtain a list of medications, including over-the-counter supplements, the patient is taking; the list may help you determine the underlying cause of hypocalcemia. Make sure you also assess the patient's ability to perform activities of daily living, which may be affected by hypocalcemia. Teach the patient about the signs and symptoms of hypocalcemia. (See *Teaching about hypocalcemia*, page 157.)

When the bottom drops out

If your patient is recovering from parathyroid or thyroid surgery, keep calcium gluconate on hand. A ready supply of the drug ensures a quick response to signs of a sudden drop in calcium levels.

If the patient develops hypocalcemia, here's what you can do:

- Monitor vital signs and assess the patient frequently. Monitor respiratory status, including rate, depth, and rhythm. Watch for stridor, dyspnea, and crowing.
- If the patient shows overt signs of hypocalcemia, keep a tracheotomy tray and a handheld resuscitation bag at the bedside in case laryngospasm occurs.
- Place your patient on a cardiac monitor, and evaluate him for changes in heart rate and rhythm. Notify the practitioner if the patient develops arrhythmias, such as ventricular tachycardia or heart block.
- Check the patient for Chvostek's and Trousseau's signs.
- Insert and maintain a patent I.V. line for calcium therapy as ordered.
- Monitor a patient receiving I.V. calcium for arrhythmias, especially if he's also taking digoxin. Calcium and digoxin have similar effects on the heart.

Administering I.V. calcium safely

Be prepared to administer parenteral calcium to a patient who has symptomatic hypocalcemia. Always clarify whether the doctor orders calcium gluconate or calcium chloride. Doses vary according to the specific drug. Note the type and dosage of each calcium preparation carefully, and follow these steps when administering it.

Preparing	Administering	Monitoring
Dilute the prescribed I.V. calcium preparation in dextrose 5% in water or normal saline (NS). The preferred solution is dextrose 5% in water. Never dilute calcium in solutions containing bicarbonate because precipitation will occur. Always assess for crystals in the solution. If present, do not use.	Always administer I.V. calcium slowly, according to the practitioner's order or your facility's established protocol. Never give it rapidly because it may result in syncope, hypotension, or cardiac arrhythmias. Initially, calcium may be given as a slow I.V. bolus. If hypocalcemia persists, the initial bolus may be followed by a slow I.V. drip using an infusion pump.	Overcorrection may lead to hypercalcemia. Watch for signs and symptoms of hypercalcemia, including anorexia, nausea, vomiting, lethargy, and confusion. Institute cardiac monitoring, and observe the patient for arrhythmias. Continuous cardiac monitoring should be used especially if the patient is receiving digoxin or has a history of arrhythmias. Observe the I.V. site for signs of infiltration; calcium can cause tissue sloughing and necrosis. Closely monitor serum calcium levels.

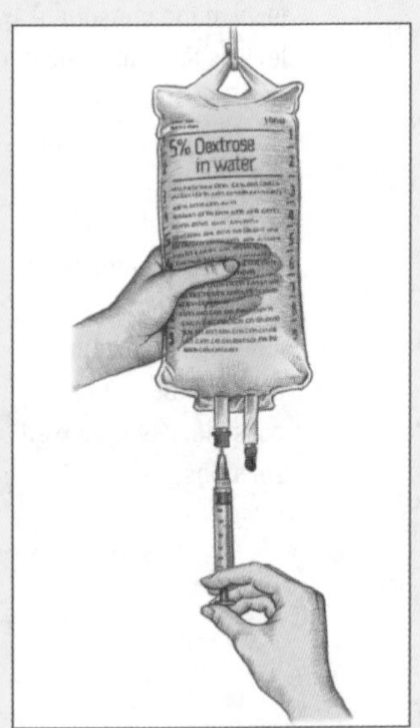

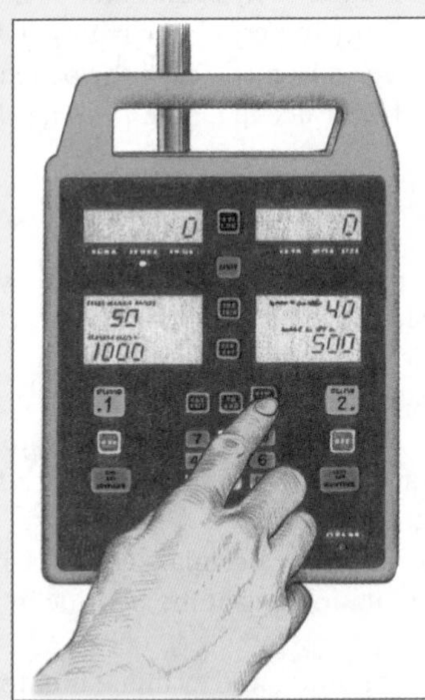

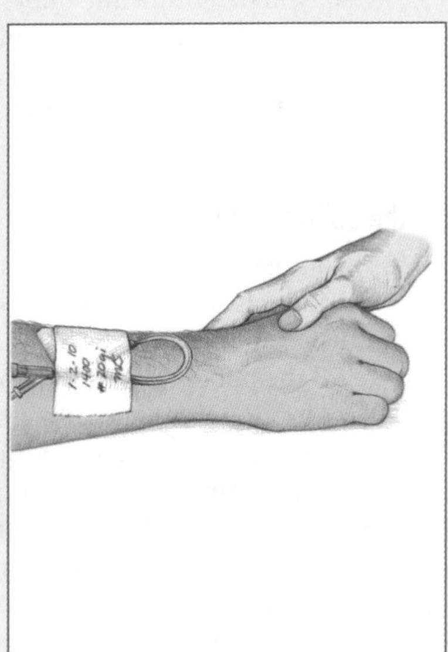

- Administer I.V. calcium replacement therapy carefully. Ensure the patency of the I.V. line because infiltration can cause tissue necrosis and sloughing.
- Administer oral replacements as ordered. Give calcium supplements 1 to 1½ hours after meals. If GI upset occurs, give the supplement with milk.
- Monitor pertinent laboratory test results, including not only calcium levels but also albumin levels and those of other

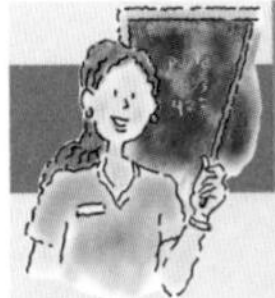

Teaching points

Teaching about hypocalcemia

When teaching a patient with hypocalcemia, be sure to cover the following topics and then evaluate your patient's learning:

- description of hypocalcemia, its causes, and treatment
- importance of a high-calcium diet
- dietary sources of calcium
- avoidance of long-term laxative use
- medications
- importance of exercise
- warning signs and symptoms (such as paresthesia and muscle weakness) and when to report them (prompt care may prevent the development of more severe symptoms)
- need to report pain during I.V. infusion of calcium
- possible use of female hormones in patients with osteoporosis.

electrolytes, such as magnesium and phosphorus. Remember to check the ionized calcium level after every 4 units of blood transfused.

- Encourage the older patient to take a calcium supplement with vitamin D as ordered and to exercise as much as he can tolerate to prevent calcium loss from bones.
- Take precautions for seizures such as padding bed side rails.
- Reorient a confused patient. Provide a calm, quiet environment.
- Teach the patient about the signs and symptoms of hypocalcemia.
- Document all care given to the patient, the patient's response to treatment, and all observations and assessments made. (See *Documenting hypocalcemia*, page 158.)

Hypercalcemia

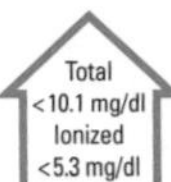

Hypercalcemia is a common metabolic emergency that occurs when serum calcium level rises above 10.1 mg/dl, ionized serum calcium level rises above 5.3 mg/dl, or the rate of calcium entry into extracellular fluid exceeds the rate of calcium excretion by the kidneys.

How it happens

Any situation that causes an increase in total serum or ionized calcium level can lead to hypercalcemia. This condition is usually

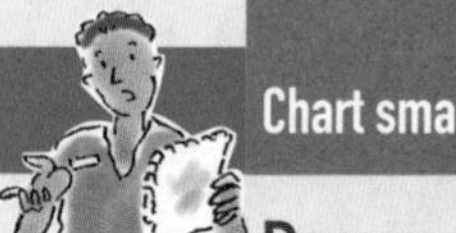

Chart smart

Documenting hypocalcemia

If your patient has hypocalcemia, make sure you document the following information:

- vital signs, including cardiac rhythm
- intake and output
- seizure activity
- safety measures
- assessments, interventions, and the patient's response
- patency and appearance of I.V. site before and after calcium infusion
- type of calcium infusion administered, the site of infusion, and rate of infusion
- pertinent laboratory results, including calcium levels
- time that you notified the practitioner
- patient teaching and teach-back.

caused by an increase in the resorption of calcium from bone. Hyperparathyroidism and cancer are the two main causes of hypercalcemia.

Blame the other hyper

With primary hyperparathyroidism, the most common cause of hypercalcemia, the body excretes more PTH than normal, which greatly strengthens the effects of the hormone. Calcium resorption from bone and reabsorption from the kidneys are also increased, as is calcium absorption from the intestines.

Malignant invasion

Cancer, the second most common cause of hypercalcemia, causes bone destruction as malignant cells invade the bones and cause the release of a hormone similar to PTH. That PTH-like substance causes an increase in serum calcium levels.

When serum calcium levels rise, the kidneys can become overwhelmed and can't excrete all that excess calcium, which in turn keeps calcium levels elevated. Patients who have squamous cell carcinoma of the lung, myeloma, Hodgkin's lymphoma, renal cell carcinoma, or breast cancer are especially prone to hypercalcemia.

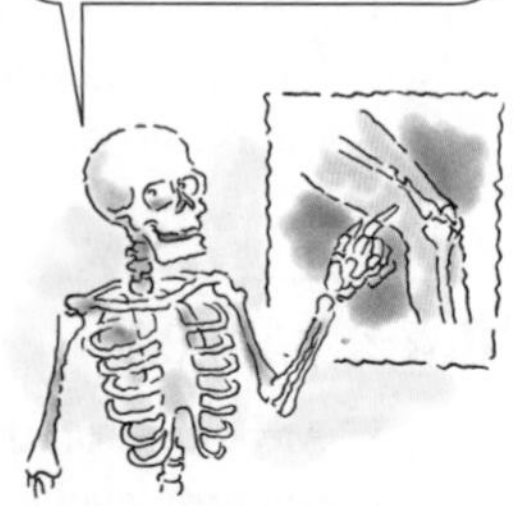
Multiple fractures or prolonged immobilization can cause an increase in calcium release from bone. Them's the breaks!

Still more causes

Hypercalcemia can also be caused by an increase in the absorption of calcium in the GI tract or by a decrease in the excretion of calcium by the kidneys. These mechanisms may occur alone or in combination.

A false high level can result from prolonged blood draws with an excessively tight tourniquet or prolonged dehydration.

Hyperthyroidism can cause an increase in calcium release as more calcium is resorbed from bone. Multiple fractures, lack of weight bearing, or prolonged immobilization can also cause an increase in calcium release from bone.

Hypophosphatemia and acidosis (which increases calcium ionization) are metabolic conditions that are linked with hypercalcemia. Certain medications are also associated with the condition. For instance, abusing antacids that contain calcium, receiving an overdose of calcium (from calcium medications given during cardiopulmonary resuscitation, for example), or ingesting excessive amounts of vitamin D or calcium supplements can prompt an increase in serum calcium levels. (See *Drugs associated with hypercalcemia.*)

Vitamin A overdose can lead to increased bone resorption of calcium, which can also result in hypercalcemia. Use of lithium or thiazide diuretics can decrease calcium excretion by the kidneys. Milk-alkali syndrome, a condition in which calcium and alkali are combined, also raises calcium levels.

What to look for

Signs and symptoms of hypercalcemia are intensified if the condition develops acutely. They're also more severe if calcium levels are greater than 14 mg/dl. Elderly patients are more likely to have symptoms from only moderate elevations in calcium levels.

Many signs and symptoms stem from the effects of excess calcium in the cells, which causes a decrease in cell membrane excitability, especially in the tissues of skeletal muscle, heart muscle, and the nervous system.

A patient with hypercalcemia may complain of fatigue or exhibit confusion, memory loss, altered mental status, depression, or personality changes. Lethargy can progress to coma in severe cases.

Drugs associated with hypercalcemia

Medications that can cause hypercalcemia include:

- antacids that contain calcium
- calcium preparations (oral or I.V.)
- lithium
- thiazide diuretics
- thyroxine
- vitamin A
- vitamin D.

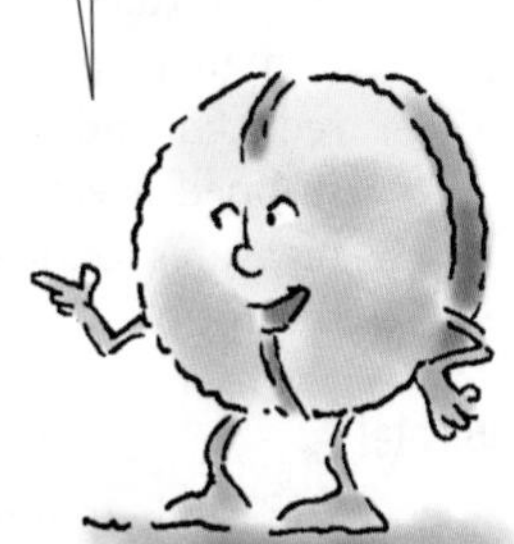

Certain drugs can increase the risk of hypercalcemia.

Tuning in to muscle tone

As calcium levels rise, muscle weakness, hyporeflexia, ataxia, and decreased muscle tone occur. Hypercalcemia may lead to hypertension.

Because heart muscle and the cardiac conduction system are affected by hypercalcemia, arrhythmias (such as bradycardia) can lead to cardiac arrest. ECGs may reveal a shortened QT interval and a shortened ST segment. Also look for digoxin toxicity if the patient is receiving digoxin.

Intestinal issues

Hypercalcemia can also lead to GI effects, which are commonly the first indications the patient notices. The patient may experience thirst, anorexia, nausea, and vomiting. Bowel sounds will decrease. Constipation can occur because of calcium's effect on smooth muscle and the subsequent decrease in GI motility. Abdominal or flank pain and paralytic ileus may result.

As the kidneys work overtime to remove excess calcium, renal problems may develop. The patient may experience polyuria and subsequent dehydration. Hypercalcemia can also cause kidney stones and other calcifications. Renal failure may be the end result. Also, the patient may develop pathologic fractures and bone pain. (See *Danger signs of hypercalcemia*.)

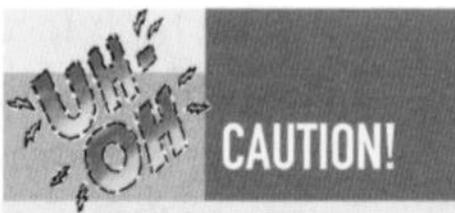

Danger signs of hypercalcemia

If you suspect hypercalcemia in a patient, these signs may indicate that the condition has become life-threatening:
- arrhythmias such as bradycardia
- cardiac arrest
- coma
- paralytic ileus
- renal failure
- stupor.

What tests show

If you suspect that your patient has hypercalcemia, look for:
- serum calcium level above 10.1 mg/dl
- ionized calcium level above 5.3 mg/dl
- digoxin toxicity (if your patient is taking digoxin)
- X-rays revealing pathologic fractures
- characteristic ECG changes (shortened QT interval, prolonged PR interval, flattened T waves, and heart block).

How it's treated

If hypercalcemia produces no symptoms, treatment may consist only of managing the underlying cause. Dietary intake of calcium may be reduced, and medications or infusions containing calcium may be stopped. Treatment for asymptomatic hypercalcemia also includes measures to increase the excretion of calcium and to decrease bone resorption of it.

Hydrate!

You can help increase excretion of calcium by hydrating the patient, which encourages diuresis. Normal saline solution is typically used for hydration in these cases. The sodium in the solution inhibits renal tubular reabsorption of calcium.

Loop diuretics such as furosemide (Lasix) and ethacrynic acid (Edecrin) also promote calcium excretion. Thiazide diuretics aren't used for hypercalcemia because they inhibit calcium excretion.

For patients with life-threatening hypercalcemia and those with renal failure, measures to increase calcium excretion may include hemodialysis or peritoneal dialysis with a solution that contains little or no calcium.

Dietary changes—cutting back on dairy products such as milk or cheese, for instance—can help treat asymptomatic hypercalcemia.

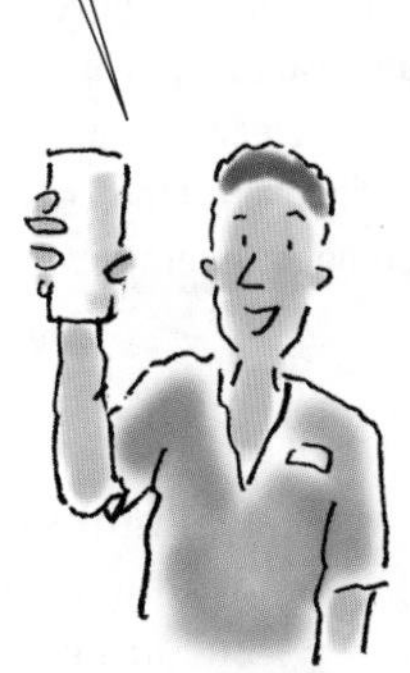

Back to the bones

Measures to inhibit bone resorption of calcium may also be used to help reduce calcium levels in extracellular fluids. Corticosteroids administered I.V. and then orally can block bone resorption and decrease calcium absorption from the GI tract.

Bisphosphonates are used to treat hypercalcemia caused by malignancy. Zoledronate inhibits bone resorption by acting on osteoclasts.

Etidronate disodium, commonly used to treat hypercalcemia, also inhibits the action of osteoclasts. This medication takes full effect in 2 to 3 days. Pamidronate disodium, which is similar to etidronate disodium, can also be used to inhibit bone resorption.

Plicamycin (mithramycin), a chemotherapeutic (antineoplastic) drug, can decrease bone resorption of calcium and is used primarily when hypercalcemia is caused by cancer. Calcitonin, a naturally occurring hormone, inhibits bone resorption as well, but its effects are short lived. (See *When treatment doesn't work.*)

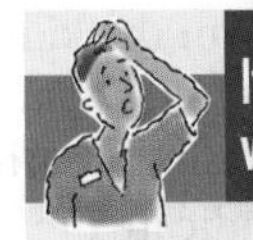

It's not working

When treatment doesn't work

If your patient doesn't seem to be responding to treatment for hypercalcemia, make sure he isn't still taking vitamin D supplements.

Keep in mind that calcitonin may be given to decrease calcium levels rapidly, but the effects are only temporary. If hypercalcemia is severe, you may give one or two doses with fluids and furosemide to provide rapid reduction of calcium levels.

How you intervene

Be sure to monitor the calcium levels of patients who are at risk for hypercalcemia, such as those who have cancer or parathyroid disorders, are immobile, or are receiving a calcium supplement. For a patient who develops hypercalcemia, take the following actions:

- Monitor vital signs and assess the patient frequently.
- Watch the patient for arrhythmias.
- Assess neurologic and neuromuscular function and level of consciousness and report changes.
- Monitor the patient's fluid intake and output.
- Monitor serum electrolyte levels, especially calcium, to determine the effectiveness of treatment and to detect new imbalances that might result from therapy.
- Insert an I.V. catheter and maintain I.V. access. Normal saline solution is usually administered at an initial rate of 200 to 300 ml/hour in the absence of edema, and then the flow rate is adjusted to maintain a urine output of approximately 100 ml/hour. Monitor the patient for signs of fluid overload such as crackles and dyspnea.

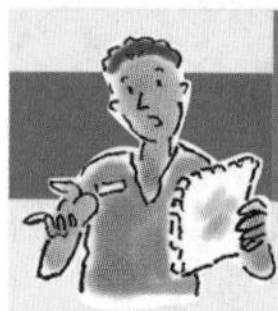

Chart smart

Documenting hypercalcemia

If your patient has hypercalcemia, make sure you document the following information:

- assessment findings, including neurologic examination and level of consciousness
- vital signs, including cardiac rhythm
- intake and output
- interventions, including I.V. therapy, and the patient's response to them
- signs and symptoms
- safety measures taken
- patient teaching done and the patient's response
- notification of the practitioner
- pertinent laboratory results, including calcium levels.

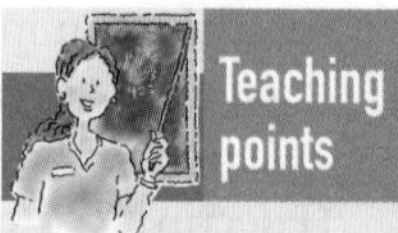

Teaching points

Teaching about hypercalcemia

When teaching a patient with hypercalcemia, be sure to cover the following topics and then evaluate your patient's learning:

- description of hypercalcemia, its causes, and treatment
- risk factors
- importance of increased fluid intake
- dietary guidelines for a low-calcium diet
- prescribed medications, including possible adverse effects
- warning signs and symptoms
- avoidance of supplements and antacids that contain calcium.

- If administering a diuretic, make sure the patient is properly hydrated first so that he doesn't experience volume depletion.
- Encourage the patient to drink 3 to 4 qt (3 to 4 L) of fluid daily, unless contraindicated, to stimulate calcium excretion from the kidneys and to decrease the risk of calculi formation. (See *Teaching about hypercalcemia.*)
- Strain the urine for calculi. Also check for flank pain, which can indicate the presence of renal calculi.
- If the patient is receiving digoxin, watch for signs and symptoms of a toxic reaction, such as anorexia, nausea, vomiting, or an irregular heart rate.
- Get the patient up and moving as soon as possible to prevent bones from releasing calcium.

A gentle touch

- Handle a patient who has chronic hypercalcemia gently to prevent pathologic fractures. Reposition bedridden patients frequently. Perform active or passive range-of-motion exercises to prevent complications from immobility.
- Provide a safe environment. Keep the side rails raised as needed, maintain the bed in its lowest position, and keep the wheels locked. Make sure the patient's belongings and call button are within reach. If the patient is confused, reorient him.
- Offer emotional support to the patient and his family throughout treatment. Overt signs of hypercalcemia can be emotionally distressing for all involved.
- Chart all care given and the patient's response. (See *Documenting hypercalcemia.*)

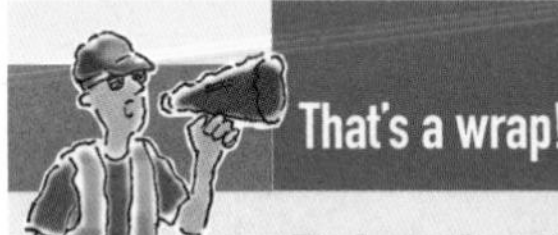

That's a wrap!

Balancing fluids review

Calcium basics

- Positively charged ion (cation)
- Ninety-nine percent in bones and teeth; 1% in extracellular fluid
- Important for bone and tooth formation, normal cell function, and neural transmission
- Affects contraction of muscles, blood clotting, and hormone balance
- Mostly bound to albumin (always look at albumin level with calcium)
- Normal total serum calcium levels: 8.9 to 10.1 mg/dl
- Normal ionized calcium levels: adults, 4.4 to 5.3 mg/dl; children, 4.4 to 6.0 mg/dl; elderly, 2.3 to 4.1 mg/dl.

Calcium balance

- Calcium level is affected by dietary intake and existing stores of calcium in the body.
- PTH is released by the parathyroid gland when calcium stores are low; it pulls calcium from bones and promotes transfer of calcium into plasma, kidney reabsorption of calcium, and absorption from intestines.
- Calcitonin, another hormone released by the thyroid, antagonizes PTH; if calcium levels are too high, calcitonin inhibits bone resorption, decreases absorption of calcium, and increases excretion of calcium by the kidneys.
- Vitamin D promotes calcium absorption from intestines, resorption from bones, and reabsorption by kidneys to increase calcium levels.
- Phosphorus is inversely related to calcium and inhibits calcium absorption from intestines; when calcium levels are low, kidneys retain calcium and excrete phosphorus.
- Serum pH has an inverse relationship with ionized calcium. If pH rises, more calcium binds with protein and ionized calcium level drops; if pH drops, less calcium binds to protein and ionized calcium level rises.

Hypocalcemia

- Major cause: hypoalbuminemia
- Also caused by poor dietary intake, malabsorption, pancreatitis, parathyroid and thyroid gland surgery, medications, kidney failure, hypomagnesemia, hyperphosphatemia, and alkalosis

Signs and symptoms

- Predominantly neuromuscular and cardiovascular
- Classic sign: tetany evidenced by Trousseau's and Chvostek's signs
- Also include anxiety; confusion; irritability; decreased cardiac output; arrhythmias; prolonged ST segment and QT intervals; fractures; muscle cramps; tremors; twitching; and paresthesia of the face, fingers, and toes

Treatment

- I.V. calcium gluconate or calcium chloride
- Possibly magnesium supplements, vitamin D supplements, and adequate dietary intake of calcium (for chronic hypocalcemia)

Hypercalcemia

- Common electrolyte disorder
- Considered a metabolic emergency

(continued)

Balancing fluids review *(continued)*

- Two major causes: primary hyperparathyroidism, which releases excess PTH, and cancer, which releases a substance similar to PTH
- Other causes: hyperthyroidism, fractures, prolonged immobilization, hypophosphatemia, acidosis, vitamin A overdose, and certain medications

Signs and symptoms

- Heart, skeletal muscle, and nervous system are most affected.
- Include confusion, lethargy, depression, altered mental status, muscle weakness, hyporeflexia, characteristic ECG changes, hypertension, bone pain, abdominal pain and constipation, nausea, vomiting, anorexia, polyuria, and extreme thirst

Treatment

- Hydration
- Decreased calcium intake
- Diuretics, corticosteroids, bisphosphonates, and plicamycin
- Hemodialysis or peritoneal dialysis (for life-threatening cases)

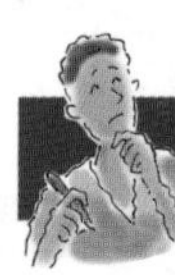

Quick quiz

1. Albumin affects calcium levels by:
   A. blocking phosphorus absorption, which prevents calcium excretion.
   B. binding with calcium, which makes calcium ineffective.
   C. inhibiting magnesium uptake, which prevents calcium absorption.
   D. affecting pH level.

Answer: B. Albumin binds with calcium and renders it ineffective.

2. Hypocalcemia involves a dysfunction of:
   A. calcitonin.
   B. antidiuretic hormone.
   C. growth hormone.
   D. PTH.

Answer: D. PTH promotes reabsorption of calcium from the bone to the serum. When secretion of PTH is decreased, hypocalcemia results.

3. If your patient is hypercalcemic, you would expect to:
   A. administer I.V. sodium bicarbonate.
   B. administer vitamin D.
   C. hydrate the patient.
   D. administer digoxin.

Answer: C. Hydrating a patient with oral or I.V. fluids increases the urine excretion of calcium and helps lower serum calcium levels.

4. Hypercalcemia would be most likely to develop in:
   A. a 60-year-old man who has squamous cell carcinoma of the lung.
   B. an 80-year-old woman who has heart failure and is taking furosemide (Lasix).
   C. a 25-year-old trauma patient who has received massive blood transfusions.
   D. a 40-year-old man with hypoalbuminemia.

Answer: A. Squamous cell carcinoma of the lung can lead to hypercalcemia.

5. You're told during shift report that your patient has a positive Chvostek's sign. You would expect his laboratory test results to reveal:
   A. a total serum calcium level below 8.9 mg/dl.
   B. a total serum calcium level above 10.1 mg/dl.
   C. an ionized calcium level above 5.3 mg/dl.
   D. an ionized calcium level between 4.4 and 5.3 mg/dl.

Answer: A. Chvostek's and Trousseau's signs are associated with hypocalcemia. A total serum calcium level below 8.9 mg/dl confirms the presence of that condition.

Scoring

☆☆☆ If you answered all five questions correctly, we're impressed! We wonder, have you been hanging out in Professor Chvostek's lab?

☆☆ If you answered four questions correctly, oh my! Have you been reading Professor Trousseau's diary, by chance?

☆ If you answered fewer than four questions correctly, that's fine. We have a great seat for you at the Chvostek-Trousseau lecture series.

References

Bansal, N., Katz, R., de Boer, I. H., Kestenbaum, B., Siscovick, D. S., Hoofnagle, A. N., . . . Ix, J. H. (2013). Influence of estrogen therapy on calcium, phosphorus, and other regulatory hormones in postmenopausal women: The MESA study. *Journal of Clinical Endocrinology and Metabolism, 98*(12), 4890–4898.

Bech, A., Reichert, L., Telting, D., & de Boer, H. (2013). Assessment of calcium balance in patients on hemodialysis, based on ionized calcium and parathyroid hormone responses. *Journal of Nephrology, 26*(5), 925–930.

Bell, D. A., Crooke, M. J., Hay, N., & Glendenning, P. (2013). Prolonged vitamin D intoxication: Presentation, pathogenesis and progress. *Internal Medicine Journal, 43*(10), 1148–1150.

Bouillon, R., Van Schoor, N. M., Gielen, E., Boonen, S., Mathieu, C., Vanderschueren, D., & Lips, P. (2013). Optimal vitamin D status: A critical analysis on the basis of evidence-based medicine. *Journal of Clinical Endocrinology and Metabolism, 98*(8), E1283–E1304.

Carter, T., & Ratnam, S. (2013). Calciphylaxis: A devastating complication of derangements of calcium-phosphorus metabolism—A case report and review of the literature. *Nephrology Nursing Journal, 40*(5), 431–435.

Cauley, J., Chlebowski, R. T., Wactawski-Wende, J., Robbins, J. A., Rodabough, R. J., Chen, Z., . . . Manson, J. E. (2013). Calcium plus vitamin D supplementation and health outcomes five years active intervention ended: The Women's Health Initiative. *Journal of Women's Health, 22*(11), 915–929.

Jamal, S. A., Vandermeer, B., Raggi, P., Mendelssohn, D. C., Chatterley, T., Dorgan, M., . . . Tsuyuki, R. T. (2013). Effect of calcium-based versus non-calcium-based phosphate binders on mortality in patients with chronic kidney disease: An updated systematic review and meta-analysis. *Lancet, 382*(9900), 1268–1277.

Jungert, A., & Neuhäuser-Berthold, M. (2013). Dietary vitamin D intake is not associated with 25-hydroxyvitamin D3 or parathyroid hormone in elderly subjects, whereas the calcium-to-phosphate ratio affects parathyroid hormone. *Nutrition Research, 33*(8), 661–667.

McCarthy, M. S., Loan, L. A., Azuero, A., & Hobbs, C. (2010). The consequences of modern military deployment on calcium status and bone health. *Nursing Clinics of North America, 45*(2), 109–122.

Mocanu, V., & Vieth, R. (2013). Three-year follow-up of serum 25-hydroxyvitamin D, parathyroid hormone, and bone mineral density in nursing home residents who had received 12 months of daily bread fortification with 125 mug of vitamin D3. *Nutrition Journal, 12*(1), 137.

Pipili, C., & Oreopoulos, D. G. (2012). Vitamin D status in patients with recurrent kidney stones. *Nephron Clinical Practice, 122*(3–4), 134–138.

Shirazi, L., Almquist, M., Malm, J., Wirfält, E., & Manjer, J. (2013). Determinants of serum levels of vitamin D: A study of lifestyle, menopausal status, dietary intake, serum calcium, and PTH. *BMC Women's Health, 13*, 33.

Chapter 9

When phosphorus tips the balance

Just the facts

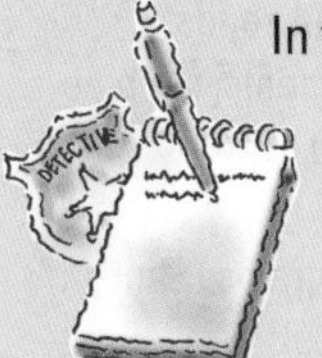

In this chapter, you'll learn:

- the role that phosphorus plays in the body
- the body's mechanisms for regulating phosphorus
- ways to assess a patient for a phosphorus imbalance
- management of hypophosphatemia and hyperphosphatemia.

A look at phosphorus

Phosphorus is the primary anion, or negatively charged ion, found in intracellular fluid. It's contained in the body as phosphate. (The two words—*phosphorus* and *phosphate*—are commonly used interchangeably.) About 85% of phosphorus exists in bone and teeth, combined in a 1:2 ratio with calcium. About 14% is in soft tissue, and less than 1% is in extracellular fluid.

Why it's important

An essential element of all body tissues, phosphorus is vital to various body functions. It plays a crucial role in cell membrane integrity (phospholipids make up the cell membranes); muscle function; neurologic function; and the metabolism of carbohydrates, fat, and protein. Phosphorus is a primary ingredient in 2,3-diphosphoglycerate (2,3-DPG), a compound in red blood cells (RBCs) that promotes oxygen delivery from RBCs to the tissues.

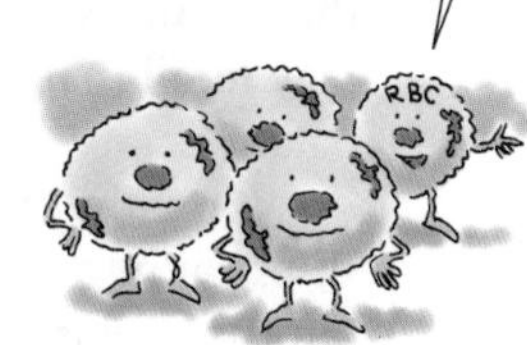
Phosphorus plays a crucial role in cell membrane integrity. Now, that's an electrolyte you can really trust!
RBC

Phosphorus also helps buffer acids and bases. It promotes energy transfer to cells through the formation of energy-storing substances such as adenosine triphosphate (ATP). It's also important for white blood cell (WBC) phagocytosis and for platelet function. Finally, with calcium, phosphorus is essential for healthy bones and teeth.

The lowdown on low phosphorus levels

Normal serum phosphorus levels in adults range from 2.5 to 4.5 mg/dl (or 1.8 to 2.6 mEq/L). In comparison, the normal phosphorus level in the cells is 100 mEq/L. Because phosphorus is located primarily within the cells, serum levels may not always reflect the total amount of phosphorus in the body. For example, it's important to distinguish between a decrease in the level of serum phosphate (hypophosphatemia) and a decrease in total body storage of phosphate (phosphate deficiency).

Dietary sources of phosphorus

Major dietary sources of phosphorus include:

- dairy products, such as milk and cheese
- dried beans
- eggs
- fish
- nuts and seeds
- organ meats, such as brain and liver
- poultry
- whole grains (Shuto et al., 2009)

How the body regulates phosphorus

The total amount of phosphorus in the body is related to dietary intake, hormonal regulation, kidney excretion, and transcellular shifts. For adults, the range for the recommended daily requirement of phosphorus is 800 to 1,200 mg. Phosphorus is readily absorbed through the gastrointestinal (GI) tract, with the amount absorbed proportional to the amount ingested. (See *Dietary sources of phosphorus.*)

Most ingested phosphorus is absorbed through the jejunum. The kidneys excrete about 90% of phosphorus as they regulate serum levels. (The GI tract excretes the rest.) If dietary intake of phosphorus increases, the kidneys increase excretion to maintain normal levels of phosphorus. A low-phosphorus diet causes the kidneys to conserve phosphorus by reabsorbing more of it in the proximal tubules.

Balancing it out with PTH

The parathyroid gland controls hormonal regulation of phosphorus levels by affecting the activity of parathyroid hormone (PTH). (See *PTH and phosphorus.*) Changes in calcium levels, rather than changes in phosphorus levels, affect the release of PTH. You may recall that phosphorus balance is closely related to calcium balance.

Normally, calcium and phosphorus have an inverse relationship. For instance, when the serum calcium level is low, the phosphorus level is high. This causes the parathyroid gland to release PTH, which causes an increase in calcium and phosphorus resorption from bone, raising both calcium and phosphorus levels. Phosphorus absorption from the intestines also increases. (Activated vitamin D—calcitriol—also enhances phosphorus absorption in the intestines.)

PTH and phosphorus

This illustration shows how PTH affects serum phosphorus (P) levels by increasing phosphorus release from bone, increasing phosphorus absorption from the intestines, and decreasing phosphorus reabsorption in the renal tubules.

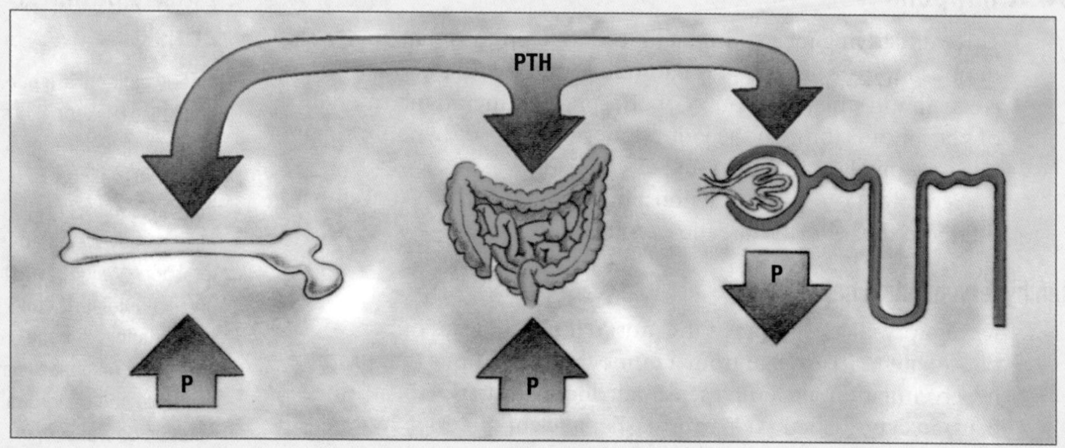

Kidneys enter the equation

PTH also acts on the kidneys to increase excretion of phosphorus. The renal effect of PTH outweighs its other effects on the serum phosphorus level, particularly that of returning the phosphorus level to normal. Reduced PTH levels allow for phosphorus reabsorption by the kidneys. As a result, serum levels rise (Connor, 2009).

Shifty business

Certain conditions cause phosphorus to move, or shift, in and out of cells. Insulin moves not only glucose but also phosphorus into the cell. Alkalosis results in the same kind of phosphorus shift. Those shifts affect serum phosphorus levels. (See *Elderly patients at risk,* page 170.)

Hypophosphatemia

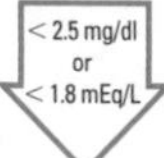

Hypophosphatemia occurs when the serum phosphorus level falls below 2.5 mg/dl (or 1.8 mEq/L). Although this condition generally indicates a deficiency of phosphorus, it can occur under various circumstances when total body phosphorus stores are normal. Severe hypophosphatemia occurs when serum phosphorus levels are less than 1 mg/dl and the body can't support its energy needs. The condition may lead to organ failure.

How it happens

Three underlying mechanisms can lead to hypophosphatemia: a shift of phosphorus from extracellular fluid to intracellular fluid, a decrease in intestinal absorption of phosphorus, and an increased loss of phosphorus through the kidneys. Some causes of hypophosphatemia may involve more than one mechanism.

Several factors may cause phosphorus to shift from extracellular fluid into the cell. Here are the most common causes.

When hyperventilation happens

Respiratory alkalosis, one of the most common causes of hypophosphatemia, can stem from a number of conditions that produce hyperventilation, including sepsis, alcohol withdrawal, heat stroke, pain, anxiety, diabetic ketoacidosis, hepatic encephalopathy, and acute salicylate poisoning. Although the mechanism that prompts respiratory alkalosis to induce hypophosphatemia is unknown, the response is a shift of phosphorus into the cells and a resulting decrease in serum phosphorus levels.

Sugar high

Hyperglycemia, an elevated serum glucose level, causes the release of insulin, which transports glucose and phosphorus into the cells. The same effect may occur in a patient with diabetes who's receiving insulin or in a significantly malnourished patient; at particular risk for malnourishment are elderly, debilitated, or alcoholic patients and those with anorexia nervosa.

Failure to add phosphorus

After initiation of enteral or parenteral feeding without sufficient phosphorus supplementation, phosphorus shifts into the cells. This shift—called *refeeding syndrome*—usually occurs 3 or more days after feedings begin. Patients recovering from hypothermia can also develop hypophosphatemia as phosphorus moves into the cells.

Abnormal absorption

Malabsorption syndromes, starvation, and prolonged or excessive use of phosphorus-binding antacids or sucralfate are among the many causes of impaired intestinal absorption of phosphorus. Because vitamin D contributes to intestinal absorption of phosphorus, inadequate vitamin D intake or synthesis can inhibit phosphorus

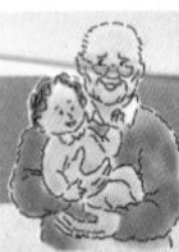

Ages and stages

Elderly patients at risk

Elderly patients are particularly at risk for altered electrolyte levels for two main reasons. First, they have a lower ratio of lean body weight to total body weight, which places them at risk for water deficit. Second, their thirst response is diminished and their renal function decreased, which makes maintaining electrolyte balance more difficult. Age-related renal changes include changes in renal blood flow and glomerular filtration rate.

Medications can also alter electrolyte levels by affecting the absorption of phosphate. So make sure you ask elderly patients if they're using such over-the-counter medications as antacids, laxatives, herbs, and teas.

Drugs associated with hypophosphatemia

The following drugs are commonly associated with hypophosphatemia:

- acetazolamide, thiazide diuretics (chlorothiazide and hydrochlorothiazide), loop diuretics (bumetanide and furosemide), and other diuretics
- antacids, such as aluminum carbonate, aluminum hydroxide, calcium carbonate, and magnesium oxide
- insulin
- laxatives.

absorption. Chronic diarrhea or laxative abuse can also result in increased GI loss of phosphorus. Decreased dietary intake rarely causes hypophosphatemia because phosphate is found in most foods.

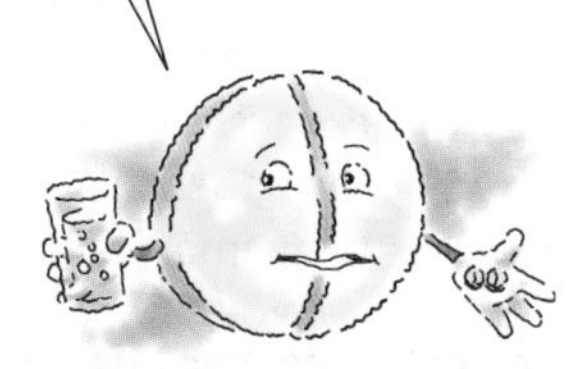

Drugs such as thiazides and loop diuretics can cause hypophosphatemia.

Calling the kidneys to account

Diuretic use is the most common cause of phosphorus loss through the kidneys. Thiazides, loop diuretics, and acetazolamide are the diuretics that most commonly cause hypophosphatemia. (See *Drugs associated with hypophosphatemia.*)

The second most common cause is diabetic ketoacidosis (DKA) in diabetic patients who have poorly controlled blood glucose levels. In DKA, high glucose levels induce an osmotic diuresis. This results in a significant loss of phosphorus from the kidneys. Ethanol affects phosphorus reabsorption in the kidneys so that more phosphorus is excreted in urine.

A buildup of PTH, which occurs with hyperparathyroidism and hypocalcemia, also leads to hypophosphatemia because PTH stimulates the kidneys to excrete phosphate. Finally, hypophosphatemia occurs in patients who have extensive burns. Although the mechanism is unclear, the condition seems to occur in response to the extensive diuresis of salt and water that typically occurs during the first 2 to 4 days after a burn injury. Respiratory alkalosis and carbohydrate administration may also play a role here.

What to look for

Mild to moderate hypophosphatemia doesn't usually cause symptoms. Noticeable effects of hypophosphatemia typically occur only in severe cases. The characteristics of severe hypophosphatemia are apparent in many organ systems. Signs and symptoms may develop acutely because of rapid decreases in phosphorus or gradually as the result of slow, chronic decreases in phosphorus.

Hypophosphatemia affects the musculoskeletal, central nervous, cardiac, and hematologic systems. Because phosphorus is required to make high-energy ATP, many of the signs and symptoms of hypophosphatemia are related to low energy stores.

Weak and weary

With hypophosphatemia, muscle weakness is the most common symptom. Other symptoms may include diplopia (double vision), malaise, and anorexia. The patient may experience a weakened hand grasp, slurred speech, or dysphagia. He also may develop myalgia (tenderness or pain in the muscles).

Respiratory failure may result from weakened respiratory muscles and poor contractility of the diaphragm. Respirations may appear shallow and ineffective. In later stages, the patient may be cyanotic. Keep in mind that it may be difficult to wean a mechanically ventilated patient with hypophosphatemia from the ventilator.

With severe hypophosphatemia, rhabdomyolysis (skeletal muscle destruction) can occur with altered muscle cell activity. Muscle enzymes such as creatine kinase are released from the cells into the extracellular fluid. Loss of bone density, osteomalacia (softening of the bones), and bone pain may also occur with prolonged hypophosphatemia. Fractures can result.

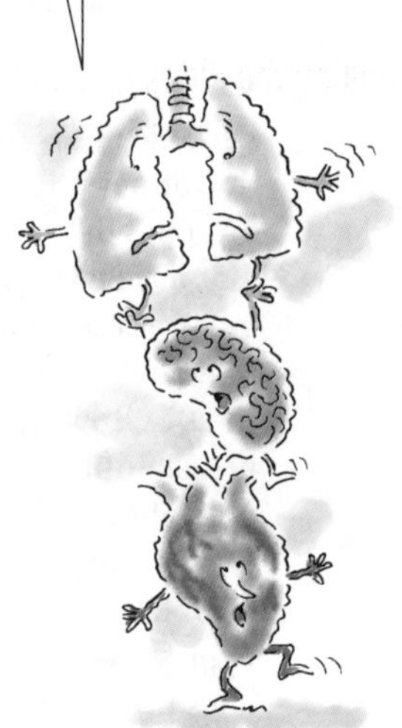

Hypophosphatemia can affect all of us. We're not feeling too steady right now!

Logical neurologic effects

Without enough phosphorus, the body can't make enough ATP, a cornerstone of energy metabolism. As a result, central nervous system cells can malfunction, causing paresthesia, irritability, apprehension, memory loss, and confusion. The neurologic effects of hypophosphatemia may progress to seizures or coma.

When the heart isn't hardy

The heart's contractility decreases because of low energy stores of ATP. As a result, the patient may develop hypotension and low cardiac output. Severe hypophosphatemia may lead to cardiomyopathy, which treatment can reverse.

Oxygen delivery drop-off

A drop in production of 2,3-DPG causes a decrease in oxygen delivery to tissues. Because hemoglobin has a stronger affinity for oxygen than for other gases, oxygen is less likely to be given up to the tissues as it circulates through the body. As a result, less oxygen is delivered to the myocardium, which can cause chest pain.

Hypophosphatemia may also cause hemolytic anemia because of changes in the structure and function of RBCs. Patients with hypophosphatemia are more susceptible to infection because of the effect of low levels of ATP in WBCs. Lack of ATP results in a decreased functioning of leukocytes. Chronic hypophosphatemia also affects platelet function, resulting in bruising and bleeding, particularly mild GI bleeding.

What tests show

These diagnostic test results may indicate hypophosphatemia or a related condition:

- serum phosphorus level of less than 2.5 mg/dl (or 1.8 mEq/L); severe hypophosphatemia, less than 1 mg/dl
- elevated creatine kinase level if rhabdomyolysis is present
- X-ray studies that reveal the skeletal changes typical of osteomalacia or bone fractures
- abnormal electrolytes (decreased magnesium levels and increased calcium levels).

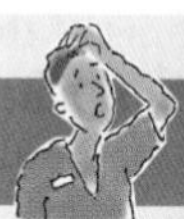

It's not working

When dietary changes aren't working

If your patient's phosphorus-rich diet hasn't raised serum phosphorus levels as you had hoped, it's time to ask these questions:

- Is a GI problem making phosphorus digestion difficult?
- Is your patient using a phosphate-binding antacid?
- Is your patient abusing alcohol?
- Is your patient using a thiazide diuretic?
- Is your patient complying with the treatment regimen for diabetes?

How it's treated

Treatment varies with the severity and cause of the condition. It includes treating the underlying cause and correcting the imbalance with phosphorus replacement and a high-phosphorus diet. The route of replacement therapy depends on the severity of the imbalance.

Milder measures

Treatment for mild to moderate hypophosphatemia includes a diet high in phosphorus-rich foods, such as eggs, nuts, whole grains, organ meats, fish, poultry, and milk products. However, if calcium is contraindicated or the patient can't tolerate milk, he should instead receive oral phosphorus supplements. Oral supplements include Neutra-Phos and Neutra-Phos-K and can be used for moderate hypophosphatemia. Dosage limitations are related to the adverse effects, most notably nausea and diarrhea. (See *When dietary changes aren't working.*)

Sterner steps

For patients with severe hypophosphatemia or a nonfunctioning GI tract, I.V. phosphorus replacement is the recommended choice. Two preparations are used: I.V. potassium phosphate and I.V. sodium phosphate. Dosage is guided by the patient's response to treatment and serum phosphorus levels.

Potassium phosphate requires slow administration (no more than 10 mEq/hour). Adverse effects of I.V. replacement for hypophosphatemia include hyperphosphatemia and hypocalcemia.

How you intervene

If your patient begins total parenteral nutrition or is otherwise at risk for developing hypophosphatemia, monitor him for signs and symptoms of this imbalance. If the patient has already developed hypophosphatemia, your nursing care should focus on careful monitoring, safety measures, and interventions to restore normal serum phosphorus levels. (See *Teaching about hypophosphatemia.*) Alert the practitioner to any changes in the patient's condition and take these other actions:

- Monitor vital signs. Remember, hypophosphatemia can lead to respiratory failure, low cardiac output, confusion, seizures, or coma.
- Assess the patient's level of consciousness and neurologic status each time you check his vital signs. Document your observations and the patient's neurologic status on a flow sheet so changes can be noted immediately. (See *Documenting hypophosphatemia.*)
- Monitor the rate and depth of respirations, especially if the patient has severe hypophosphatemia. Report signs of hypoxia, such as confusion, restlessness, increased respiratory rate and, in later stages, cyanosis. If possible, take steps to prevent hyperventilation because it worsens respiratory alkalosis and can lower phosphorus levels. Follow arterial blood gas results and pulse oximetry levels to monitor the effectiveness of ventilation. If the patient is on a ventilator, wean him off slowly.
- Monitor the patient for evidence of heart failure related to reduced myocardial functioning. Signs and symptoms include crackles, shortness of breath, decreased blood pressure, and elevated heart rate.
- Monitor the patient's temperature at least every 4 hours. Check WBC counts. Follow strict sterile technique in changing dressings. Report signs of infection.
- Assess the patient frequently for evidence of decreasing muscle strength, such as weak hand grasps or slurred speech, and document your findings regularly.
- Administer prescribed phosphorus supplements. Keep in mind that oral supplements may cause diarrhea. To improve their taste, mix them with juice. Vitamin D may also be ordered with the oral phosphate supplements to increase absorption.
- Insert an I.V. line as ordered, and keep it patent. Infuse phosphorus solutions slowly using an infusion device to control the rate. During infusions, watch for signs of hypocalcemia, hyperphosphatemia, and I.V. infiltration; potassium phosphate can cause tissue sloughing and necrosis. Monitor serum phosphate levels every 6 hours.
- Administer an analgesic, if ordered.
- If ordered, make sure the patient maintains bed rest for safety. Keep the bed in its lowest position, with the wheels locked and the side rails raised. If the patient is at risk for seizures,

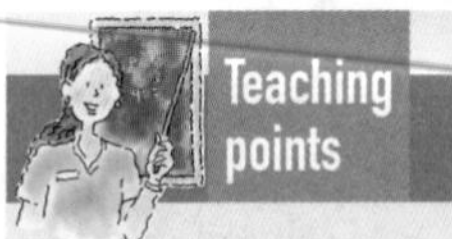

Teaching about hypophosphatemia

When teaching a patient with hypophosphatemia, be sure to cover the following topics and then evaluate your patient's learning:

- description of hypophosphatemia and its risk factors, prevention, and treatment
- medications ordered
- need to consult with a dietitian
- need for a high-phosphorus diet (1 qt of cow's milk per day provides the average amount of phosphate required)
- avoidance of phosphate-binding antacids
- warning signs and symptoms and when to report them
- need to maintain follow-up appointments.

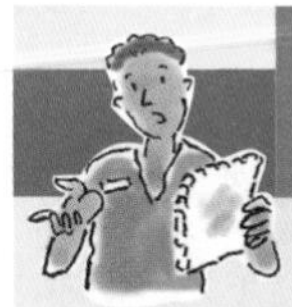

Chart smart

Documenting hypophosphatemia

If your patient has hypophosphatemia, make sure you document the following information:

- vital signs
- neurologic status, including level of consciousness, restlessness, and apprehension
- muscle strength
- respiratory assessment
- serum electrolyte levels and other pertinent laboratory data
- notification of the practitioner
- I.V. therapy, including condition of I.V. site, medication, dose, and the patient's response
- seizures, if any
- your interventions and the patient's response
- safety measures to protect the patient
- patient teaching.

pad the side rails and keep an artificial airway at the patient's bedside.

- Orient the patient as needed. Keep clocks, calendars, and familiar personal objects within his sight.
- Inform the patient and his family that confusion caused by a low phosphorus level is only temporary and will likely decrease with therapy.
- Record the patient's fluid intake and output.
- Closely monitor serum electrolyte levels, especially calcium and phosphorus levels, as well as other pertinent laboratory test results. Report abnormalities.
- Assist the patient with ambulation and activities of daily living, if needed, and keep essential objects near the patient to prevent accidents.

Hyperphosphatemia

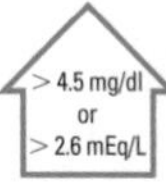

Hyperphosphatemia occurs when serum phosphorus levels exceed 4.5 mg/dl (or 2.6 mEq/L) and usually reflects the kidneys' inability to excrete excess phosphorus. The condition commonly occurs along with an increased release of phosphorus from damaged cells. Severe hyperphosphatemia occurs when the serum phosphorus levels reach 6 mg/dl or higher.

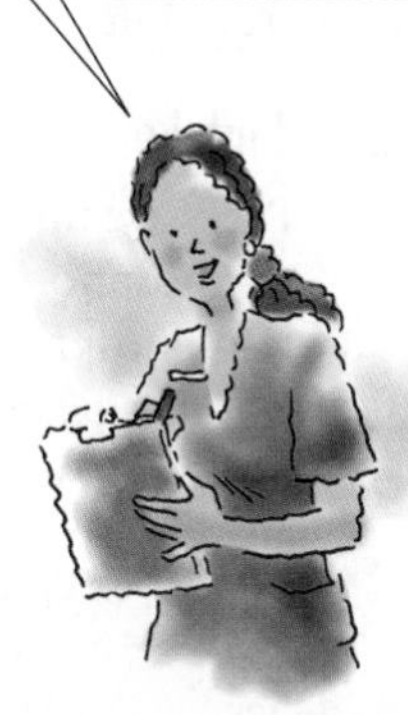
Hyperphosphatemia is usually related to the kidneys' inability to excrete excess phosphorus.

How it happens

Hyperphosphatemia can result from a number of underlying mechanisms, including impaired renal excretion of phosphorus, a shift of phosphorus from the intracellular fluid to the extracellular fluid, and an increase in dietary intake of phosphorus.

Kidney filter failure

Normally, renal excretion of phosphorus equals the amount the GI tract absorbs daily. Hyperphosphatemia most commonly results from renal failure due to the kidneys' inability to excrete excess phosphorus.

When glomerular filtration rate drops below 30 ml/minute, the kidneys can't filter excess phosphorus adequately. Because the kidneys are responsible for most of the excretion of phosphorus, their inability to filter phosphorus leads to an elevated serum phosphorus level (Spaia, 2011).

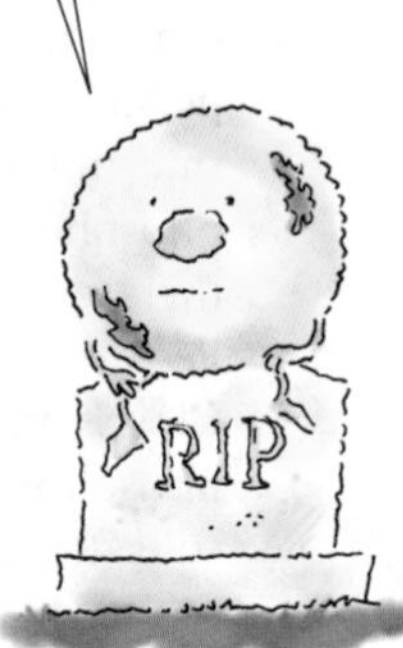
Cell destruction can release intracellular phosphorus into extracellular fluid. What a tragic ending . . .
RIP

PTH problem

A risk after thyroid or parathyroid surgery, hypoparathyroidism impairs synthesis of PTH. When less PTH is synthesized, less phosphorus is excreted from the kidneys. The result? Elevated serum phosphorus levels.

Shift work

Several conditions can cause phosphorus to shift from the intracellular fluid to the extracellular fluid. Acid-base imbalances, such as respiratory acidosis and DKA, are common examples. Anything that causes cellular destruction can also result in a transcellular shift of phosphorus.

Destruction of cells can trigger the release of intracellular phosphorus into extracellular fluid, causing serum phosphorus levels to rise. Chemotherapy, for example, causes significant cell destruction, as do muscle necrosis and rhabdomyolysis, conditions that can stem from infection, heat stroke, and trauma.

Increased intake

Excessive intake of phosphorus can result from overadministration of phosphorus supplements or of laxatives or enemas that contain phosphorus (such as Fleet enemas). (See *Drugs associated with hyperphosphatemia.*)

In infants, excessive intake of vitamin D can result in increased absorption of phosphorus and lead to elevated serum phosphorus levels. (See *Cow's milk and hyperphosphatemia.*)

Drugs associated with hyperphosphatemia

The following drugs may cause hyperphosphatemia:

- enemas such as Fleet enemas
- laxatives containing phosphorus or phosphate
- oral phosphorus supplements (Neutra-Phos)
- parenteral phosphorus supplements (sodium phosphate, potassium phosphate)
- vitamin D supplements.

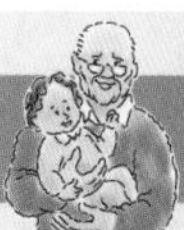

Ages and stages

Cow's milk and hyperphosphatemia

Infants who are fed cow's milk are predisposed to hyperphosphatemia because cow's milk contains more phosphorus than breast milk. In addition, infants have naturally high phosphorus levels.

What to look for

Hyperphosphatemia causes few clinical problems by itself. However, phosphorus and calcium levels have an inverse relationship: If one is high, the other is low. Because of this seesaw relationship, hyperphosphatemia may lead to hypocalcemia, which can be life-threatening. Signs and symptoms of acute hyperphosphatemia are usually caused by the effects of hypocalcemia.

The patient may develop paresthesia in the fingertips and around the mouth, which may increase in severity and spread proximally along the limbs and to the face. Severe muscle spasm, cramps, pain, and weakness may prevent the patient from performing normal activities. The patient may exhibit hyperreflexia and positive Chvostek's and Trousseau's signs. These signs are due to low calcium levels and may progress to tetany and neurologic disorders.

Neurologic signs and symptoms include decreased mental status, delirium, and seizures. Electrocardiogram (ECG) changes include a prolonged QT interval and ST segment. The patient may also experience hypotension, heart failure, anorexia, nausea, and vomiting. Bone development may also be affected.

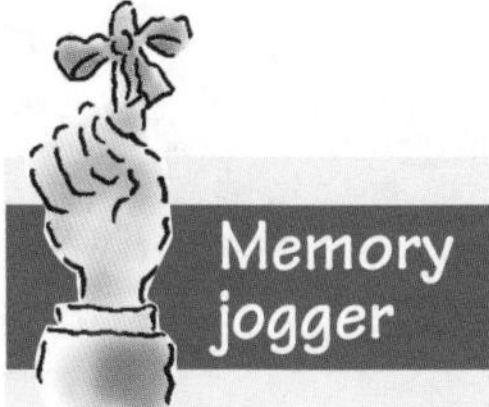

Memory jogger

To remember some of the signs and symptoms of hyperphosphatemia, think of the word **CHEMO** (keeping in mind that chemotherapy can lead to hyperphosphatemia):

Cardiac irregularities

Hyperreflexia

Eating poorly

Muscle weakness

Oliguria.

Calcification cues

When phosphorus levels rise, phosphorus binds with calcium, forming an insoluble compound called *calcium phosphate.* Organ dysfunction can result when calcium phosphate precipitates, or is deposited, in the heart, lungs, kidneys, or other soft tissues. This process, called *calcification,* usually occurs as a result of chronically elevated phosphorus levels. (See *A look at calcification,* page 178.)

With calcification, the patient may experience arrhythmias, an irregular heart rate, and decreased urine output. Corneal haziness, conjunctivitis, cataracts, and impaired vision may occur, and papular eruptions may develop on the skin.

A look at calcification

When serum phosphorus levels are high, phosphorus binds with calcium to form an insoluble compound called *calcium phosphate.* The compound is deposited in the heart, lungs, kidneys, eyes, skin, and other soft tissues where it interferes with normal organ and tissue function. This illustration shows some of the organs affected and the effect calcification has on these organs.

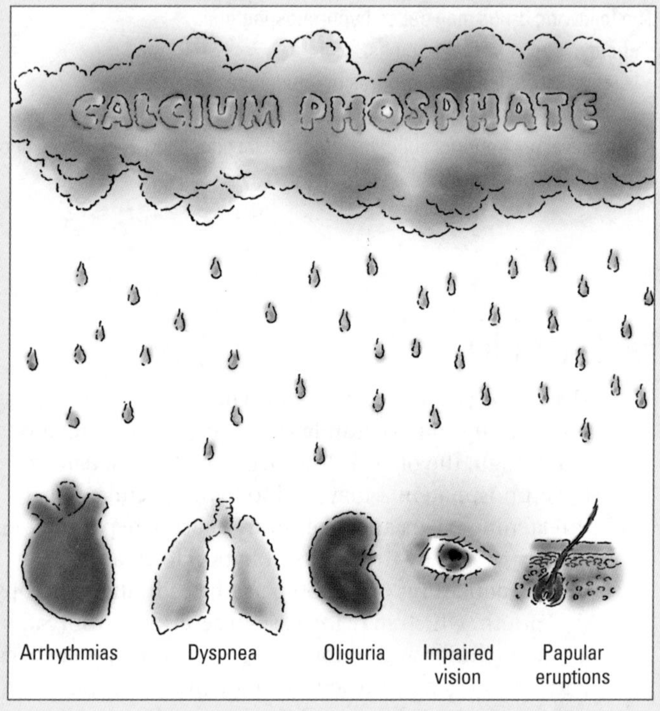

What tests show

The following diagnostic tests results may indicate hyperphosphatemia or a related condition such as hypocalcemia:

- serum phosphorus level above 4.5 mg/dl (or 2.6 mEq/L)
- serum calcium level below 8.5 mg/dl
- X-ray studies that reveal skeletal changes due to osteodystrophy (defective bone development) in chronic hyperphosphatemia
- increased blood urea nitrogen (BUN) and creatinine levels, which reflect worsening renal function
- ECG changes characteristic of hypocalcemia (such as a prolonged QT interval).

How it's treated

An elevated serum phosphorus level may be treated with drugs and other therapeutic measures. Treatment aims to correct the underlying disorder, if one exists, and correct hypocalcemia.

Going low phospho

If a patient's elevated serum phosphorus level results from excessive phosphorus intake, the condition may be easily remedied by reducing phosphorus intake. Therapeutic measures include reducing dietary intake of phosphorus and eliminating the use of phosphorus-based laxatives and enemas. (See *When dietary changes aren't enough*.)

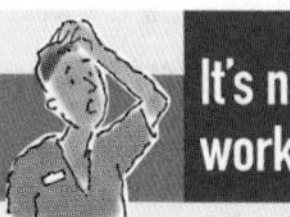

It's not working

When dietary changes aren't enough

If your patient's low-phosphorus diet hasn't changed his serum phosphorus level, it's time to ask these questions:

- Is the patient taking medications (such as phosphorus-binding antacids) as directed?
- Is the patient continuing to use laxatives or enemas that contain phosphate?
- Are the patient's kidneys functioning?
- Has the underlying cause of hyperphosphatemia been corrected?

Altering absorption

Drug therapy may help decrease absorption of phosphorus in the GI system. Such therapy may include aluminum, magnesium, or calcium gel or phosphate-binding antacids. Although widely used, such calcium salts as calcium carbonate and calcium acetate may cause hypercalcemia, so the patient will need careful dosing. Polymeric phosphate binders such as sevelamer hydrochloride may also be given. A patient with underlying renal insufficiency or renal failure should not receive magnesium antacids because they may cause hypermagnesemia. A patient with end-stage renal disease may receive lanthanum carbonate, a noncalcium, nonaluminum phosphate binder.

Keep in mind that a mildly elevated phosphorus level may benefit a patient with renal failure. Higher phosphorus levels (on the higher side of the normal range) allow more oxygen to move from the RBCs to tissues, which can help prevent hypoxemia and limit the effects of chronic anemia on oxygen delivery.

Treat what's underneath

Treatment of the underlying cause of hyperphosphatemia, including conditions such as respiratory acidosis or DKA, can lower serum phosphorus levels. In a patient with diabetes, administering insulin causes phosphorus to shift back into the cells, which can result in decreased serum phosphorus levels.

Situation: severe

Patients with severe hyperphosphatemia may receive I.V. saline solution to promote renal excretion of phosphorus. However, this treatment requires the patient to have functional kidneys and the ability to tolerate the increased load of sodium and fluid. Patients may also receive proximal diuretics such as acetazolamide to increase renal excretion of phosphorus.

As a final therapeutic intervention, hemodialysis or peritoneal dialysis may be initiated if the patient has chronic renal failure or an extreme case of acute hyperphosphatemia with symptomatic hypocalcemia.

How you intervene

Keep an eye out for patients at risk for hyperphosphatemia, and monitor them carefully. Also, use care when administering phosphorus in I.V. infusions, enemas, and laxatives because the extra phosphorus may cause hyperphosphatemia.

If your patient has already developed hyperphosphatemia, your care should focus on careful monitoring, safety measures, and interventions to restore normal serum phosphorus levels. Follow these steps to provide care for the patient:

- Monitor vital signs.
- Watch for signs and symptoms of hypocalcemia, such as paresthesia in the fingers or around the mouth, hyperactive reflexes, or muscle cramps. If any of these occur, immediately notify the doctor. (See *Teaching about hyperphosphatemia.*) Also notify the practitioner if you detect signs or symptoms of calcification, including oliguria, visual impairment, conjunctivitis, irregular heart rate or palpitations, and papular eruptions.
- Monitor fluid intake and output. If urine output falls below 30 ml/hour, immediately notify the practitioner. Decreased urine output can seriously affect renal clearance of excess serum phosphorus.
- Closely monitor serum electrolyte levels, especially calcium and phosphorus. Report changes immediately. Also, monitor BUN and serum creatinine levels because hyperphosphatemia can impair renal tubules when calcification occurs.
- Keep a flow sheet of daily laboratory test results for a patient at risk. Include BUN and serum phosphorus, calcium, and creatinine levels as well as fluid intake and output. Keep the flow

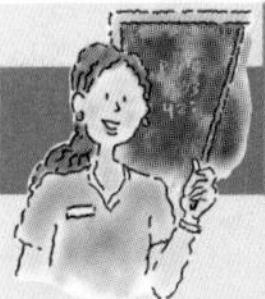

Teaching points

Teaching about hyperphosphatemia

When teaching a patient with hyperphosphatemia, be sure to cover the following topics and then evaluate your patient's learning:

- causes and treatment
- prescribed medications
- avoidance of preparations that contain phosphorus, such as laxatives, enemas, and supplements
- avoidance of high-phosphorus foods, such as dairy products, organ meats, fish, poultry, eggs, and nuts and seeds
- warning signs and symptoms
- referrals to a dietitian and social services, if indicated.

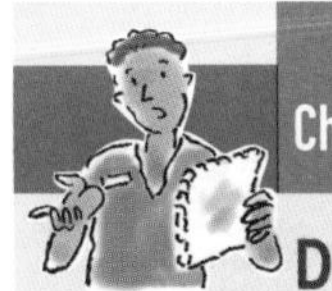

Chart smart

Documenting hyperphosphatemia

If your patient has hyperphosphatemia, make sure you document the following information:

- all assessment findings
- intake and output
- I.V. therapy and medications given
- muscle spasms, cramps, pain, and muscle strength
- paresthesia in the fingertips and around the mouth
- visual disturbances
- safety measures to protect patient
- notification of the practitioner
- your interventions, including patient teaching, and the patient's response.

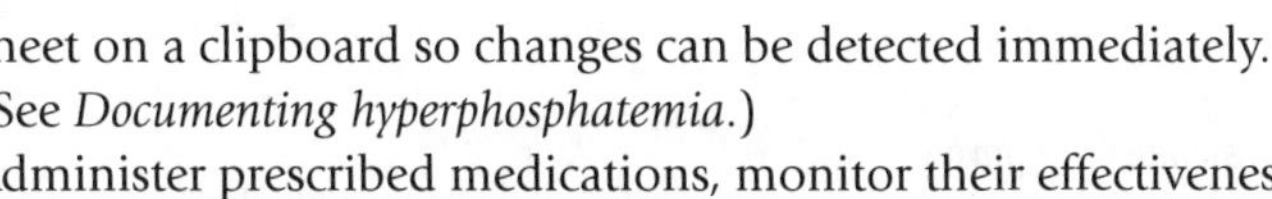

sheet on a clipboard so changes can be detected immediately. (See *Documenting hyperphosphatemia.*)

- Administer prescribed medications, monitor their effectiveness, and assess the patient for possible adverse reactions. Give antacids with meals to increase their effectiveness in binding phosphorus.
- Prepare the patient with severe hyperphosphatemia for possible dialysis.
- If a patient's condition results from chronic renal failure or if his treatment includes a low-phosphorus diet, consult a dietitian to help the patient comply with dietary restrictions. Dietary phosphorus should be restricted to 0.6 to 0.9 g/day.

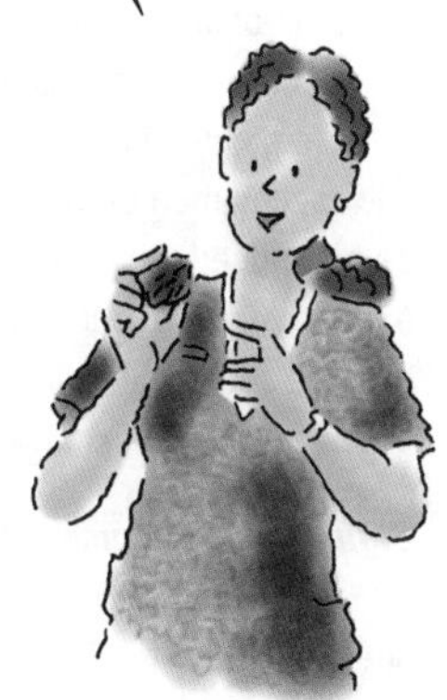

Consult a dietitian for the patient with dietary restrictions. The patient may need to cut back on such high-phosphorus foods as walnuts.

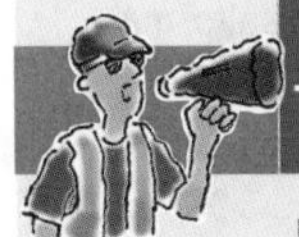

That's a wrap!

Phosphorus imbalances review

Phosphorus basics

- Primary anion in intracellular fluid
- About 85% found in bones and teeth, combined with calcium in a 1:2 ratio
- Crucial to cell membrane integrity, muscle and neurologic function, and metabolism of carbohydrates, fats, and proteins
- Promotes oxygen delivery from RBCs to tissues
- Buffers acids and bases, promotes energy transfer by forming ATP, and is essential for healthy bones and teeth
- Normal range: 2.5 to 4.5 mg/dl (1.8 to 2.6 mEq/L)

Phosphorus balance

- Dietary intake and renal excretion maintain normal levels; if intake increases, renal excretion also increases.

(continued)

Phosphorus imbalances review *(continued)*

- The parathyroid gland controls hormonal regulation of phosphorus levels by affecting PTH.
- PTH release is affected by calcium level; PTH causes the kidneys to increase excretion of phosphorus if the calcium level is high and to reabsorb phosphorus if the calcium level is low.
- Balance is affected by certain conditions that cause transcellular shift of phosphorus; for example, insulin moves glucose and phosphorus into cells; alkalosis causes the same kind of shift.

Hypophosphatemia

- Severe hypophosphatemia: serum phosphorus levels less than 1 mg/dl; may lead to organ failure
- Three underlying mechanisms:
  - Shift of phosphorus into intracellular fluid
  - Decrease in intestinal absorption
  - Increased excretion from kidneys
- Most common causes: respiratory alkalosis, hyperglycemia, refeeding syndrome, malabsorption syndrome, excessive use of phosphorus-binding antacids, diarrhea, laxative abuse, diuretics, DKA hyperparathyroidism, hypocalcemia, and extensive burns

Signs and symptoms

- Most commonly occur as a result of severe hypophosphatemia that affects the musculoskeletal, central nervous, cardiac, and hematologic systems
- Most common: muscle weakness
- Slurred speech, dysphagia, cardiomyopathy, hypotension, decreased cardiac output, rhabdomyolysis, cyanosis, and respiratory failure

Treatment

For mild to moderate conditions

- Oral supplements
- Increased dietary intake

For severe conditions

- I.V. phosphorus (potassium phosphate or sodium phosphate)

Hyperphosphatemia

- Severe: 6 mg/dl or higher
- Usually caused by impaired renal excretion of phosphorus
- Other causes: hypoparathyroidism (usually after thyroid or parathyroid surgery), resulting in reduced PTH levels and reduced phosphate excretion
- Conditions causing shift of phosphorus into extracellular fluid: respiratory acidosis, DKA, cell destruction caused by chemotherapy, necrosis, rhabdomyolysis, trauma, heat stroke, and infection
- Also caused by overadministration of phosphorus supplements or phosphorus-containing laxatives and enemas and excessive intake of vitamin D

Signs and symptoms

- Usually caused by hypocalcemia
- Include paresthesia, muscle cramps, muscle weakness, tetany, positive Trousseau's and Chvostek's signs, decreased mental status, hyperreflexia, anorexia, nausea and vomiting, and calcification (which causes arrhythmias, irregular heart rate, decreased urine output, conjunctivitis, cataracts, impaired vision, and papular eruptions)

Treatment

- Aimed at correcting underlying problem
- Includes low-phosphorus diet and drugs to decrease absorption of phosphorus (aluminum, calcium salts, magnesium [except in those with renal failure], or phosphate-binding antacids)

For severe hyperphosphatemia

- I.V. saline solution
- Proximal diuretics to promote excretion
- Dialysis if necessary

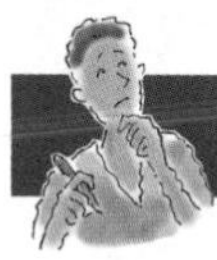

Quick quiz

1. If your patient has hyperphosphatemia, he or she may also have the secondary electrolyte disturbance:
   A. hypermagnesemia.
   B. hypocalcemia.
   C. hypernatremia.
   D. hyperkalemia.

Answer: B. Phosphorus and calcium have an inverse relationship: If serum phosphorus levels are increased, then serum calcium levels are decreased.

2. For a patient with hyperphosphatemia and renal failure, avoid giving the phosphate-binding antacid:
   A. aluminum hydroxide.
   B. calcium carbonate.
   C. calcium acetate.
   D. magnesium oxide.

Answer: D. Administering an antacid that contains magnesium to a patient with renal failure can result in hypermagnesemia.

3. Many of the signs and symptoms of hypophosphatemia are related to:
   A. low energy stores.
   B. hypercalcemia.
   C. extensive diuresis.
   D. hypocalcemia.

Answer: A. The body needs phosphorus to make ATP, which provides all the cells—especially muscles—with energy.

4. The binding of phosphorus and calcium in a patient with hyperphosphatemia can lead to:
   A. increased calcium release by the kidneys.
   B. widespread calcification of tissues.
   C. decreased calcium uptake by the pituitary gland.
   D. increased production of PTH.

Answer: B. Hyperphosphatemia results in hypocalcemia. The calcium and phosphorus bind together and are deposited in the tissues, resulting in calcification.

5. It might be difficult to wean your patient from mechanical ventilation if he has a serum phosphorus level:
   A. higher than 8 mg/dl.
   B. between 4.5 and 6.0 mg/dl.
   C. between 2 and 4 mg/dl.
   D. lower than 1 mg/dl.

Answer: D. Severe hypophosphatemia can lead to respiratory muscle weakness and impaired contractility of the diaphragm, which compromises the patient's ability to breathe spontaneously.

Scoring

☆☆☆ If you answered all five questions correctly, you're phosphabulous! Keep up the good work.

☆☆ If you answered four questions correctly, way to go! You're a natural when it comes to phosphorus balance.

☆ If you answered fewer than four questions correctly, that's okay. Take a break to renew your mental power and then review the chapter again.

References

Akizawa, T., Kameoka, C., Kaneko, Y., & Kawasaki, S. (2013). Long-term treatment of hyperphosphatemia with bixalomer in Japanese hemodialysis patients. *Therapeutic Apheresis and Dialysis, 17*(6), 612–619.

Assadi, F. (2010). Hypophosphatemia: An evidence-based problem-solving approach to clinical cases. *Iranian Journal of Kidney Diseases, 4*(3), 195–201.

Block, G. A., Wheeler, D. C., Persky, M. S., Kestenbaum, B., Ketteler, M., Spiegel, D. M., . . . Chertow, G. M. (2012). Effects of phosphate binders in moderate CKD. *Journal of the American Society of Nephrology, 23*(8), 1407–1415.

Brooks, M. (2013). FDA clears new phosphate binder velphoro. *Medscape Medical News*. Retrieved from http://www.medscape.com/viewarticle/815337

Connolly, G. M., Cunningham, R., McNamee, P. T., Young, I. S., & Maxwell, A. P. (2009). Elevated serum phosphate predicts mortality in renal transplant recipients. *Transplantation, 87*(7), 1041–1044.

Connor, A. (2009). Novel therapeutic agents and strategies for the management of chronic kidney disease mineral and bone disorder. *Postgraduate Medical Journal, 85*(1003), 274–279.

Hansen, D., Rasmussen, K., Danielsen, H., Meyer-Hofmann, H., Bacevicius, E., Lauridsen, T.G., . . . Brandi, L. (2011). No difference between alfacalcidol and paricalcitol in the treatment of secondary hyperparathyroidism in hemodialysis patients: A randomized crossover trial. *Kidney International, 80*(8), 841–850.

Ichikawa, S., Sorenson, A. H., Austin, A. M., Mackenzie, D. S., Fritz, T. A., Moh, A., . . . Econs, M. J. (2009). Ablation of the Galnt3 gene leads to low-circulating intact fibroblast growth factor 23 (Fgf23) concentrations and hyperphosphatemia despite increased Fgf23 expression. *Endocrinology, 150* (6), 2543–2550.

Isakova, T., Gutiérrez, O. M., Chang, Y., Shah, A., Tamez, H., Smith, K., . . . Wolf, M. (2009). Phosphorus binders and survival on hemodialysis. *Journal of the American Society of Nephrology, 20* (2), 388–396.

Ketteler, M. (2011). Phosphate metabolism in CKD stages 3-5: Dietary and pharmacological control. *International Journal of Nephrology, 2011*, 970245.

Kling, J. (2013). New phosphate binder for renal failure lowers pill burden. *Medscape Medical News*. Retrieved from http://www.medscape.com/viewarticle/805262

Kreisl, T. N., Kimn, L., Moore, K., Duic, P., Royce, C., Stroud, I., . . . Fine, H. A. (2009). Phase II trial of single-agent bevacizumab followed by bevacizumab plus irinotecan at tumor progression in recurrent glioblastoma. *Journal of Clinical Oncology, 27*(5), 740–745.

Lammoglia, J. J., & Mericq, V. (2009). Familial tumoral calcinosis caused by a novel FGF23 mutation: Response to induction of tubular renal acidosis with acetazolamide and the non-calcium phosphate binder sevelamer. *Hormone Research, 71*(3), 178–184.

Razzaque, M. S. (2009). FGF23-mediated regulation of systemic phosphate homeostasis: Is Klotho an essential player? *American Journal of Physiology. Renal Physiology, 296*(3), F470–F476.

Schubert, L., & DeLuca, H. F. (2010). Hypophosphatemia is responsible for skeletal muscle weakness of vitamin D deficiency. *Archives of Biochemistry and Biophysics, 500*(2), 157–161.

Segawa, H., Onitsuka, A., Kuwahata, M., Hanabusa, E., Furutani, J., Kaneko, I., . . . Miyamoto, K. (2009). Type IIc sodium-dependent phosphate transporter regulates calcium metabolism. *Journal of the American Society of Nephrology, 20*(1), 104–113.

Shuto, E., Taketani, Y., Tanaka, R., Harada, N., Isshiki, M., Sato, M., . . . Takeda, E. (2009). Dietary phosphorus acutely impairs endothelial function. *Journal of the American Society of Nephrology, 20*(7), 1504–1512.

Shutto, Y., Shimada, M., Kitajima, M., Yamabe, H., Saitoh, Y., Saitoh, H., & Razzaque M. S. (2013). Inadequate awareness among chronic kidney disease patients regarding food and drinks containing artificially added phosphate. *PLoS One, 8*(11), e78660.

Spaia, S. (2011). Phosphate binders: Sevelamer in the prevention and treatment of hyperphosphataemia in chronic renal failure. *Hippokratia, 15*(Suppl 1), 22–26.

Vemuri, N., Michelis, M. F., & Matalon, A. (2011). Conversion to lanthanum carbonate monotherapy effectively controls serum phosphorus with a reduced tablet burden: A multicenter open-label study. *BMC Nephrology, 12*, 49.

Verdonck, J., Geuens, G., Delaere, P., Vander Poorten, V., Evenepoel, P., & Debruyne, E. (2009). Surgical findings and post-operative parathormone levels in patients with secondary hyperparathyroidism. *B-ENT, 5*(3), 143–148.

Chapter 10

When chloride tips the balance

Just the facts

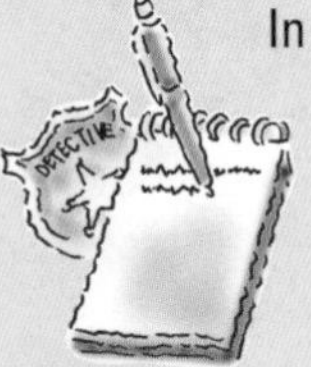

In this chapter, you'll learn:

- the importance of chloride in the body
- the relationship between chloride and sodium
- the body's mechanisms for regulating chloride
- ways to recognize and treat high and low chloride levels.

A look at chloride

Chloride is the most abundant anion (negatively charged ion) in extracellular fluid. It moves in and out of the cells with sodium and potassium and combines with major cations (positively charged ions) to form sodium chloride, hydrochloric acid, potassium chloride, calcium chloride, and other important compounds. High levels of chloride exist in cerebrospinal fluid (CSF), but the anion can also be found in bile and in gastric and pancreatic juices.

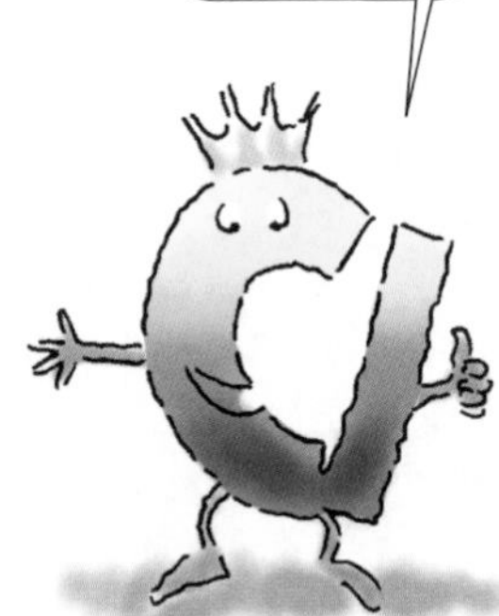

When it comes to anions in extracellular fluid, I rule!

Why it's important

Because of its negative charge, chloride travels with positively charged sodium and helps maintain serum osmolality and water balance. Chloride and sodium also work together to form CSF. The choroid plexus, a tangled mass of tiny blood vessels inside the ventricles of the brain, depends on these two electrolytes to attract water and form the fluid component of CSF.

In the stomach, the gastric mucosa secretes chloride as hydrochloric acid, providing the acid medium necessary for digestion and enzyme activation. Chloride also helps maintain acid-base balance and helps transport carbon dioxide in the red blood cells.

On the level

Serum chloride levels normally range between 98 and 108 mEq/L. Values may vary slightly depending on the laboratory doing the analysis. By comparison, the chloride level inside a cell is 4 mEq/L. Chloride levels remain relatively stable with age. Because chloride balance is closely linked with sodium balance, the levels of both electrolytes usually change in direct proportion to one another.

Dietary sources of chloride

Dietary sources of chloride include:

- canned vegetables
- eggs
- fresh fruits and vegetables, especially high concentration in tomatoes, celery, lettuce, and olives
- milk
- processed meats
- salty foods
- table or sea salt.

How the body regulates chloride

Chloride regulation depends on intake and excretion of chloride and reabsorption of chloride ions in the kidneys. The daily chloride requirement for adults is 1.8 to 2.3 g/day per the National Institutes of Health (NIH) guidelines. Most diets provide sufficient chloride in the form of salt (usually as sodium chloride) or processed foods. (See *Dietary sources of chloride.*)

Most chloride is absorbed in the intestines, with only a small portion lost in feces. Chloride is produced mainly in the stomach in the form of hydrochloric acid, so chloride levels can be influenced by gastrointestinal (GI) disorders.

Best buddies

Because chloride and sodium are closely linked, a change in one electrolyte level causes a comparable change in the other. Chloride levels can also be indirectly affected by aldosterone secretion, which causes the renal tubules to reabsorb sodium. As positively charged sodium ions are reabsorbed, negatively charged chloride ions are passively reabsorbed because of their electrical attraction to sodium.

Battling acids and bases

Regulation of chloride levels also involves acid-base balance. Chloride is reabsorbed and excreted in direct opposition to bicarbonate. When chloride levels change, the body attempts to keep its positive-negative balance by making corresponding changes in the levels of bicarbonate (another negatively charged ion) in the kidneys. (Remember, bicarbonate is alkaline.)

When chloride levels decrease, the kidneys retain bicarbonate and bicarbonate levels increase. When chloride levels increase, the kidneys excrete bicarbonate and bicarbonate levels decrease. Therefore, changes in chloride and bicarbonate levels can lead to acidosis or alkalosis. (See *Chloride and bicarbonate,* page 188.)

Chloride regulation is related to acid-base balance.

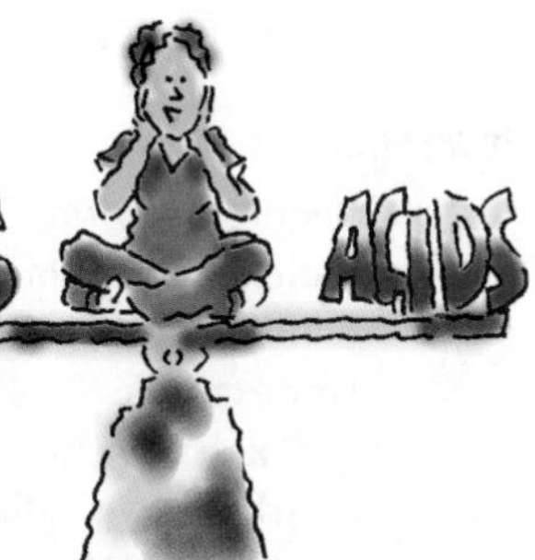

Chloride and bicarbonate

Chloride (Cl) and bicarbonate (HCO_3^-) have an inverse relationship. When the level of one goes up, the level of the other goes down.

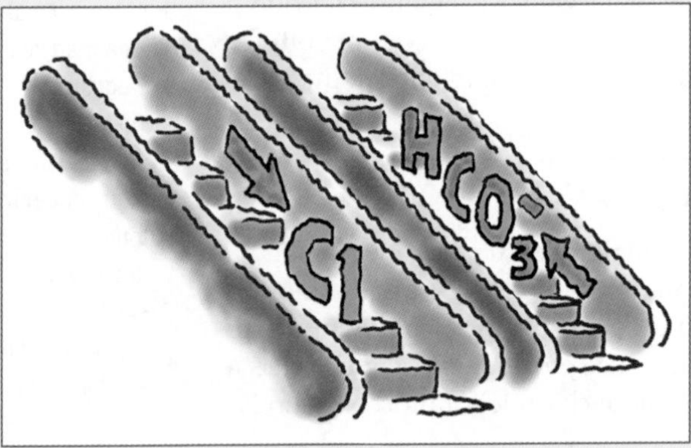

Hypochloremia

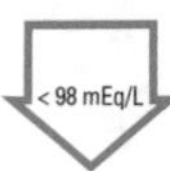

Hypochloremia is a deficiency of chloride in extracellular fluid. This occurs when serum chloride levels fall below 98 mEq/L. When serum chloride levels drop, levels of sodium, potassium, calcium, and other electrolytes may also be affected. If much more chloride than sodium is lost, hypochloremic alkalosis may occur.

How it happens

Serum chloride levels drop when chloride intake or absorption decreases or when chloride losses increase. Losses may occur through the skin (chloride is found in sweat), the GI tract, or the kidneys. Changes in sodium levels or acid-base balance also alter chloride levels.

Down with intake

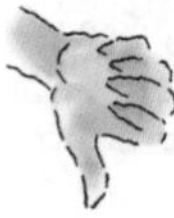

Reduced chloride intake may occur in infants being fed chloride-deficient formula and in people on salt-restricted diets. Patients dependent on I.V. fluids are also at risk if the fluids lack chloride (for example, D_5W).

Excessive chloride losses can occur with prolonged vomiting, diarrhea, severe diaphoresis, burns, Addison's disease, gastric surgery, nasogastric (NG) suctioning, and other GI tube drainage. Severe vomiting can cause a loss of hydrochloric acid from the stomach,

Dangerous development

Here's how hypochloremia can lead to hypochloremic metabolic alkalosis.

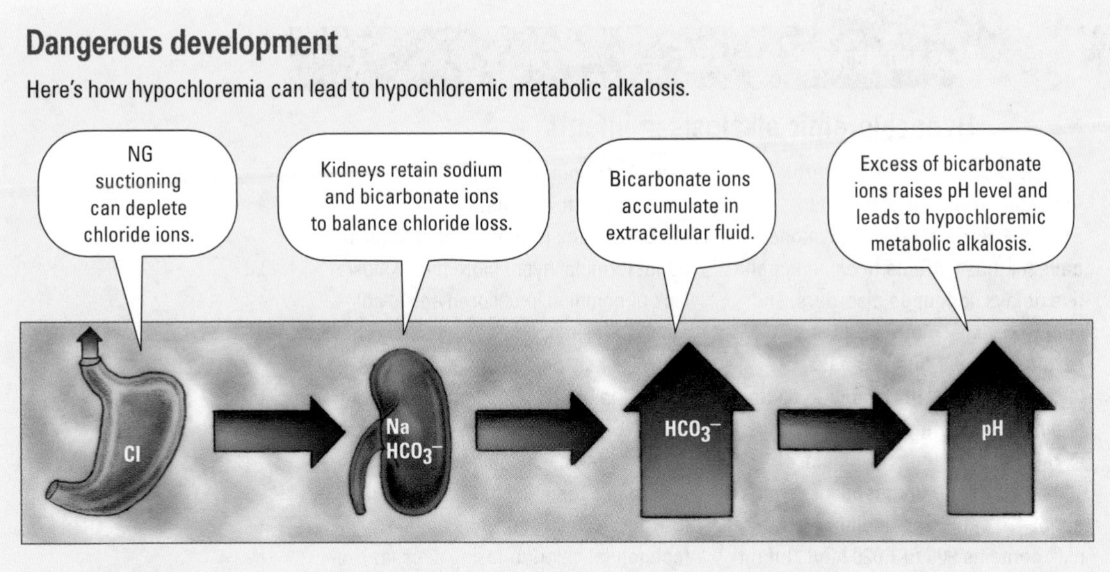

NG suctioning can deplete chloride ions.
Kidneys retain sodium and bicarbonate ions to balance chloride loss.
Bicarbonate ions accumulate in extracellular fluid.
Excess of bicarbonate ions raises pH level and leads to hypochloremic metabolic alkalosis.
Cl
Na
HCO3⁻
HCO3⁻
pH

an acid deficit in the body, and subsequent metabolic alkalosis. Patients with cystic fibrosis can also lose more chloride than normal. Any prolonged and untreated hypochloremic state can result in a state of hypochloremic alkalosis. (See *Dangerous development*.)

Hypochloremic alkalosis can affect infants and children as well as adults. (See *Hypochloremic alkalosis in infants*, page 190.) People at risk for hypochloremia include those with prolonged vomiting from pyloric obstruction and those with draining fistulas and ileostomies, which can cause a loss of chloride from the GI tract.

Drugs associated with hypochloremia

Drugs that can cause hypochloremia include:

- loop diuretics (such as furosemide)
- osmotic diuretics (such as mannitol)
- thiazide diuretics (such as hydrochlorothiazide)
- bicarbonate
- corticosteroids
- laxatives
- theophylline.

Decreaser drugs

Various drugs may decrease chloride, including bicarbonate, corticosteroids, laxatives, and theophylline. Diuretics, such as furosemide (Lasix), ethacrynic acid (Edecrin), and hydrochlorothiazide can also cause an excessive loss of chloride from the kidneys. (See *Drugs associated with hypochloremia*.)

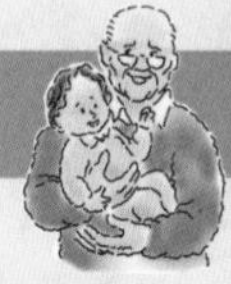

Ages and stages

Hypochloremic alkalosis in infants

Before 1980, some infants were fed chloride-deficient formulas. Hypochloremic alkalosis developed, causing those infants to exhibit cognitive delays, language disorders, and impaired visual motor skills. As a result, the U.S. Congress passed a law requiring infant formula to contain a minimum chloride content of 55 to 65 mg/100 kcal and a maximum of 150 mg/100 kcal. Breast milk contains about 420 mg/L, and undiluted cow's milk contains 900 to 1,020 mg/L. Infant formula contains 10.6 to 13.5 mEq/L; formula for older infants (follow-up formula), 14 to 19.2 mEq/L.

Despite the regulation of chloride in infant formula, hypochloremic alkalosis isn't uncommon in children and is commonly seen in neonates. Hypochloremic alkalosis may be caused by diuretic therapy in bronchopulmonary dysplasia or by NG suctioning. It may also be seen in infants with chloride-wasting syndromes resulting from renal causes (Bartter's syndrome), intestinal causes (congenital chloride-losing diarrhea), or chloride loss from cystic fibrosis.

Wait, there's more

Other causes of hypochloremia include sodium and potassium deficiency or metabolic alkalosis; conditions that affect acid-base or electrolyte balance, such as untreated diabetic ketoacidosis, water intoxication, and Addison's disease; and rapid removal of ascitic fluid (which contains sodium) during paracentesis. Also, patients who have heart failure may develop hypochloremia because serum chloride levels are diluted by excess fluid in the body.

What to look for

Patients who have hypochloremia may exhibit signs and symptoms of acid-base and electrolyte imbalances. You may notice signs of hyponatremia, hypokalemia, or metabolic alkalosis. Alkalosis results in a high pH and to compensate, respirations become slow and shallow as the body tries to retain carbon dioxide and restore a normal pH level.

The nerves also become more excitable, so look for tetany, hyperactive deep tendon reflexes, and muscle hypertonicity. (See *Danger signs of hypochloremia.*) The patient may have muscle cramps, twitching, fever, weakness and be agitated or irritable. If hypochloremia goes unrecognized, it can become life-threatening. As the chloride imbalance worsens (along with other imbalances), the patient may suffer arrhythmias, seizures, coma, or respiratory arrest.

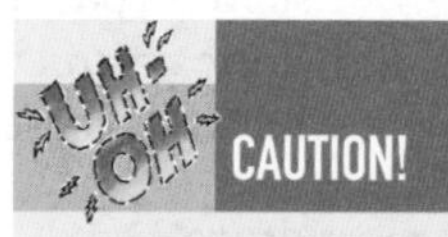

CAUTION!

Danger signs of hypochloremia

Suspect that your patient with hypochloremia is really in trouble if he exhibits any of these late-developing danger signs:

- seizures
- coma
- arrhythmias
- respiratory arrest.

What tests show

These diagnostic test results are associated with hypochloremia:

- serum chloride level below 98 mEq/L
- serum sodium level below 135 mEq/L (indicates hyponatremia)
- serum pH greater than 7.45 and serum bicarbonate level greater than 26 mEq/L (indicates metabolic alkalosis).

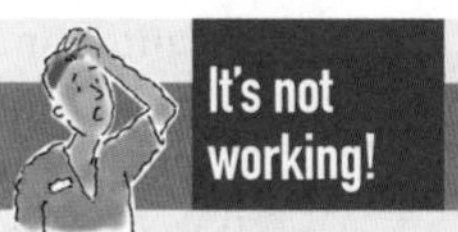

When treatment doesn't work

If treatment for hypochloremia doesn't seem to be working, make sure the patient isn't drinking large amounts of tap water, which can cause him to excrete large amounts of chloride. Review the causes of hypochloremia to identify new or coexisting conditions that might be causing chloride loss.

How it's treated

Treatment for hypochloremia focuses on correcting the underlying cause. Chloride may be replaced through fluid administration or drug therapy. Treatment may be necessary for associated metabolic alkalosis or other electrolyte imbalances.

Chloride may be given orally—for example, in a salty broth. If the patient can't take oral supplements, he may receive I.V. medications or normal saline solution. To avoid hypernatremia (high sodium level) or to treat hypokalemia, potassium chloride may be administered I.V.

Addressing the alkalosis

Treatment for associated metabolic alkalosis usually addresses the underlying causes, such as diaphoresis, vomiting or other GI losses, or renal losses. Rarely, metabolic alkalosis may be treated by administering ammonium chloride, an acidifying agent that's used when alkalosis is caused by chloride loss. Drug dosage depends on the severity of the alkalosis. The effects of ammonium chloride last only 3 days. After that, the kidneys begin to excrete the extra acid. (See *When treatment doesn't work.*)

How you intervene

Monitor patients at risk for hypochloremia, such as those receiving diuretic therapy or NG suctioning. When caring for a patient with hypochloremia, you'll also want to take these actions:

- Monitor level of consciousness (LOC), muscle strength, and movement. Notify the doctor if the patient's condition worsens.
- Monitor vital signs, especially respiratory rate and pattern, and observe for worsening respiratory function. Also, monitor cardiac rhythm because hypokalemia may be present with hypochloremia. Have emergency equipment handy in case the patient's condition deteriorates.

- Monitor and record serum electrolyte levels, especially chloride, sodium, potassium, and bicarbonate. Also assess arterial blood gas (ABG) results for acid-base imbalance.
- If the patient is alert and can swallow without difficulty, offer foods high in chloride, such as tomato juice or salty broth. Don't let the patient fill up on tap water. (See *Teaching about hypochloremia.*)
- Insert an I.V. line as ordered, and keep it patent. Administer chloride and potassium replacements as ordered.
- If administering ammonium chloride, assess the patient for pain at the infusion site and adjust the rate as needed. This drug is metabolized by the liver, so don't give it to patients with severe hepatic disease.
- Use normal saline solution, not tap water, to flush the patient's NG tube.
- Accurately measure and record intake and output, including the volume of vomitus and gastric contents from suction and other GI drainage tubes.
- Provide a safe environment. Help the patient ambulate, and keep his personal items and call button within reach. Institute seizure precautions as needed.
- Provide a quiet environment, explain interventions, and reorient the patient as needed.
- Document all care and the patient's response. (See *Documenting hypochloremia.*)

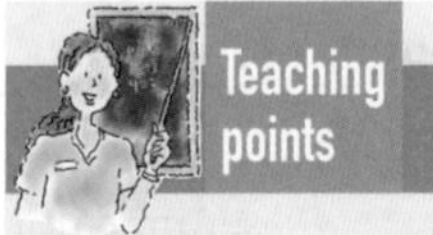

Teaching points

Teaching about hypochloremia

When teaching a patient with hypochloremia, be sure to cover the following topics and then evaluate your patient's learning:

- signs and symptoms, complications, and risk factors
- warning signs and symptoms to report to the practitioner
- dietary supplements
- medications if prescribed
- importance of replenishing lost fluids from vomiting or diarrhea.

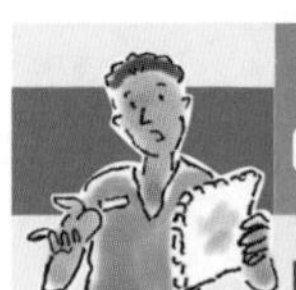

Chart smart

Documenting hypochloremia

If your patient has hypochloremia, make sure you document the following information:

- vital signs, including cardiac and respiratory rhythm
- intake and output
- serum electrolyte levels and ABG results
- your assessment, including LOC, seizure activity, and respiratory status
- time of notification of the practitioner
- I.V. therapy, along with other interventions, and the patient's response
- safety measures implemented
- patient teaching performed and the patient's response.

Hyperchloremia

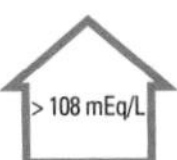

Hyperchloremia, an excess of chloride in extracellular fluid, occurs when serum chloride levels exceed 108 mEq/L. This condition is associated with other acid-base imbalances, such as metabolic acidosis, and rarely occurs alone.

How it happens

Because chloride regulation and sodium regulation are closely related, hyperchloremia may also be associated with hypernatremia. Chloride and bicarbonate have an inverse relationship, so an excess of chloride ions may be linked to a decrease in bicarbonate. Excess serum chloride results from increased chloride intake or absorption, from acidosis, or from chloride retention by the kidneys.

Up with intake and absorption

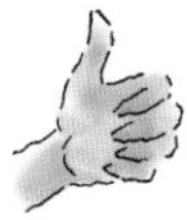

Increased intake of chloride in the form of sodium chloride can cause hyperchloremia, especially if water loss from the body occurs at the same time. The water loss raises the chloride level even more. Increased chloride absorption by the bowel can occur in patients who have had anastomoses joining the ureter and intestines.

Conditions that alter electrolyte and acid-base balance and cause metabolic acidosis include dehydration, renal tubular acidosis, diabetes insipidus, renal failure, respiratory alkalosis, salicylate toxicity, hyperparathyroidism, hyperaldosteronism, and hypernatremia.

Drug-related retention

Several medications can also contribute to hyperchloremia. For example, direct ingestion of ammonium chloride or other drugs that contain chloride or cause chloride retention can lead to hyperchloremia. Ion exchange resins that contain sodium, such as Kayexalate, can cause chloride to be exchanged for potassium in the bowel. When chloride follows sodium into the bloodstream, serum chloride levels rise. Carbonic anhydrase inhibitors, such as acetazolamide, also promote chloride retention in the body by increasing bicarbonate ion loss. (See *Drugs associated with hyperchloremia.*)

Increased sodium intake can lead to hyperchloremia. So advise your patient to stop shaking all that salt on me!

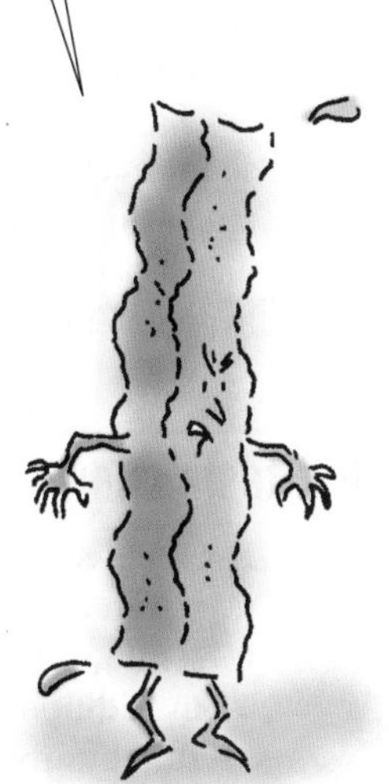

Drugs associated with hyperchloremia

Drugs that can cause hyperchloremia include:

- acetazolamide
- ammonium chloride
- androgens and estrogens
- cortisone
- phenylbutazone
- salicylates (overdose)
- sodium polystyrene sulfonate (Kayexalate)
- diuretics such as triamterene.

What to look for

Hyperchloremia rarely produces signs and symptoms on its own. Instead, the major indications are essentially those of metabolic acidosis, including tachypnea, lethargy, thirst, weakness, dehydration, hypotension diminished cognitive ability, and deep, rapid respirations (Kussmaul's respirations).

Left untreated, acidosis can lead to arrhythmias, decreased cardiac output, a further decrease in LOC, and even coma. Metabolic acidosis related to a high chloride level is called *hyperchloremic metabolic acidosis*. (See *Anion gap and metabolic acidosis*.)

If a patient has an increased serum chloride level, his serum sodium level is probably high as well, which can lead to fluid retention. He also may be agitated and have dyspnea, tachycardia, hypertension, or pitting edema—signs of hypernatremia and hypervolemia.

What tests show

The following diagnostic test results typically occur in hyperchloremia:

- serum chloride level greater than 108 mEq/L
- serum sodium level greater than 145 mEq/L.

In addition, the patient may have a serum pH level less than 7.35, a serum bicarbonate level less than 22 mEq/L, and a normal anion gap (8 to 14 mEq/L). These findings suggest metabolic acidosis.

How it's treated

Treatment for hyperchloremia includes correcting the underlying cause as well as restoring fluid, electrolyte, and acid-base balance. (See *Diuretics to the rescue*.) A dehydrated patient may receive fluids to dilute the chloride and speed renal excretion of chloride ions. The patient's sodium and chloride intake may also be restricted.

If the patient has normal liver function, he may receive an infusion of lactated Ringer's solution to convert lactate to bicarbonate in the liver, thereby increasing the base bicarbonate level and correcting acidosis. In severe hyperchloremia, the patient may need I.V. sodium bicarbonate to raise serum bicarbonate levels. Because bicarbonate and chloride compete for sodium, I.V. sodium bicarbonate therapy can lead to renal excretion of chloride ions and correction of acidosis.

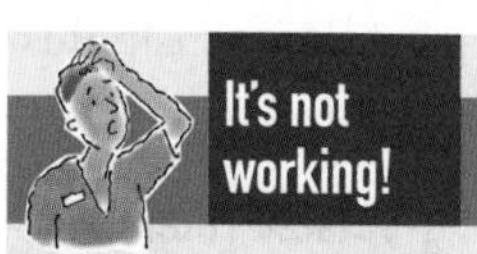

Diuretics to the rescue

If the patient doesn't respond to therapy, the doctor may order diuretics to eliminate chloride. Although other electrolytes are also lost, chloride level should decrease with this treatment.

Anion gap and metabolic acidosis

Hyperchloremia increases the likelihood that a patient will develop hyperchloremic metabolic acidosis. The illustration below shows the relationship between chloride and bicarbonate in the development of that form of acidosis.

How it happens

A normal anion gap in a patient with metabolic acidosis indicates the acidosis is most likely caused by a loss of bicarbonate ions by the kidneys or GI tract. In such cases, a corresponding increase in chloride ions also occurs.

Acidosis can also result from an accumulation of chloride ions in the form of acidifying salts. A corresponding decrease in bicarbonate ions occurs at the same time. In this illustration, the chloride level is high (> 108 mEq/L) and the bicarbonate level is low (< 22 mEq/L).

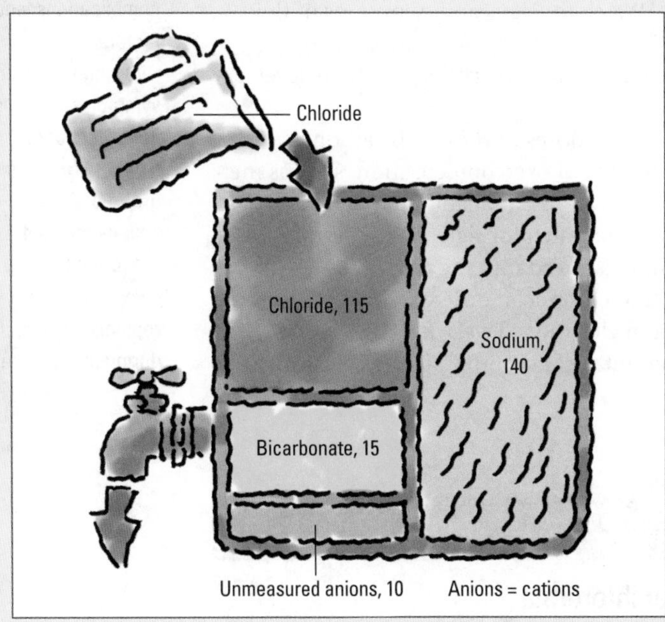

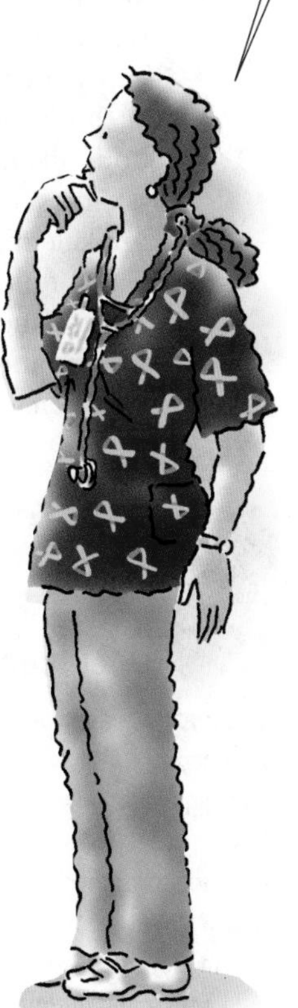
I see . . . chloride can increase in response to the kidneys' excretion of bicarbonate.

How you intervene

Try to prevent hyperchloremia by monitoring high-risk patients. If your patient develops a chloride imbalance, follow these steps:

- Monitor vital signs, including cardiac and respiratory rhythm.
- If the patient is confused, reorient him as needed, and provide a safe, quiet environment to prevent injury. Teach the patient's family to do the same. (See *Teaching about hyperchloremia.*)
- Continually assess the patient, paying particular attention to the neurologic, cardiac, and respiratory examinations. Immediately report changes to the practitioner.
- Look for changes in the respiratory pattern that may indicate a worsening of acid-base imbalance.
- Insert an I.V. and maintain its patency. Administer I.V. fluids and medications as ordered. Watch for signs and symptoms of fluid overload.
- Evaluate muscle strength and adjust the patient's activity level accordingly.
- If the patient is receiving high doses of sodium bicarbonate, watch for signs and symptoms of overcompensation, such as metabolic alkalosis, which may cause central and peripheral nervous system overstimulation. Also, watch for signs and symptoms of hypokalemia as potassium is forced into the cells.
- Restrict fluids, sodium, and chloride, if ordered.
- Monitor and record serum electrolyte levels and ABG results.
- Monitor and record fluid intake and output. (See *Documenting hyperchloremia.*)

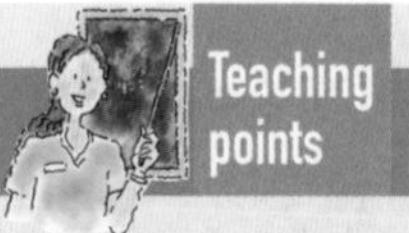

Teaching points

Teaching about hyperchloremia

When teaching a patient with hyperchloremia, be sure to cover the following topics and then evaluate your patient's learning:

- signs and symptoms, complications, and risk factors
- warning signs and symptoms to report to the practitioner
- dietary restrictions if ordered
- medications if prescribed
- importance of replenishing lost fluids during hot weather.

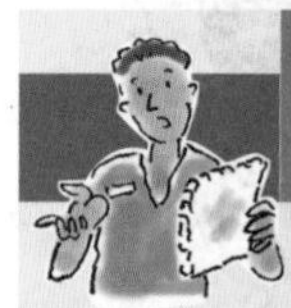

Chart smart

Documenting hyperchloremia

If your patient has hyperchloremia, make sure you document the following information:

- vital signs, including cardiac rhythm
- LOC
- muscle strength
- activity level
- serum electrolyte and ABG levels
- fluid intake and output
- safety precautions taken
- your assessments and interventions and the patient's response
- patient teaching and response.

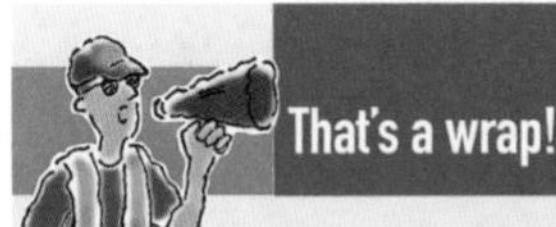

That's a wrap!

Chloride imbalances review

Chloride basics

- Most abundant anion in extracellular fluid
- Moves with sodium and potassium
- Helps maintain serum osmolality and water balance
- Can combine with sodium, helping the choroid plexus to attract water and form CSF
- Is also found in bile and gastric and pancreatic juices in the form of hydrochloric acid, which aids digestion and enzyme activation
- Helps maintain acid-base balance and carbon dioxide transport in red blood cells
- Normal range: 98 to 108 mEq/L

Chloride balance

- Regulation depends on intake and excretion of chloride and reabsorption of chloride ions by the kidneys.
- Chloride is absorbed in the intestines; GI disorders may affect balance.
- Sodium levels are closely linked with chloride and affected by aldosterone secretion.
- The inverse relationship to bicarbonate affects acid-base balance.

Hypochloremia

- Can be caused by:
  - poor chloride intake because of a salt-restricted diet, chloride-deficient infant formula, or I.V. fluid replacement without electrolyte supplementation
  - excessive losses from the GI tract, skin, or kidneys
  - sodium or potassium deficiency or metabolic alkalosis, diabetic ketoacidosis, Addison's disease, diuretics, rapid removal of ascitic fluid, and heart failure

Signs and symptoms

- Hyperactive deep tendon reflexes
- Muscle hypertonicity and cramps
- Signs and symptoms of acid-base imbalance (alkalosis) and electrolyte imbalances (hyponatremia and hypokalemia)
- Tetany

Treatment

- Increased dietary intake
- Treatment of underlying cause of metabolic alkalosis
- I.V. saline solution with either sodium chloride or potassium chloride

Hyperchloremia

- Rarely occurs on its own; often associated with other acid-base imbalances (such as metabolic acidosis)
- Chloride and sodium closely related; hypernatremia may cause hyperchloremia
- Bicarbonate and chloride inversely related; hyperchloremia may occur if bicarbonate decreases
- Also may result from increased chloride and decreased water intake, decreased absorption of chloride from intestines, and certain medications

Signs and symptoms

- Associated with metabolic acidosis (which rarely produces signs and symptoms on its own), such as tachypnea, lethargy, changes in cognition, and weakness

(continued)

Chloride imbalances review *(continued)*

Severe metabolic acidosis
- Arrhythmias
- Kussmaul's respirations
- Decreased cardiac output
- Decreased LOC that may progress to coma

Treatment
- I.V. fluids to speed renal excretion of chloride
- Restricted sodium and chloride intake
- I.V. sodium bicarbonate for severe hyperchloremia

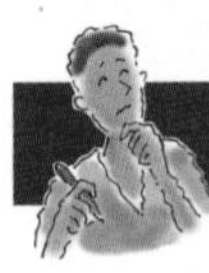

Quick quiz

1. Chloride is primarily produced by the:
   A. brain.
   B. kidneys.
   C. heart.
   D. stomach.

Answer: D. The chloride ion is largely produced by gastric mucosa and occurs in the form of hydrochloric acid.

2. If the level of bicarbonate ions increases, the level of chloride ions:
   A. increases.
   B. decreases.
   C. stays the same.
   D. isn't affected.

Answer: B. Chloride ions and bicarbonate ions have an inversely proportional relationship. If one level rises, the other level drops.

3. In a postoperative patient who has a chloride imbalance, you would also expect to see a change in the electrolyte:
   A. calcium.
   B. potassium.
   C. sodium.
   D. phosphate.

Answer: C. Sodium and chloride move together through the body, so an imbalance in one usually causes an imbalance in the other.

4. If a patient has a low serum chloride level, what acid-base imbalance would you expect to see?
   A. Respiratory acidosis
   B. Metabolic acidosis
   C. Metabolic alkalosis
   D. Respiratory alkalosis

Answer: C. A drop in chloride ions causes the body to retain bicarbonate—a base—and results in hypochloremic metabolic alkalosis.

5. Deep, rapid breathing may indicate a:
   A. serum chloride level greater than 108 mEq/L.
   B. serum chloride less than 98 mEq/L.
   C. pH greater than 7.45.
   D. normal chloride levels.

Answer: A. Deep, rapid breathing, or Kussmaul's respirations, is the body's attempt to blow off excess acid in the form of carbon dioxide. When this occurs, suspect metabolic acidosis, a condition associated with a serum chloride level greater than 108 mEq/L.

Scoring

☆☆☆ If you answered all five questions correctly, incredible! You're the salt of the Earth when it comes to chloride imbalances.

☆☆ If you answered four questions correctly, super! You're obviously in the loop about chloride imbalances.

☆ If you answered fewer than four questions correctly, that's okay. Your chloride intake from the chapter is a little low, but the imbalance can be easily corrected by reviewing the chapter.

References

Berend, K. (2010). Misconceptions about hyperchloremic acidosis. *Journal of Critical Care, 25*(3), 532; author reply 532–533. doi:10.1016/j.jcrc.2010.06.006

Berend, K., van Hulsteijn, L. H., & Gans, R. O. (2012). Chloride: The queen of electrolytes? *European Journal of Internal Medicine, 23*(3), 203–211. doi:10.1016/j.ejim.2011.11.013

Boniatti, M., Cardoso, P. R., Castilho, R. K., & Vieira, S. R. (2011). Is hyperchloremia associated with mortality in critically ill patients? A prospective cohort study. *Journal of Critical Care, 26*(2), 175–179. doi:10.1016/j.jcrc.2010.04.013

Bruce, J. M., Harrington, C. J., Foster, S., & Westervelt, H. J. (2009). Common blood laboratory values are associated with cognition among older inpatients referred for neuropsychological testing. *Clinical Neuropsychology, 23*(6), 909–925. doi:10.1080/13854040902795026

Gheorghe, C., Dadu, R., Blot, C., Barrantes, F., Vazquez, R., Berianu, F., . . . Manthous, C. A. (2010). Hyperchloremic metabolic acidosis following resuscitation of shock. *Chest, 138*(6), 1521–1522. doi:10.1378/chest.10-1458

Lepane, C., Peleman, R., & Kinzie, J. (2012). Chronic diarrhea with hyperchloremic acidosis and hypokalemia. *Gastroenterology, 142*(1), e22–e23. doi:10.1053/j.gastro.2011.01.065

McCallum, L., Jeemon, P., Hastie, C. E., Patel, R. K., Williamson, C., Redzuan, A. M., . . . Padmanabhan, S. (2013). Serum chloride is an independent predictor of mortality in hypertensive patients. *Hypertension, 62*(5), 836–843. doi:10.1161/HYPERTENSIONAHA.113.01793

McCluskey, S. A., Karkouti, K., Wijeysundera, D., Minkovich, L., Tait, G., & Beattie, W. S. (2013). Hyperchloremia after noncardiac surgery is independently associated with increased morbidity and mortality: A propensity-matched cohort study. *Anesthesia and Analgesia, 117*(2), 412–421. doi:10.1213/ANE.0b013e318293d81e

McIntosh, E., & Andrews, P. J. (2013). Is sodium chloride worth its salt? *Critical Care, 17*(3), 150.

MedlinePlus. (2013). *Chloride in diet.* Retrieved from http://www.nlm.nih.gov/medlineplus/ency/article/002417.htm

Miyahara, J., Aramaki S., & Yokochi, K. (2009). Dietary chloride deficiency due to new liquid nutritional products. *Pediatrics International, 51*(2), 197–200. doi:10.1111/j.1442-200X.2008.02670.x

Seifter, J. R. (2011). Acid-base disorders. In L. Goldman & A. I. Schafer (Eds.), *Cecil Medicine* (24th ed., ch. 120). Philadelphia, PA: Saunders.

Tani, M., Morimatsu, H., Takatsu, F., & Morita, K. (2012). The incidence and prognostic value of hypochloremia in critically ill patients. *Scientific World Journal, 2012*, 474185. doi:10.1100/2012/474185

Tutay, G. J., Capraro, G., Spirko, B., Garb, J., & Smithline, H. (2013). Electrolyte profile of pediatric patients with hypertrophic pyloric stenosis. *Pediatric Emergency Care, 29*(4), 465–468. doi:10.1097/PEC.0b013e31828a3006

Yan, M. T., Yang, S. S., Chu, H. Y., & Lin, S. H. (2009). Ataxia associated with spurious hyperchloremia: The one behind the scene. *American Journal of Emergency Medicine, 27*(6), 752.e1–752.e3. doi:10.1016/j.ajem.2008.09.044

Chapter 11

When acids and bases tip the balance

Just the facts

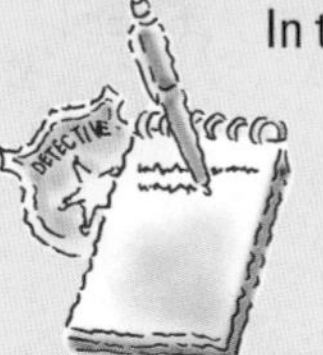

In this chapter, you'll learn:

- the body's mechanisms for maintaining acid-base balance
- conditions that trigger acid-base imbalances
- ways to differentiate the four respiratory and metabolic acid-base imbalances
- proper care for the patient with an acid-base imbalance.

A look at acid-base imbalances

The body constantly works to maintain a balance (homeostasis) between acids and bases. Without that balance, cells can't function properly. As cells use nutrients to produce the energy they need to function, two by-products are formed—carbon dioxide and hydrogen. Acid-base balance depends on the regulation of free hydrogen ions. The concentration of hydrogen ions in body fluids determines the extent of acidity or alkalinity, both of which are measured in pH. Remember, pH levels are inversely proportionate to hydrogen ion concentration, which means that when hydrogen concentration increases, pH decreases (acidosis). Conversely, when hydrogen concentration decreases, pH increases (alkalosis). (For more information about pH, see chapter 3, Balancing acids and bases.)

The body works hard to balance acids and bases—not an easy task!

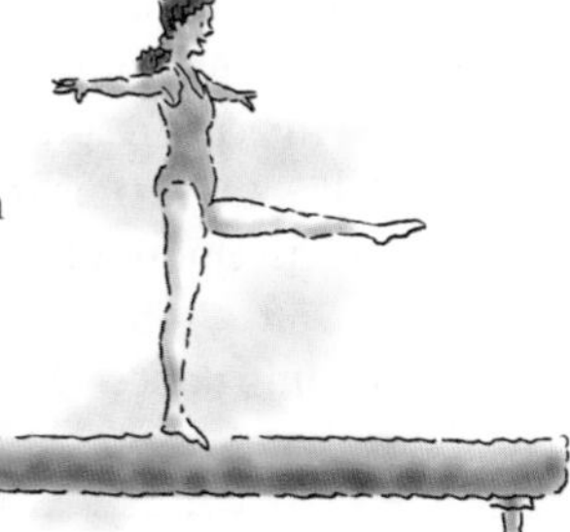

Gas gives good answers

Blood gas measurements remain the major diagnostic tool for evaluating acid-base states. An arterial blood gas (ABG) analysis includes these tests: pH, which measures the hydrogen ion concentration and is an indication of the blood's acidity or alkalinity; partial pressure of arterial carbon dioxide ($Paco_2$), which reflects the adequacy of ventilation by the lungs; and bicarbonate level, which reflects the activity of the kidneys in retaining or excreting bicarbonate. (See *The ABCs of ABGs.*)

The ABCs of ABGs

This chart lists normal ABG levels for adult patients.

pH	7.35 to 7.45
$Paco_2$	35 to 45 mm Hg
Bicarbonate	22 to 26 mEq/L

Normal fix-me-ups

Most of the time, the body's compensatory mechanisms restore acid-base balance—or at least prevent the life-threatening consequences of an imbalance. Those compensatory mechanisms include chemical buffers, certain respiratory reactions, and certain kidney reactions.

For example, the body compensates for a primary respiratory disturbance such as respiratory acidosis by inducing metabolic alkalosis. Unfortunately, not all attempts to compensate are equal. The respiratory system is efficient and can compensate for metabolic disturbances quickly, whereas the metabolic system, working through the kidneys, can take hours or days to compensate for an imbalance, therefore intervention in necessary in order to further patient deterioration. This chapter takes a closer look at each of the four major acid-base imbalances.

Respiratory acidosis

A compromise in any of the three essential parts of breathing—ventilation, perfusion, or diffusion—may result in respiratory acidosis. This acid-base disturbance is characterized by alveolar hypoventilation, meaning the pulmonary system is unable to rid the body of enough carbon dioxide to maintain a healthy pH balance. This occurs because of decreased respiration or inadequate gas exchange.

The lack of efficient carbon dioxide release leads to hypercapnia in which $Paco_2$ is greater than 45 mm Hg. The condition can be acute, resulting from sudden failure in ventilation, or chronic, resulting from chronic pulmonary disease.

In acute respiratory acidosis, pH drops below normal (lower than 7.35). In chronic respiratory acidosis, commonly due to chronic obstructive pulmonary disease (COPD), pH stays within normal limits (7.35 to 7.45) because the kidneys have had time to compensate for the imbalance. (More on that complex phenomenon later.)

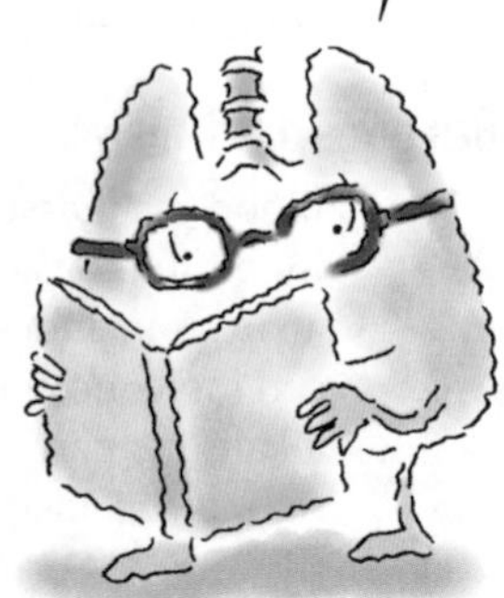
Says here, a compromise in any of the three essential parts of breathing may result in respiratory acidosis.

How it happens

When a patient hypoventilates, carbon dioxide builds up in the bloodstream and pH drops below normal—respiratory acidosis. The kidneys try to compensate for a drop in pH by conserving bicarbonate (base) ions, or generating them in the kidneys, which in turn raises the pH. (See *What happens in respiratory acidosis.*)

What happens in respiratory acidosis

This series of illustrations shows how respiratory acidosis develops at the cellular level.

1. When pulmonary ventilation decreases, retained carbon dioxide (CO_2) combines with water (H_2O) to form carbonic acid (H_2CO_3) in larger-than-normal amounts. The carbonic acid dissociates to release free hydrogen ions (H^+) and bicarbonate ions (HCO_3^-). The excessive carbonic acid causes a drop in pH. *Look for a $Paco_2$ level above 45 mm Hg and a pH level below 7.35.*

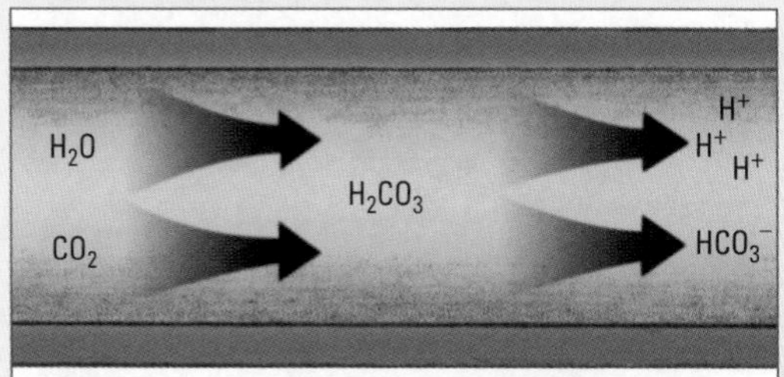

2. As the pH level falls, hemoglobin (Hb) release oxygen (O_2). The altered Hb, now strongly alkaline, picks up H^+ and CO_2, thus eliminating some of the free H^+ and excess CO_2. *Look for decreased arterial oxygen saturation.*

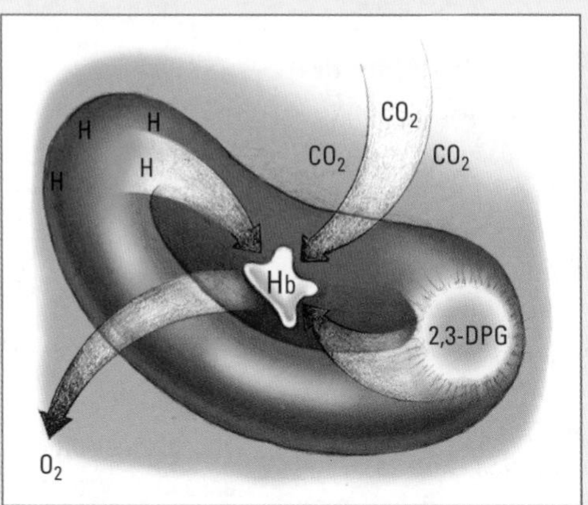

3. Whenever $Paco_2$ increases, CO_2 builds up in all tissues and fluids, including cerebrospinal fluid and the respiratory center in the medulla. The CO_2 reacts with H_2O to form H_2CO_3, which then breaks into free H^+ and HCO_3^-. The increased amount of CO_2 and free H^+ stimulate the respiratory center to increase the respiratory rate. An increased respiratory rate expels more CO_2 and helps to reduce the CO_2 level in blood and tissues. *Look for rapid, shallow respirations and a decreasing $Paco_2$.*

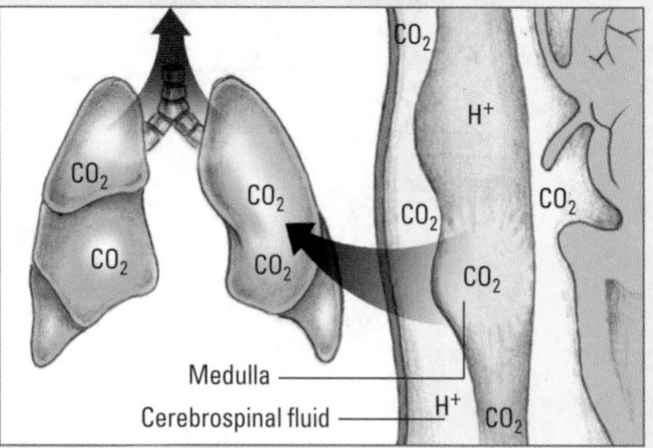

4. Eventually, CO_2 and H^+ cause cerebral blood vessels to dilate, which increases blood flow to the brain. That increased flow can cause cerebral edema and depress central nervous system activity. *Look for headache, confusion, lethargy, nausea, diaphoresis, tachycardia, and vomiting.*

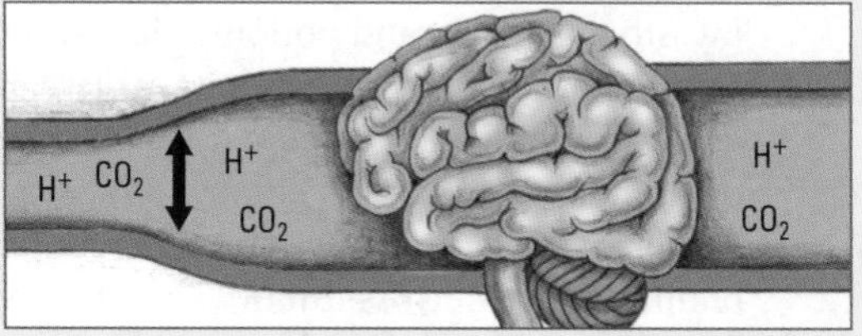

(continued)

What happens in respiratory acidosis *(continued)*

5. As respiratory mechanisms fail, the increasing $Paco_2$ stimulates the kidneys to conserve HCO_3^- and sodium ions (Na) and to excrete H^+, some in the form of ammonium (NH_4). The additional HCO_3^- and Na combine to form extra sodium bicarbonate ($NaHCO_3^-$), which is then able to buffer more free H^+. *Look for increased acid content in the urine; increased serum pH and HCO_3^- levels; and shallow, depressed respirations.*

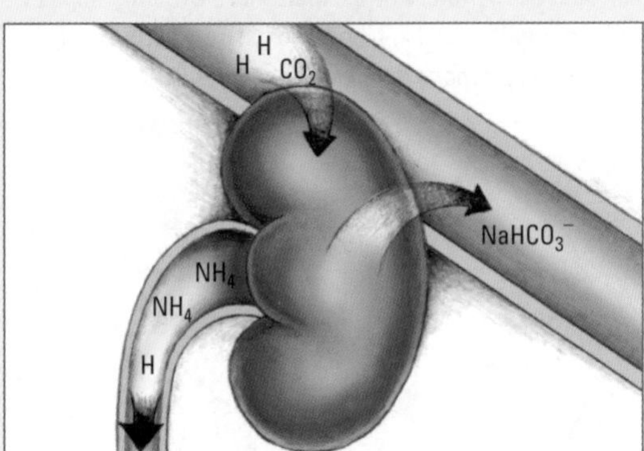

6. As the concentration of H^+ overwhelms the body's compensatory mechanisms, the H^+ move into the cells, and potassium ions (K) move out. A concurrent lack of O_2 causes an increase in the anaerobic production of lactic acid, which further skews the acid-base balance and critically depresses neurologic and cardiac functions. *Look for hyperkalemia, arrhythmias, increased $Paco_2$, decreased Pao_2, decreased pH, and decreased level of consciousness.*

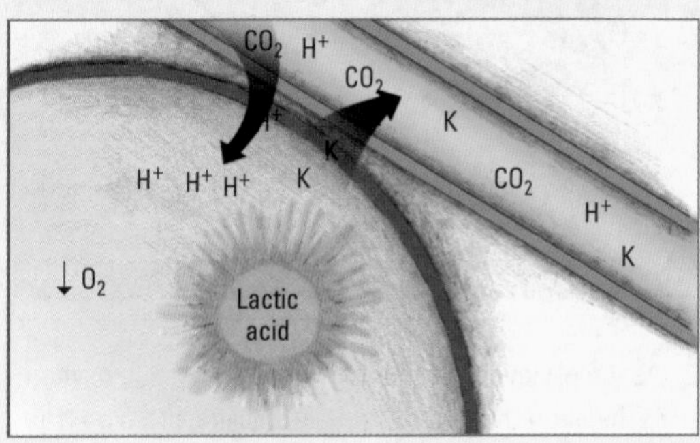

Respiratory acidosis can result from neuromuscular problems, depression of the respiratory center in the brain, lung disease, obesity, postoperative pain, or an airway obstruction.

That breathless feeling

In certain neuromuscular diseases—such as Guillain-Barré syndrome, myasthenia gravis, and poliomyelitis—the respiratory muscles fail to respond properly to the respiratory drive, resulting in respiratory acidosis. Diaphragmatic paralysis, which commonly occurs with spinal cord injury, works the same way to cause respiratory acidosis.

Hypoventilation from central nervous system (CNS) trauma or brain lesions—such as tumors, vascular disorders, or infections—may impair the patient's ventilatory drive. Obesity (as in pickwickian syndrome) or primary hypoventilation (as in Ondine's curse) may contribute to this imbalance as well. Also, certain drugs—including anesthetics, hypnotics, opioids, and sedatives—can depress the respiratory center of the brain, leading to hypercapnia. (See *Drugs associated with respiratory acidosis*.)

Drugs associated with respiratory acidosis

The following drugs are associated with respiratory acidosis:

- anesthetics
- hypnotics
- opioids
- sedatives.

Scanty surface

Lung diseases that decrease the amount of pulmonary surface area available for gas exchange can prompt respiratory acidosis. Less surface area decreases the amount of gas exchange that can occur, thus impeding carbon dioxide exchange. Examples of pulmonary problems that can decrease surface area include respiratory infections, COPD, acute asthma attacks, chronic bronchitis, late stages of adult respiratory distress syndrome, pulmonary edema, conditions in which there's increased dead space in the lungs (hypoventilation), and physiologic or anatomic shunts.

Chest wall trauma (leading to pneumothorax or flail chest) can also cause respiratory acidosis. The ventilatory drive remains intact, but the chest wall mechanics of the collapsed lung don't allow for sufficient alveolar ventilation to meet the body's needs. Chest wall mechanics can also be impeded as a result of the rib cage distortion caused by fibrothorax or kyphoscoliosis.

Danger! Obstruction ahead

Respiratory acidosis can also be caused by airway obstruction, which leads to carbon dioxide retention in the lungs. Airway obstruction can occur as a result of retained secretions, tumors, anaphylaxis, laryngeal spasm, or lung diseases that interfere with alveolar ventilation. Keep in mind that children are particularly prone to airway obstruction, as are elderly and debilitated patients, who may not be able to effectively clear secretions. Other factors also increase an infant's risk of developing acidosis. (See *Infants and acidosis*.)

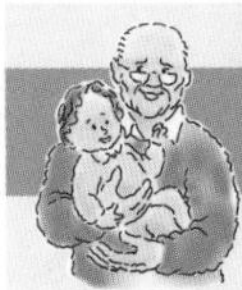

Ages and stages

Infants and acidosis

Infants commonly have problems with acid-base imbalances, particularly acidosis. Because of low residual lung volume, any alteration in respiration can rapidly and dramatically change partial pressure of arterial carbon dioxide, leading to acidosis.

Infants also have a high metabolic rate, which yields large amounts of metabolic wastes and acids that must be excreted by the kidneys. Along with their immature buffer system, these age-related differences leave infants prone to acidosis.

Risky business

Treatments can also induce respiratory acidosis. For instance, mechanical ventilation that underventilates a patient can cause carbon dioxide retention. A postoperative patient is at risk for respiratory acidosis if fear of pain prevents him from participating in pulmonary hygiene measures, such as using the incentive spirometer and coughing and deep breathing. Also, analgesics or sedatives can depress the medulla (which controls respirations), leading to inadequate ventilation and subsequent respiratory acidosis.

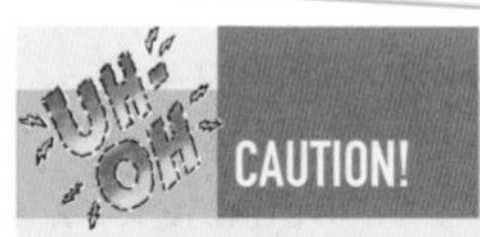

Signs and symptoms of respiratory acidosis

The following assessment findings commonly occur in patients with respiratory acidosis:

- apprehension
- confusion
- decreased deep tendon reflexes
- diaphoresis
- dyspnea, with rapid, shallow respirations
- headache
- nausea
- restlessness
- tachycardia
- tremors
- vomiting
- warm, flushed skin.

What to look for

Signs and symptoms of respiratory acidosis depend on the cause of the condition. The patient may complain of a headache because carbon dioxide dilates cerebral blood vessels. (See *Signs and symptoms of respiratory acidosis.*)

CNS depression may result in an altered level of consciousness (LOC), ranging from restlessness, confusion, and apprehension to somnolence and coma. If acidosis remains untreated, a fine flapping tremor and depressed reflexes may develop. The patient may also report nausea and vomiting, and the skin may be warm and flushed.

A breakdown in breathing

Most patients with respiratory acidosis have rapid, shallow respirations; they may be dyspneic and diaphoretic. Auscultation reveals diminished or absent breath sounds over the affected area. However, if acidosis stems from CNS trauma or lesions or drug overdose, the respiratory rate is greatly decreased.

In a patient with acidosis, hyperkalemia, and hypoxemia, you may note tachycardia and ventricular arrhythmias. Cyanosis is a late sign of the condition. Resulting myocardial depression may lead to shock and, ultimately, cardiac arrest.

What tests show

Several test results help confirm a diagnosis of respiratory acidosis and guide treatment:

- ABG analysis is the key test for detecting respiratory acidosis. Typically, pH is below 7.35, and $Paco_2$ is above 45 mm Hg. The bicarbonate level varies, depending on how long the acidosis has been present. In a patient with acute respiratory acidosis, bicarbonate may be normal; in a patient with chronic respiratory acidosis, it may be above 26 mEq/L. (See *ABG results in respiratory acidosis.*)
- Chest X-rays can help pinpoint some causes, such as COPD, pneumonia, pneumothorax, and pulmonary edema.

ABG results in respiratory acidosis

This chart shows typical ABG findings in uncompensated and compensated respiratory acidosis.

	Uncompensated	Compensated
pH	< 7.35	Normal
$Pa{CO_2}$ (mm Hg)	> 45	> 45
Bicarbonate (mEq/L)	Normal	> 26

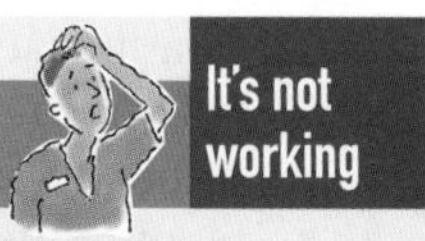

When hypoventilation can't be corrected

If hypoventilation can't be corrected, expect your patient to have an artificial airway inserted and then receive mechanical ventilation. Be aware that he may require bronchoscopy to remove retained secretions.

- Serum electrolyte levels with potassium greater than 5 mEq/L typically indicate hyperkalemia. In acidosis, potassium leaves the cell, so expect serum level to be elevated.
- Drug screening may confirm a suspected overdose.

How it's treated

Treatment of respiratory acidosis focuses on improving ventilation and lowering $Pa{CO_2}$. If respiratory acidosis stems from nonpulmonary conditions, such as neuromuscular disorders or a drug overdose, treatment aims to correct or improve the underlying cause.

Treatment for respiratory acidosis with a pulmonary cause includes:

- a bronchodilator to open constricted airways
- supplemental oxygen as needed
- drug therapy to treat hyperkalemia
- antibiotic therapy to treat infection
- chest physiotherapy to remove secretions from the lungs
- removal of a foreign body from the patient's airway if needed (See *When hypoventilation can't be corrected.*)
- pain medication to control pain to promote effective breathing.

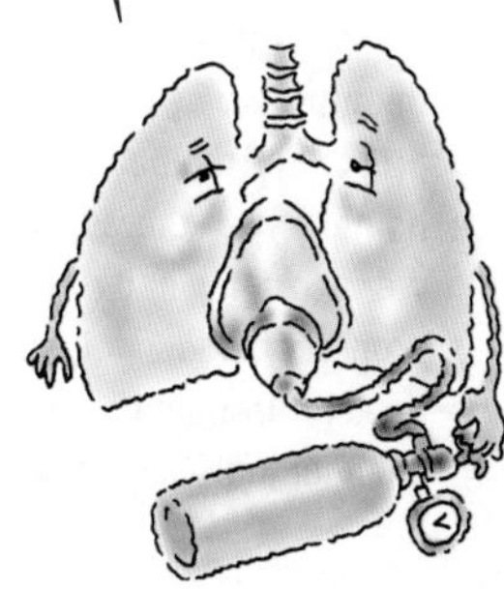

The patient with respiratory acidosis that stems from a pulmonary cause may need supplemental oxygen.

How you intervene

If your patient develops respiratory acidosis, maintain a patent airway. Help remove any foreign bodies from his airway and establish an artificial airway. Provide adequate humidification to keep the patient's secretions moist. Also, follow these measures:

- Monitor vital signs, and assess cardiac rhythm. Respiratory acidosis can cause tachycardia, alterations in respiratory rate and rhythm, hypotension, and arrhythmias.

- Continue to assess respiratory patterns, and report changes quickly. Prepare for mechanical ventilation if indicated.
- Institute measures to prevent ventilator-associated pneumonia.
- Monitor the patient's neurologic status, and report significant changes. Also monitor cardiac function because respiratory acidosis may progress to shock and cardiac arrest.
- Report any variations in ABG levels, pulse oximetry, or serum electrolyte levels.
- Give medications, such as an antibiotic or a bronchodilator, as prescribed. (See *Teaching about respiratory acidosis*.)

Oxygen: Too much of a good thing

- Administer oxygen as ordered. Generally, patients with COPD should receive lower concentrations of oxygen. The medulla of a patient with COPD is accustomed to high carbon dioxide levels. A lack of oxygen, called the *hypoxic drive*, stimulates those patients to breathe. Too much oxygen diminishes that drive and depresses respiratory efforts.
- Perform tracheal suctioning, incentive spirometry, postural drainage, and coughing and deep breathing exercises as indicated.
- Make sure the patient takes in enough fluids, both oral and I.V., and maintain accurate intake and output records. (See *Documenting respiratory acidosis*.)
- Provide reassurance to the patient and family.
- Keep in mind that any sedatives you give to the patient can decrease his respiratory rate.
- Institute safety measures as needed to protect a confused patient.

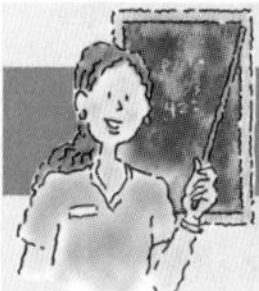

Teaching points

Teaching about respiratory acidosis

When teaching a patient with respiratory acidosis, be sure to cover the following topics and then evaluate your patient's learning:

- description of the condition and how to prevent it
- reasons for repeated ABG analyses
- deep-breathing exercises
- prescribed medications
- home oxygen therapy if indicated
- warning signs and symptoms and when to report them
- proper technique for using bronchodilators, if appropriate
- need for frequent rest
- need for increased caloric intake if appropriate.

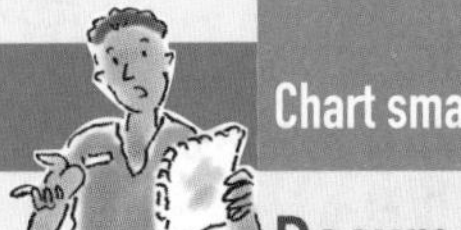

Chart smart

Documenting respiratory acidosis

If your patient has respiratory acidosis, make sure you document the following information:

- vital signs and cardiac rhythm
- intake and output
- your assessment findings and interventions and the patient's response
- notification of the practitioner
- medications administered
- oxygen therapy and ventilator settings
- character of pulmonary secretions
- serum electrolyte levels and ABG results
- patient teaching.

As you reevaluate your patient's condition, consider these questions:

- Have the patient's respiratory rate and LOC returned to normal?
- Does auscultation of the patient's chest reveal reduced adventitious breath sounds?
- Have tachycardia and ventricular arrhythmias been stabilized?
- Have the patient's cyanosis and dyspnea diminished?
- Have the patient's ABG results and serum electrolyte levels returned to normal?
- Do chest X-rays show improvement in the condition of the patient's lungs?

Respiratory alkalosis

The opposite of respiratory acidosis, respiratory alkalosis results from alveolar hyperventilation and hypocapnia. In respiratory alkalosis, increased elimination of carbon dioxide occurs; therefore, pH is greater than 7.45 and $Paco_2$ is less than 35 mm Hg. Acute respiratory alkalosis results from a sudden increase in ventilation. Chronic respiratory alkalosis may be difficult to identify because of renal compensation.

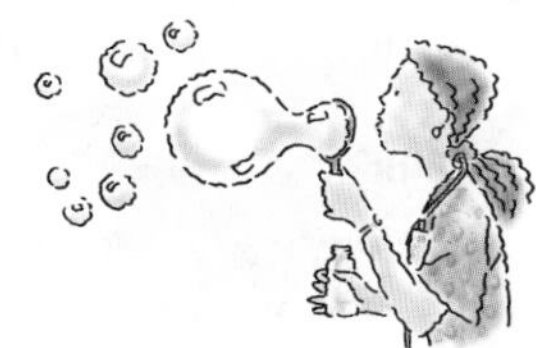
Conditions that increase respiratory rate or depth can cause the lungs to "blow off" carbon dioxide, causing alkalosis. Blowing bubbles seems to fit the bill.

How it happens

Any clinical condition that increases respiratory rate or depth can cause the lungs to eliminate, or "blow off," carbon dioxide. Because carbon dioxide is an acid, eliminating it causes a decrease in $Paco_2$ along with an increase in pH—alkalosis.

Hyperventilation (gasp!)

The most common cause of acute respiratory alkalosis is hyperventilation stemming from anxiety or panic attack. It may also occur during cardiopulmonary resuscitation when rescuers hyperventilate the patient at 30 to 40 breaths per minute. Pain can have the same effect. Hyperventilation is also an early sign of salicylate intoxication and can occur with the use of nicotine, xanthines such as aminophylline, and other drugs. (See *Drugs associated with respiratory alkalosis*.)

Hypermetabolic states—such as fever, liver failure, and sepsis (especially gram-negative sepsis)—can lead to respiratory alkalosis. Conditions that affect the respiratory control center in the medulla are also a danger. For example, the higher progesterone levels during pregnancy may stimulate this center, whereas stroke or trauma may injure it, both resulting in respiratory alkalosis.

Drugs associated with respiratory alkalosis

Drugs associated with respiratory alkalosis include:

- catecholamines
- nicotine
- salicylates
- xanthines such as aminophylline.

Hypoxia (pant!)

Acute hypoxia, secondary to high altitude, pulmonary disease, severe anemia, pulmonary embolus, or hypotension, can cause respiratory alkalosis. Such conditions may overstimulate the respiratory center and cause the patient to breathe faster and deeper. Overventilation during mechanical ventilation causes the lungs to blow off more carbon dioxide, resulting in respiratory alkalosis.

What to look for

An increase in the rate and depth of respirations is a primary sign of respiratory alkalosis. It's also common for the patient to have tachycardia. The patient may appear anxious and restless as well as complain of lightheadedness, muscle weakness, fear, or difficulty breathing. (See *What happens in respiratory alkalosis*.)

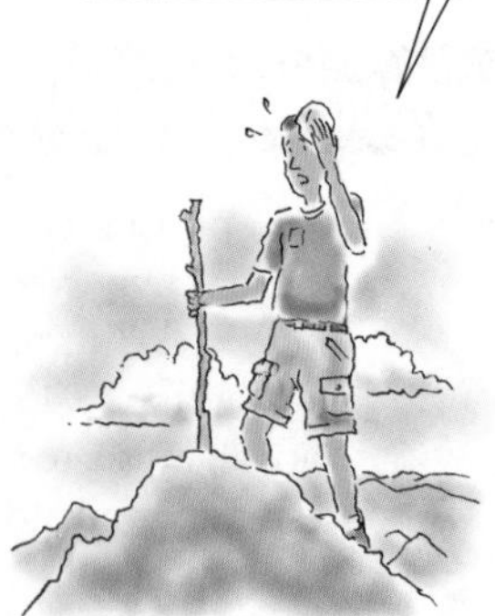

Being at a high altitude can definitely lead to acute hypoxia!

In extremis

In extreme alkalosis, confusion or syncope may occur. Because of the lack of carbon dioxide in the blood and its effect on cerebral blood flow and the respiratory center, you may see alternating periods of apnea and hyperventilation. The patient may complain of tingling in the fingers and toes.

What happens in respiratory alkalosis

This series of illustrations shows how respiratory alkalosis develops at the cellular level.

1. When pulmonary ventilation increases above the amount needed to maintain normal carbon dioxide (CO_2) levels, excessive amounts of CO_2 are exhaled. This causes hypocapnia (a fall in $Paco_2$), which leads to a reduction in carbonic acid (H_2CO_3) production, a loss of hydrogen ions (H^+) and bicarbonate ions (HCO_3^-), and a subsequent rise in pH. *Look for a pH level above 7.45, a $Paco_2$ level below 35 mm Hg, and an HCO_3^- level below 22 mEq/L.*

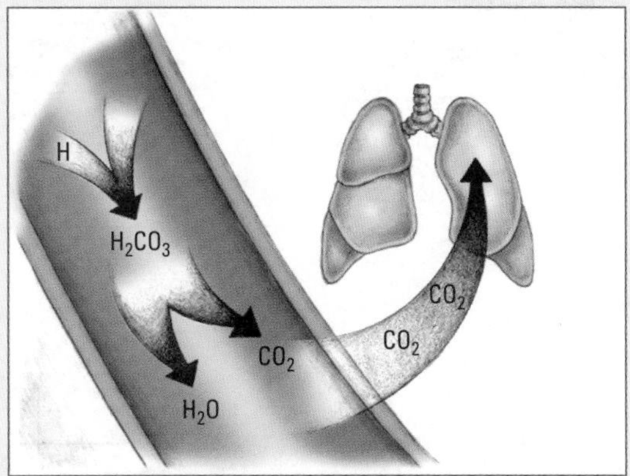

2. In defense against the rising pH, H^+ are pulled out of the cells and into the blood in exchange for potassium ions (K). The H^+ entering the blood combine with HCO_3^- to form H_2CO_3, which lowers pH. *Look for a further decrease in HCO_3^- levels, a fall in pH, and a fall in serum potassium levels (hypokalemia).*

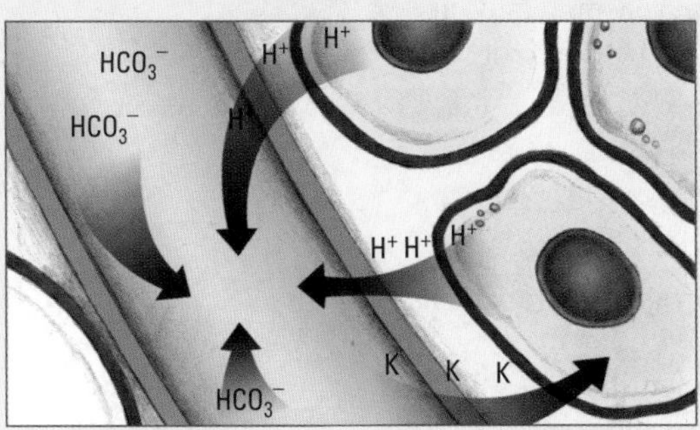

3. Hypocapnia stimulates the carotid and aortic bodies and the medulla, which causes an increase in heart rate without an increase in blood pressure. *Look for angina, electrocardiogram changes, restlessness, and anxiety.*

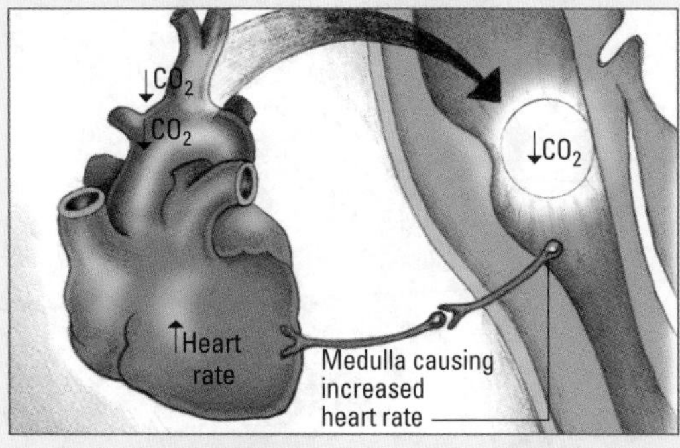

4. Simultaneously, hypocapnia produces cerebral vasoconstriction, which prompts a reduction in cerebral blood flow. Hypocapnia also overexcites the medulla, pons, and other parts of the autonomic nervous system. *Look for increasing anxiety, fear, diaphoresis, dyspnea, alternating periods of apnea and hyperventilation, dizziness, and tingling in the fingers or toes.*

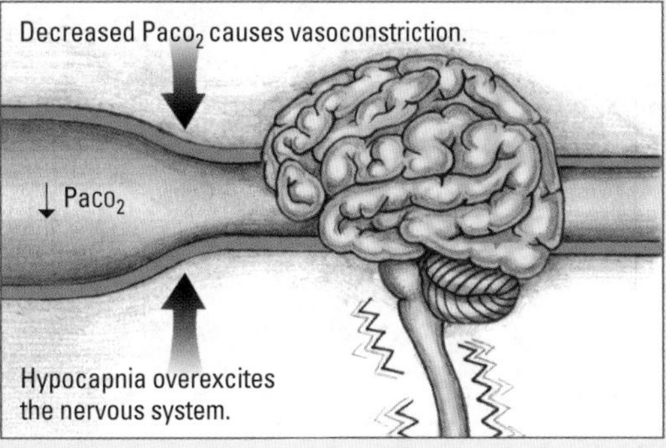

(continued)

What happens in respiratory alkalosis *(continued)*

5. When hypocapnia lasts more than 6 hours, the kidneys increase secretion of HCO_3^- and reduce excretion of H^+. Periods of apnea may result if the pH remains high and the $Paco_2$ remains low. *Look for slowed respiratory rate, hypoventilation, and Cheyne-Stokes' respirations.*

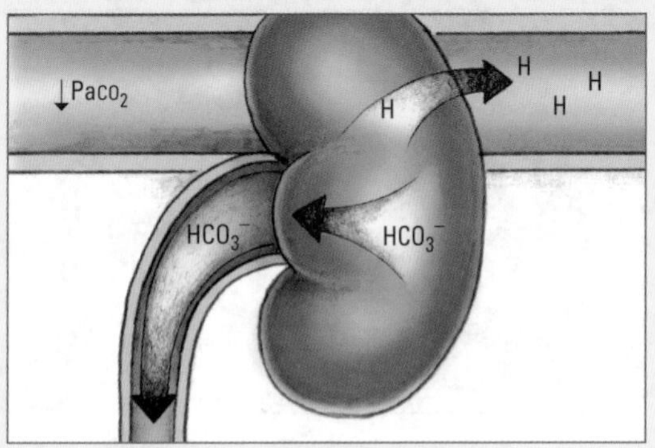

6. Continued low $Paco_2$ increases cerebral and peripheral hypoxia from vasoconstriction. Severe alkalosis inhibits calcium (Ca) ionization, which in turn causes increased nerve excitability and muscle contractions. Eventually, the alkalosis overwhelms the CNS and the heart. *Look for decreasing LOC, hyperreflexia, carpopedal spasm, tetany, arrhythmias, seizures, and coma.*

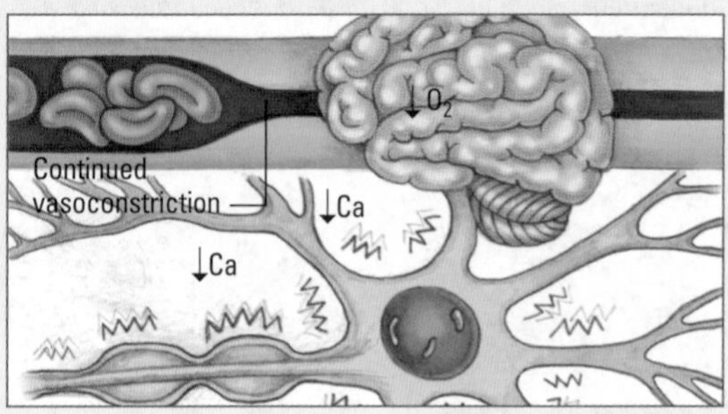

ECG exposé

You may see electrocardiogram (ECG) changes, including a prolonged PR interval, a flattened T wave, a prominent U wave, and a depressed ST segment. (For more information, see chapter 6, When potassium tips the balance.)

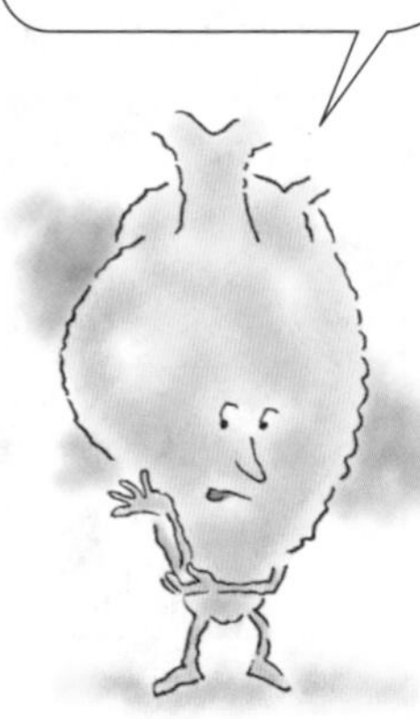

As calcium levels continue to drop, you may see serious effects, including arrhythmias. I am *not* happy about this!

Signs of trouble

Signs and symptoms worsen as calcium levels drop because of vasoconstriction of peripheral and cerebral vessels resulting from hypoxia. You may see hyperreflexia, carpopedal spasm, tetany, arrhythmias, a progressive decrease in the patient's LOC, seizures, or coma. (See *Signs and symptoms of respiratory alkalosis*.)

What tests show

Several diagnostic test results may help detect respiratory alkalosis and guide treatment:

- ABG analysis is the key diagnostic test for identifying respiratory alkalosis. Typically, pH is above 7.45 and $Paco_2$ is below 35 mm Hg. The bicarbonate level may be normal (22 to 26 mEq/L) when

ABG results in respiratory alkalosis

This chart shows typical ABG findings in uncompensated and compensated respiratory alkalosis.

	Uncompensated	Compensated
pH	> 7.45	Normal
$Paco_2$ (mm Hg)	< 35	< 35
Bicarbonate (mEq/L)	Normal	< 22

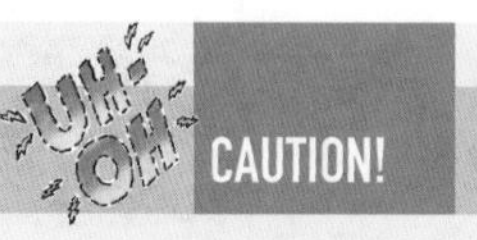

Signs and symptoms of respiratory alkalosis

The following assessment findings commonly occur in patients with respiratory alkalosis:

- anxiety
- diaphoresis
- dyspnea (increased respiratory rate and depth)
- ECG changes
- hyperreflexia
- paresthesia
- restlessness
- tachycardia
- tetany.

alkalosis is acute but usually falls below 22 mEq/L when alkalosis is chronic. (See *ABG results in respiratory alkalosis*.)

- Serum electrolyte levels may point to a metabolic disorder that is causing compensatory respiratory alkalosis. Hypokalemia may be evident, signaled by decreased LOC. The ionized serum calcium level may be decreased in those with severe respiratory alkalosis.
- ECG findings may indicate arrhythmias or the changes associated with hypokalemia or hypocalcemia.
- Toxicology screening may reveal salicylate poisoning.

How it's treated

Treatment focuses on correcting the underlying disorder, which may require removing the causative agent, such as a salicylate or other drug, or taking steps to reduce fever and eliminate the source of sepsis. If acute hypoxemia is the cause, the patient will need oxygen therapy. If anxiety is the cause, the patient may receive a sedative or an anxiolytic. If the patient is having pain, the patient may receive an analgesic.

It's in the bag

To counteract hyperventilation, the patient can breathe into a paper bag or into cupped hands. This forces the patient to breathe exhaled carbon dioxide, thereby raising the carbon dioxide level. If a patient's respiratory alkalosis is medically induced, mechanical ventilator settings may be adjusted by decreasing the tidal volume or the number of breaths per minute.

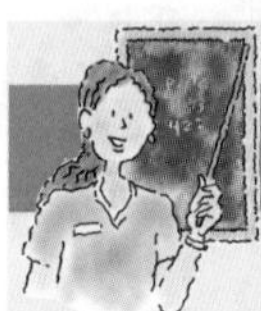

Teaching points

Teaching about respiratory alkalosis

When teaching a patient with respiratory alkalosis, be sure to cover the following topics and then evaluate your patient's learning:

- explanation of the condition and its treatment
- warning signs and symptoms and when to report them
- anxiety-reducing techniques if appropriate
- controlled-breathing exercises if appropriate
- prescribed medications.

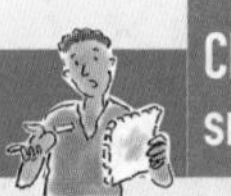

Chart smart

Documenting respiratory alkalosis

If your patient has respiratory alkalosis, make sure you document the following information:

- vital signs
- intake and output
- I.V. therapy
- interventions, including measures taken to alleviate anxiety
- patient's response to interventions
- serum electrolyte levels and ABG results
- safety measures
- notification of the practitioner
- patient teaching.

How you intervene

Monitor patients at risk for developing respiratory alkalosis. If your patient develops the condition, take these actions:

- Allay anxiety whenever possible to prevent hyperventilation. Recommend activities that promote relaxation. Help the patient breath into a paper bag or cupped hands if necessary.
- Monitor vital signs. Report changes in neurologic, neuromuscular, or cardiovascular functioning.
- Monitor ABG and serum electrolyte levels, and immediately report any variations. Remember, twitching and arrhythmias may point to alkalosis and electrolyte imbalances.
- If the patient is receiving mechanical ventilation, check ventilator settings frequently. Monitor ABG levels after making changes in settings.
- Provide undisturbed rest periods after the patient's respiratory rate returns to normal; hyperventilation may result in severe fatigue.
- Stay with the patient during periods of extreme stress and anxiety. Offer reassurance, and maintain a calm, quiet environment. (See *Teaching about respiratory alkalosis*.)
- Institute safety measures and seizure precautions as needed.
- Document all care. (See *Documenting respiratory alkalosis*.)

Metabolic acidosis

Metabolic acidosis is caused by an increase in hydrogen ion production and is characterized by a pH below 7.35 and a bicarbonate level below 22 mEq/L. This disorder depresses the CNS. Left untreated, it may lead to ventricular arrhythmias, coma, and cardiac arrest.

How it happens

The underlying mechanisms in metabolic acidosis are a loss of bicarbonate from extracellular fluid, an accumulation of metabolic acids, or a combination of the two. If the patient's anion gap (measurement of the difference between the amount of sodium and the amount of bicarbonate in the blood) is greater than 14 mEq/L, then the acidosis is a result of an accumulation of metabolic acids (unmeasured anions).

If metabolic acidosis is associated with a normal anion gap (8 to 14 mEq/L), loss of bicarbonate may be the cause. (See *What happens in metabolic acidosis*, pages 216 and 217.)

Acids ante up, bases bottom out

Metabolic acidosis is characterized by a gain in acids or a loss of bases from the plasma. The condition may be related to an overproduction of ketone bodies. This occurs when the body has used up its glucose supplies and draws on its fat stores for energy, converting fatty acids to ketone bodies. Conditions that cause an overproduction of ketone bodies include diabetes mellitus, chronic alcoholism, severe malnutrition or starvation, poor dietary intake of carbohydrates, hyperthyroidism, and severe infection with accompanying fever.

Lactic acidosis can cause or worsen metabolic acidosis and can occur secondary to shock, heart failure, pulmonary disease, hepatic disorders, seizures, or strenuous exercise.

Kidney culprit

Metabolic acidosis can also stem from a decreased ability of the kidneys to excrete acids, as occurs in renal insufficiency or renal failure with acute tubular necrosis.

Gut reactions

Metabolic acidosis also occurs with excessive gastrointestinal (GI) losses from diarrhea, intestinal malabsorption, a draining fistula of the pancreas or liver, or a urinary diversion to the ileum. Other causes include hyperaldosteronism and use of a potassium-sparing diuretic such as acetazolamide, which inhibits the secretion of acid.

Poison pills

At particular risk for metabolic acidosis are patients with poisoning or a toxic reaction to a drug. This can occur following inhalation of toluene or ingestion of a salicylate (such as aspirin or an aspirin-containing medication), methanol, ethylene glycol, paraldehyde, hydrochloric acid, or ammonium chloride.

What happens in metabolic acidosis

This series of illustrations shows how metabolic acidosis develops at the cellular level.

1. As hydrogen ions (H^+) start to accumulate in the body, chemical buffers (plasma bicarbonate [HCO_3^-] and proteins) in the cells and extracellular fluid bind with them. *No signs are detectable at this stage.*

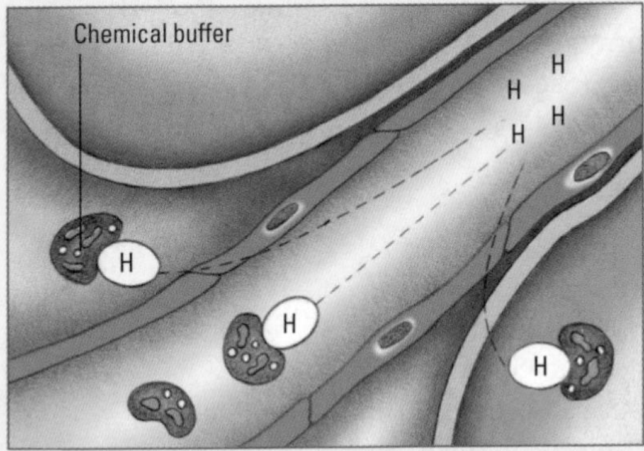

2. Excess H^+ that can't bind with the buffers decrease pH and stimulate chemoreceptors in the medulla to increase respiratory rate. Increased respiratory rate lowers $Paco_2$, which allows more H^+ to bind with HCO_3^-. Respiratory compensation occurs within minutes but isn't sufficient to correct the imbalance. *Look for a pH level below 7.35; an HCO_3^- level below 22 mEq/L; a decreasing $Paco_2$ level; and rapid, deeper respirations.*

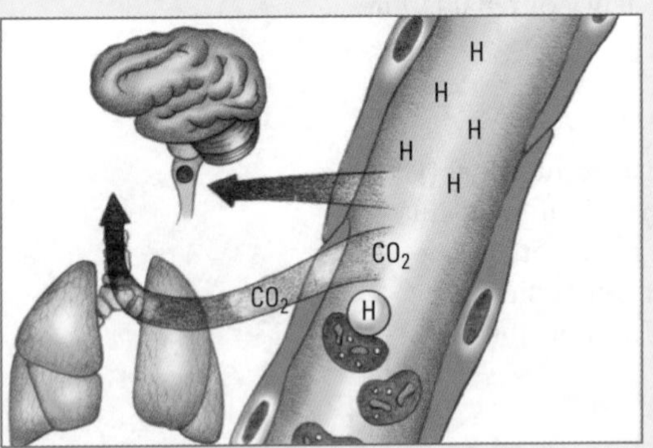

3. Healthy kidneys try to compensate for acidosis by secreting excess H^+ into the renal tubules. Those ions are buffered by phosphate or ammonia and then are excreted into the urine in the form of a weak acid. *Look for acidic urine.*

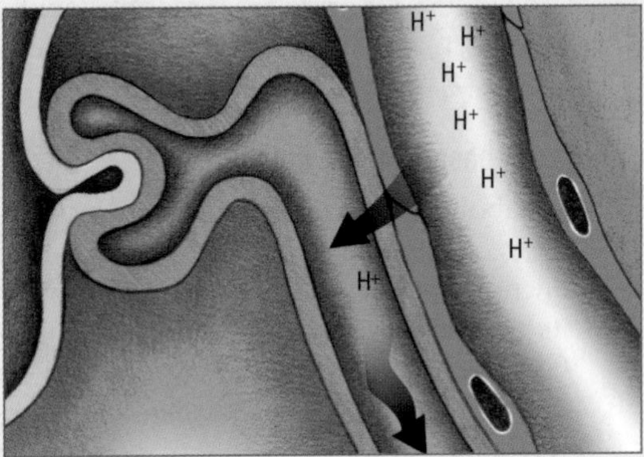

4. Each time a H^+ is secreted into the renal tubules, a sodium ion (Na) and an HCO_3^- are absorbed from the tubules and returned to the blood. *Look for pH and HCO_3^- levels that slowly return to normal.*

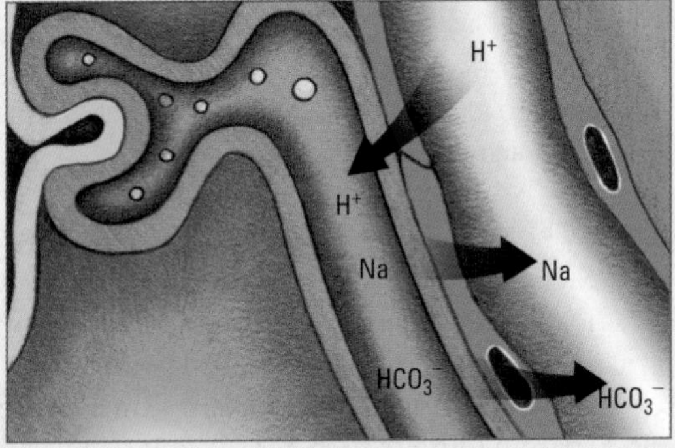

(continued)

What happens in metabolic acidosis *(continued)*

5. Excess H^+ in the extracellular fluid diffuse into cells. To maintain the balance of the charge across the membrane, the cells release potassium ions (K) into the blood. *Look for signs and symptoms of hyperkalemia, including colic and diarrhea, weakness or flaccid paralysis, tingling and numbness in the extremities, bradycardia, a tall T wave, a prolonged PR interval, and a wide QRS complex.*

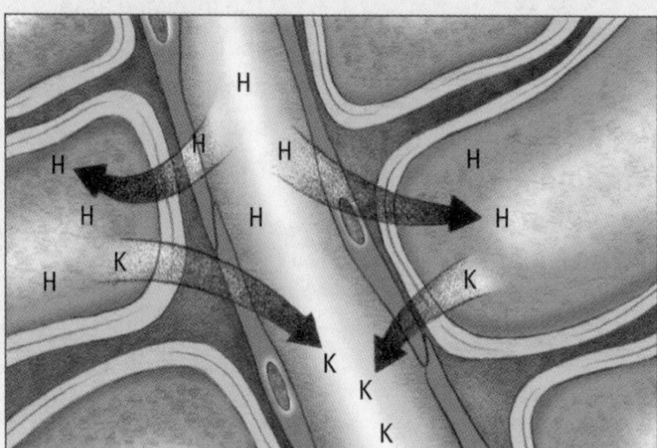

6. Excess H^+ alter the normal balance of K, Na, and calcium ions (Ca), leading to reduced excitability of nerve cells. *Look for signs and symptoms of progressive CNS depression, including lethargy, dull headache, confusion, stupor, and coma.*

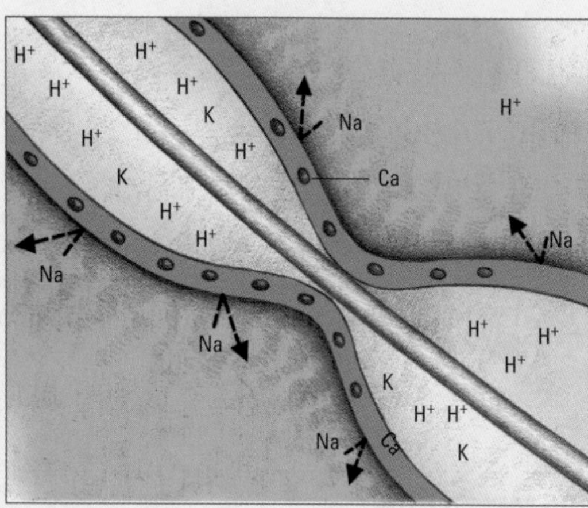

What to look for

Metabolic acidosis typically produces respiratory, neurologic, and cardiac signs and symptoms. As acid builds up in the bloodstream, the lungs compensate by blowing off carbon dioxide.

Hyperventilation, especially increased depth of respirations, is the first clue to metabolic acidosis. Called *Kussmaul's respirations*, the breathing is rapid and deep. A patient with diabetes who experiences Kussmaul's respirations may have a fruity breath odor. The odor stems from catabolism of fats and excretion of acetone through the lungs.

So depressing

As pH drops, the CNS is further depressed, as is myocardial function. Cardiac output and blood pressure drop, and arrhythmias may occur if the patient also has hyperkalemia.

Initially, the skin is warm and dry as a result of peripheral vasodilation but, as shock develops, the skin becomes cold and clammy. The patient may complain of weakness and a dull headache as the cerebral vessels dilate.

ABG results in metabolic acidosis

This chart shows typical ABG findings in uncompensated and compensated metabolic acidosis.

	Uncompensated	Compensated
pH	< 7.35	Normal
Pa_{CO_2} (mm Hg)	Normal	< 35
Bicarbonate (mEq/L)	< 22	< 22

The patient's LOC may deteriorate from confusion to stupor and coma. A neuromuscular examination may show diminished muscle tone and deep tendon reflexes. Metabolic acidosis also affects the GI system, causing anorexia, nausea, and vomiting. (See *Signs and symptoms of metabolic acidosis.*)

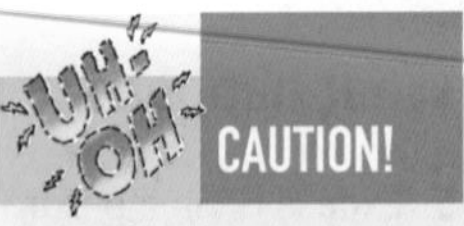
UH-OH
CAUTION!

Signs and symptoms of metabolic acidosis

The following assessment findings commonly occur in patients with metabolic acidosis:

- confusion
- decreased deep tendon reflexes
- dull headache
- hyperkalemic signs and symptoms, including abdominal cramping, diarrhea, muscle weakness, and ECG changes
- hypotension
- Kussmaul's respirations
- lethargy
- warm, dry skin
- nausea
- fruity breath
- coma.

What tests show

Several test results may help diagnose and treat metabolic acidosis:

- ABG analysis is the key diagnostic test for detecting metabolic acidosis. Typically, pH is below 7.35. Pa_{CO_2} may be less than 35 mm Hg, indicating compensatory attempts by the lungs to rid the body of excess carbon dioxide. (See *ABG results in metabolic acidosis.*)
- Serum potassium levels are usually elevated as hydrogen ions move into the cells and potassium moves out to maintain electroneutrality.
- Blood glucose and serum ketone levels rise in patients with diabetic ketoacidosis (DKA).
- Plasma lactate levels rise in patients with lactic acidosis. (See *A look at lactic acidosis.*)
- The anion gap is increased. This measurement is calculated by subtracting the amount of negative ions (chloride plus bicarbonate) from the amount of the positive ion (sodium). Sometimes, the amount of potassium ion is added to the amount of positive ion, but the amount of potassium ion is usually so small that the calculation doesn't change. The normal anion gap is 8 to 14 mEq/L.
- ECG changes associated with hyperkalemia—such as tall T waves, prolonged PR intervals, and wide QRS complexes—may be found.

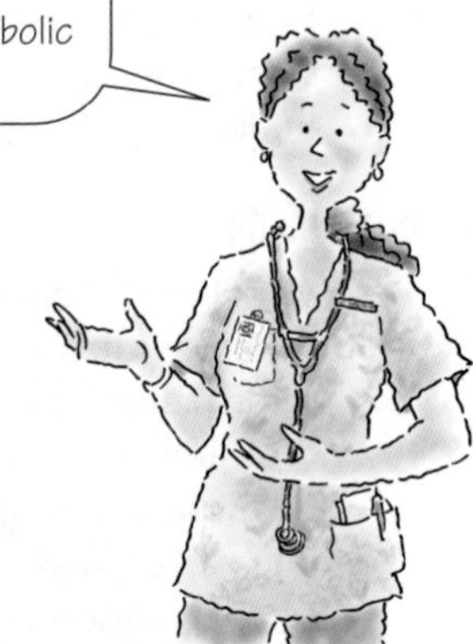
Several tests may help diagnose and treat metabolic acidosis.

A look at lactic acidosis

Lactate, produced as a result of carbohydrate metabolism, is metabolized by the liver. The normal lactate level is 0.93 to 1.65 mEq/L. With tissue hypoxia, however, cells are forced to switch to anaerobic metabolism and more lactate is produced. When lactate accumulates in the body faster than it can be metabolized, lactic acidosis occurs. It can happen any time the demand for oxygen in the body is greater than its availability.

The causes of lactic acidosis include septic shock, cardiac arrest, pulmonary disease, seizures, and strenuous exercise.

The latter two cause transient lactic acidosis. Hepatic disorders can also cause lactic acidosis because the liver can't metabolize lactate.

Treatment

Treatment focuses on eliminating the underlying cause. If pH is below 7.1, sodium bicarbonate or another alkalinizing agent such as tromethamine may be given. Use caution when administering such agents because alkalosis may result.

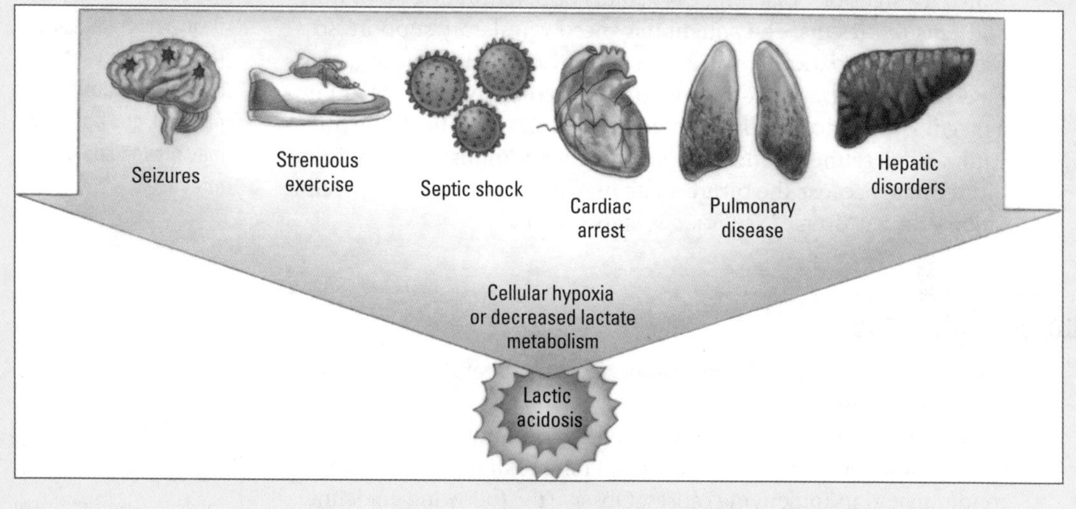

How it's treated

Treatment aims to correct the acidosis as quickly as possible by addressing both the symptoms and the underlying cause. Respiratory compensation is usually the first line of therapy, including mechanical ventilation if needed.

Put potassium in its place

For patients with diabetes, expect to administer rapid-acting insulin to reverse DKA and drive potassium back into the cell. For any patient with metabolic acidosis, monitor serum potassium levels. Even though the patient initially has high serum potassium levels, the levels drop as acidosis is corrected, and the patient may end up with hypokalemia. Any other electrolyte imbalances should be evaluated and corrected.

Bump up the bicarbonate

Expect to administer I.V. sodium bicarbonate to neutralize blood acidity in patients with bicarbonate loss and a pH lower than 7.1. Fluids are replaced parenterally as required. Dialysis may be initiated in patients with renal failure or a toxic reaction to a drug. Such patients may receive an antibiotic to treat sources of infection or an antidiarrheal to treat diarrhea-induced bicarbonate loss.

Always on the alert

Watch for signs of worsening CNS status or deteriorating laboratory and ABG test results. The patient may need ventilatory support, so prepare for intubation. A patient with renal failure may need dialysis, especially when this condition is complicated by diabetes. Maintain a patent I.V. line to administer emergency drugs, and flush the line with normal saline solution before and after administering sodium bicarbonate because the bicarbonate may inactivate or cause precipitation of many drugs. (See *Acidosis and dopamine*.)

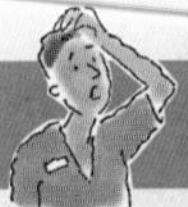

It's not working

Acidosis and dopamine

If you're administering dopamine to a patient and it isn't raising his blood pressure as you expected, investigate your patient's pH. A pH level below 7.1 (as can happen in severe metabolic acidosis) causes resistance to vasopressor therapy. Correct the pH level, and dopamine may prove to be more effective.

How you intervene

If your patient is at risk for metabolic acidosis, careful monitoring can help prevent it from developing.

If your patient already has metabolic acidosis, nursing care includes immediate emergency interventions and long-term treatment of the condition and its underlying causes. Observe the following guidelines:

- Monitor vital signs, and assess cardiac rhythm.
- Prepare for mechanical ventilation or dialysis as required.
- Closely monitor the patient's neurologic status because changes can occur rapidly. Notify the practitioner of any changes in the patient's condition.
- Insert an I.V. line as ordered, and maintain patent I.V. access. Have a large-bore catheter in place for emergency situations. Administer I.V. fluid, a vasopressor, an antibiotic, and other medications as prescribed.
- Administer sodium bicarbonate as ordered. Remember to flush the I.V. line with normal saline solution before and after giving bicarbonate because the chemical can inactivate many drugs or cause them to precipitate. Keep in mind that too much bicarbonate can cause metabolic alkalosis and pulmonary edema.

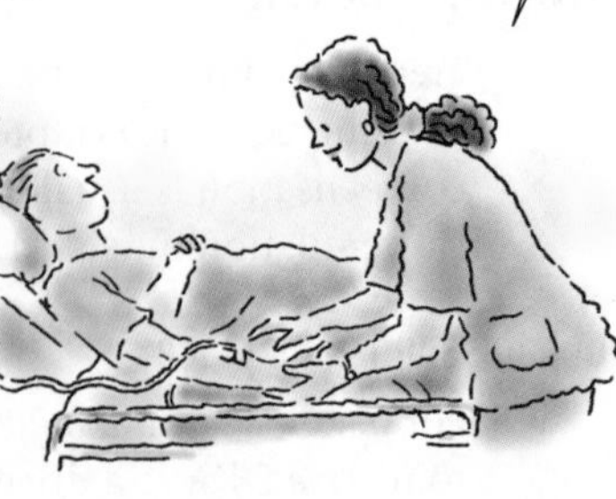
If your patient has metabolic acidosis, insert an I.V. line as ordered, and maintain patent I.V. access.

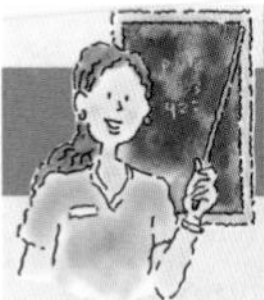

Teaching points

Teaching about metabolic acidosis

When teaching a patient with metabolic acidosis, be sure to cover the following topics and then evaluate your patient's learning:

- basics of the condition and its treatment
- testing of blood glucose levels if indicated
- need for strict adherence to antidiabetic therapy if appropriate
- avoidance of alcohol
- warning signs and symptoms and when to report them
- prescribed medications
- avoidance of ingestion of toxic substances.

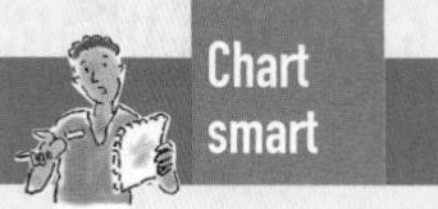

Documenting metabolic acidosis

If your patient has metabolic acidosis, make sure you document the following information:

- assessment findings, including results of neurologic examinations
- intake and output
- notification of the practitioner
- prescribed medications and I.V. therapy and patient's response
- safety measures implemented
- serum electrolyte levels and ABG results
- ventilator or dialysis data
- vital signs and cardiac rhythm
- patient teaching.

- Position the patient to promote chest expansion and ease breathing. If the patient is stuporous, turn him frequently. (See *Teaching about metabolic acidosis*.)
- Take steps to help eliminate the underlying cause. For example, administer insulin and I.V. fluids as prescribed to reverse DKA.
- Watch for any secondary changes, such as declining blood pressure, that hypovolemia may cause.
- Monitor the patient's renal function by recording intake and output. (See *Documenting metabolic acidosis*.)
- Watch for changes in serum electrolyte levels, and monitor ABG results throughout treatment to check for overcorrection.
- Orient the patient as needed. If he's confused, take steps to ensure his or her safety, such as keeping the bed in the lowest position.
- Investigate reasons for the patient's ingestion of toxic substances.

Q & A time

Physical examination and further diagnostic tests may provide more information about your patient's metabolic acidosis. As you reevaluate the patient's condition, consider these questions:

- Has the patient's LOC returned to normal?
- Have vital signs stabilized?
- Have ABG results, blood glucose levels, and serum electrolyte levels improved?
- Is cardiac output normal?
- Has the patient regained a normal sinus rhythm (or his previously stable underlying rhythm)?
- Is the patient ventilating adequately?

Metabolic alkalosis

Metabolic alkalosis is caused by a decrease in hydrogen ion production, characterized by a blood pH above 7.45, and accompanied by a bicarbonate level above 26 mEq/L. In acute metabolic alkalosis, bicarbonate may be as high as 50 mEq/L. With early diagnosis and prompt treatment, the prognosis for effective treatment is good. Left untreated, metabolic alkalosis can result in coma, arrhythmias, and death.

Left untreated, metabolic alkalosis can result in coma, arrhythmias, and death.

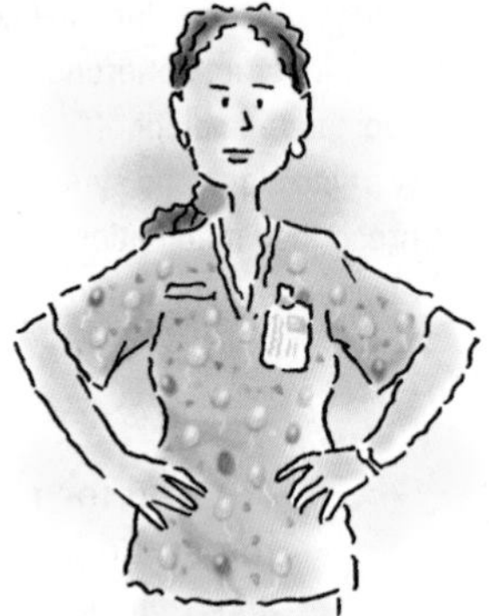

How it happens

In metabolic alkalosis, the underlying mechanisms include a loss of hydrogen ions (acid), a gain in bicarbonate, or both. A $Paco_2$ level greater than 45 mm Hg (possibly as high as 60 mm Hg) indicates that the lungs are compensating for alkalosis. Renal compensation is more effective but slower. Metabolic alkalosis is commonly associated with hypokalemia, particularly from the use of thiazides, furosemide, ethacrynic acid, and other diuretics that deplete potassium stores. In hypokalemia, the kidneys conserve potassium. At the same time, the kidneys also increase the excretion of hydrogen ions, which prompts alkalosis from the loss of acid. Metabolic alkalosis may also occur with hypochloremia and hypocalcemia. (See *What happens in metabolic alkalosis*.)

GI grief

Metabolic alkalosis can result from many causes, the most common of which is excessive acid loss from the GI tract. Vomiting causes loss of hydrochloric acid from the stomach. Children who have pyloric stenosis can develop this disorder. Alkalosis also results from prolonged nasogastric (NG) suctioning, presenting a risk for surgical patients and patients with GI disorders.

Diuretic danger

Diuretic therapy presents another risk of metabolic alkalosis. Thiazide and loop diuretics can lead to a loss of hydrogen, potassium, and chloride ions from the kidneys. Hypokalemia causes the kidneys to excrete hydrogen ions as they try to conserve potassium. Potassium moves out of the cells as hydrogen moves in, resulting in alkalosis.

With the fluid loss from diuresis, the kidneys attempt to conserve sodium and water. For sodium to be reabsorbed, hydrogen ions must be excreted. In a process known as *contraction alkalosis*, bicarbonate is reabsorbed and metabolic alkalosis results.

What happens in metabolic alkalosis

This series of illustrations shows how metabolic alkalosis develops at the cellular level.

1. As bicarbonate ions (HCO_3^-) start to accumulate in the body, chemical buffers (in extracellular fluid and cells) bind with them. *No signs are detectable at this stage.*

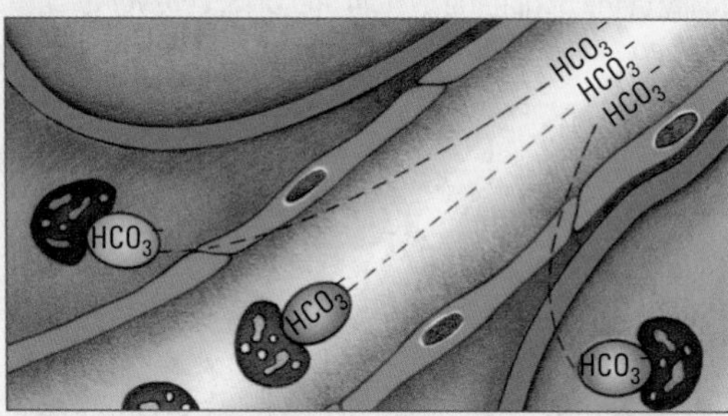

2. Excess HCO_3^- that doesn't bind with chemical buffers elevates serum pH levels, which in turn depresses chemoreceptors in the medulla. Depression of those chemoreceptors causes a decrease in the respiratory rate, which increases $Paco_2$. The additional carbon dioxide (CO_2) combines with water (H_2O) to form carbonic acid (H_2CO_3). *Note:* Lowered oxygen levels limit respiratory compensation. *Look for a serum pH level above 7.45; an HCO_3^- level above 26 mEq/L; a rising $Paco_2$; and slow, shallow respirations.*

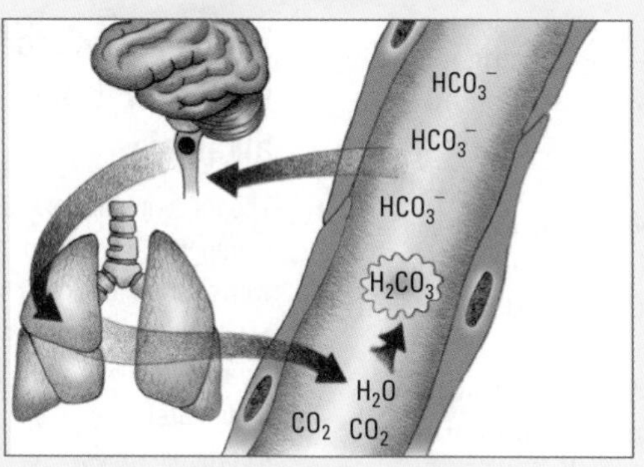

3. When the HCO_3^- level exceeds 28 mEq/L, the renal glomeruli can no longer reabsorb excess amounts. The excess HCO_3^- is excreted in urine; hydrogen ions (H^+) are retained. *Look for alkaline urine and pH and HCO_3^- levels that slowly return to normal.*

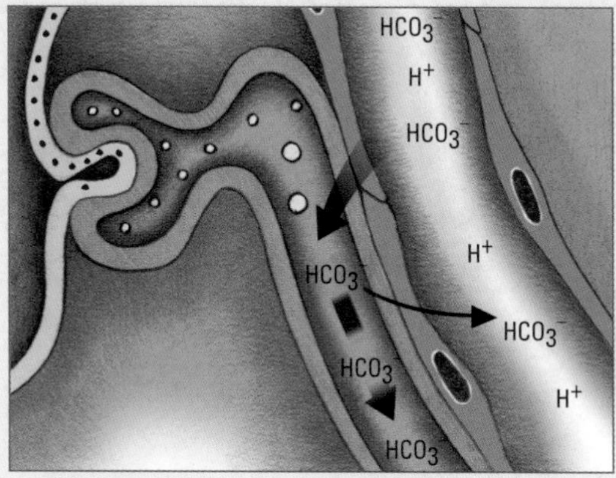

4. To maintain electrochemical balance, the kidneys excrete excess sodium ions (Na), H_2O, and HCO_3^-. *Look for polyuria initially, then signs and symptoms of hypovolemia, including thirst and dry mucous membranes.*

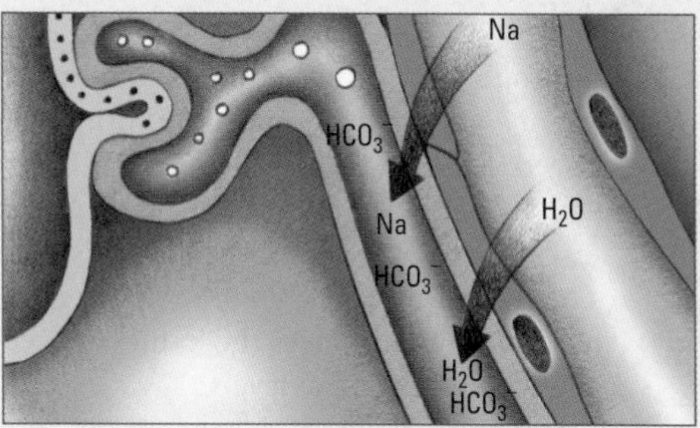

(continued)

What happens in metabolic alkalosis *(continued)*

5. Lowered H^+ levels in the extracellular fluid causes the ions to diffuse out of the cells. To maintain the balance of charge across the cell membrane, extracellular potassium ions (K) move into the cells. *Look for signs and symptoms of hypokalemia, including anorexia, muscle weakness, and loss of reflexes.*

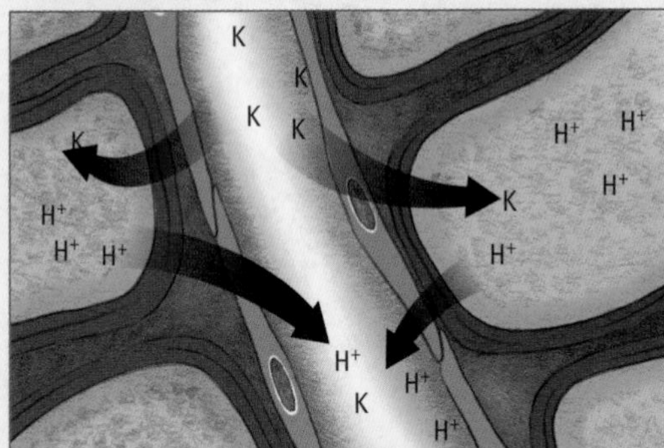

6. As H^+ levels decline, calcium (Ca) ionization decreases. That decrease in ionization makes nerve cells more permeable to Na. The movement of Na into nerve cells stimulates neural impulses and produces overexcitability of the peripheral system and CNS. *Look for tetany, belligerence, irritability, disorientation, and seizures.*

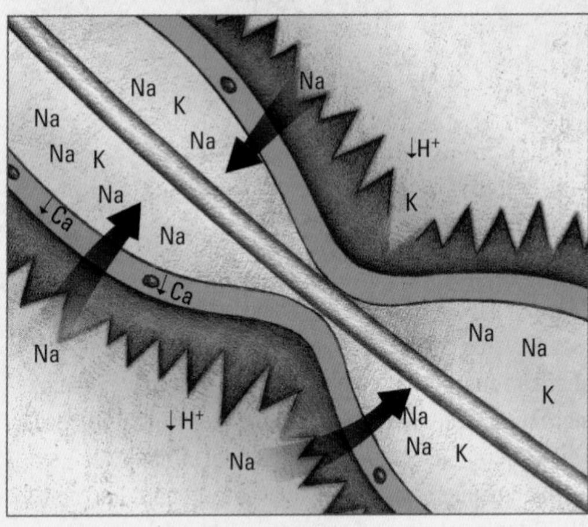

More metabolic mishaps

Cushing's disease can lead to metabolic alkalosis by causing retention of sodium and chloride and urinary loss of potassium and hydrogen. Rebound alkalosis following correction of organic acidosis, such as after cardiac arrest and administration of sodium bicarbonate, can also cause metabolic alkalosis. Posthypercapnic alkalosis occurs when chronic carbon dioxide retention is corrected by mechanical ventilation and the kidneys haven't yet corrected the chronically high bicarbonate levels.

Metabolic alkalosis can also result from kidney disease, such as renal artery stenosis, or from multiple transfusions. Certain drugs, such as corticosteroids and antacids that contain sodium bicarbonate, can also lead to metabolic alkalosis. (See *Drugs associated with metabolic alkalosis.*) Continuous NG tube suction can also cause metabolic alkalosis due to the removal of acid and electrolytes.

Drugs associated with metabolic alkalosis

The following drugs are commonly associated with metabolic alkalosis:

- antacids (sodium bicarbonate, calcium carbonate)
- corticosteroids
- thiazide and loop diuretics.

What to look for

Initially, your patient may have slow, shallow respirations as hypoventilation, a compensatory mechanism, occurs. However, this mechanism is limited because hypoxemia soon develops, which stimulates ventilation. The signs and symptoms of metabolic alkalosis are commonly associated with an underlying condition. Characteristic hypokalemic or hypocalcemic ECG changes may occur, as well as signs of hypotension.

A neurologic nightmare

Metabolic alkalosis results in neuromuscular excitability, which causes muscle twitching, weakness, and tetany. The patient develops hyperactive reflexes. He may also experience numbness and tingling of the fingers, toes, and mouth area. Neurologic symptoms include apathy and confusion. Seizures, stupor, and coma may result if severe.

Keep track of these tracts

If hypokalemia affects the GI tract, the patient is likely to experience anorexia, nausea, and vomiting. If it affects the genitourinary (GU) tract—that is, if the kidneys are affected—polyuria may result. If left untreated, metabolic alkalosis can result in arrhythmias and death. (See *Signs and symptoms of metabolic alkalosis*.)

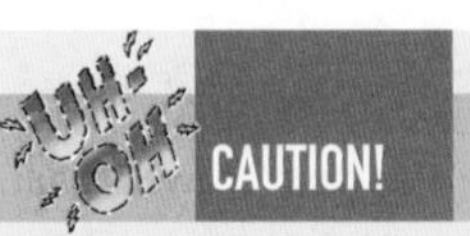

Signs and symptoms of metabolic alkalosis

The following assessment findings commonly occur in patients with metabolic alkalosis:

- anorexia
- apathy
- confusion
- cyanosis
- hypotension
- loss of reflexes
- muscle twitching
- nausea
- paresthesia
- polyuria
- vomiting
- weakness
- seizures
- coma.

What tests show

These tests may be helpful in the diagnosis and treatment of metabolic alkalosis:

- ABG analysis may reveal a blood pH above 7.45 and a bicarbonate level above 26 mEq/L. If the underlying cause is excessive acid loss, the bicarbonate level may be normal. The $Pa{CO_2}$ level may be above 45 mm Hg, indicating respiratory compensation. (See *ABG results in metabolic alkalosis*, page 226.)
- Serum electrolyte levels usually indicate low potassium, calcium, and chloride levels. Bicarbonate levels are elevated.
- ECG changes may occur, such as a low T wave that merges with the P wave.

ABG results in metabolic alkalosis

This chart shows typical ABG findings in uncompensated and compensated metabolic alkalosis.

	Uncompensated	Compensated
pH	> 7.45	Normal
$Paco_2$ (mm Hg)	Normal	> 45
Bicarbonate (mEq/L)	> 26 or normal	> 26 or normal

How it's treated

Treatment aims to correct the acid-base imbalance by providing the patient's body sufficient time to rid itself of excess bicarbonate and increase its hydrogen concentration. Treatment may include:

- I.V. administration of ammonium chloride or arginine monohydrochloride; rarely done but sometimes necessary in severe cases
- discontinuation of thiazide diuretics and NG suctioning
- administration of an antiemetic to treat underlying nausea and vomiting
- addition of acetazolamide (Diamox) to inhibit calcium and increase renal excretion of bicarbonate.

How you intervene

If your patient is at risk for metabolic alkalosis, careful monitoring can help prevent its development.

If your patient already has metabolic alkalosis, follow these guidelines:

- Monitor vital signs, including cardiac rhythm and respiratory pattern.
- Assess the patient's LOC when taking the health history or by talking with the patient while you're performing the physical examination. For instance, apathy and confusion may be evident in a patient's conversation.
- Administer oxygen as ordered to treat hypoxemia.

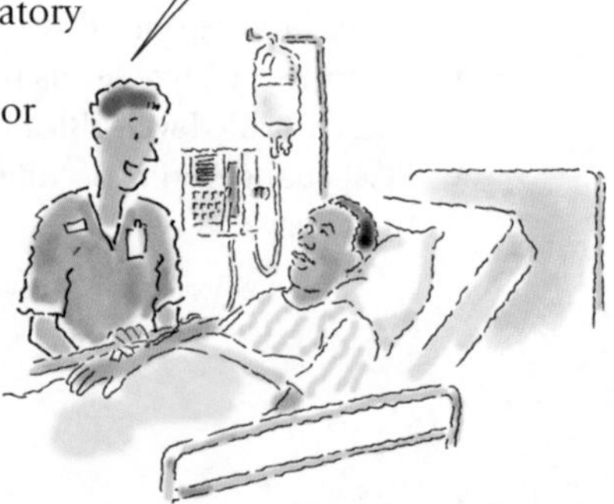
In a patient with metabolic alkalosis, assess LOC when taking the health history or performing the physical exam.

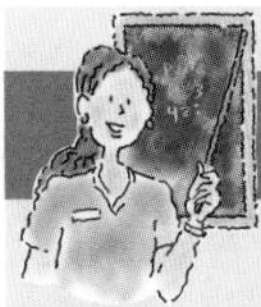

Teaching points

Teaching about metabolic alkalosis

When teaching a patient with metabolic alkalosis, be sure to cover the following topics and then evaluate your patient's learning:

- basics of the condition and its treatment
- need to avoid overuse of alkaline agents and diuretics
- prescribed medications, especially adverse effects of potassium-wasting diuretics or potassium chloride supplements
- warning signs and symptoms and when to report them.

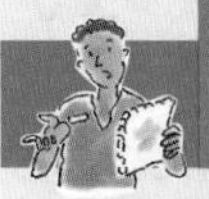

Chart smart

Documenting metabolic alkalosis

If your patient has metabolic alkalosis, make sure you document the following information:

- vital signs
- I.V. therapy
- interventions and the patient's response
- medications
- intake and output
- oxygen therapy
- notification of the practitioner
- safety measures
- serum electrolyte levels and ABG results
- patient teaching performed and the patient's response.

- Institute seizure precautions when needed, and explain them to the patient and family. (See *Teaching about metabolic alkalosis*.)
- Maintain patent I.V. access as ordered.
- Administer diluted potassium solutions with an infusion device.
- Monitor intake and output. (See *Documenting metabolic alkalosis*.)
- Infuse 0.9% ammonium chloride no faster than 1 L over 4 hours. Faster administration may cause hemolysis of red blood cells. Don't administer the drug to a patient who has hepatic or renal disease.
- Irrigate an NG tube with normal saline solution instead of tap water to prevent loss of gastric electrolytes.
- Assess laboratory test results, such as ABG and serum electrolyte levels. Notify the practitioner of any changes.
- Watch closely for signs of muscle weakness, tetany, or decreased activity.

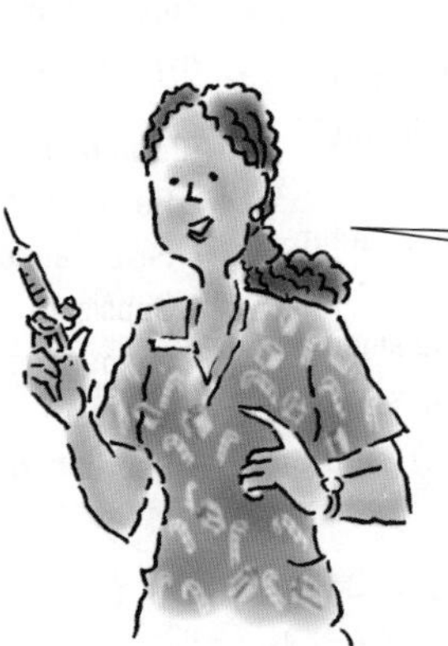
Every little bit helps. Irrigating NG tubes with normal saline solution instead of tap water helps prevent loss of gastric electrolytes.

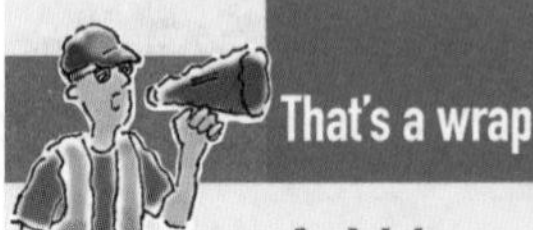

That's a wrap!

Acid-base imbalances review

Acid-base basics

- Acid-base balance depends on the regulation of free hydrogen ions.
- Balance is maintained by chemical buffers, respiratory reactions, and kidney reactions.
- ABG analysis is the major diagnostic tool for evaluating acid-base states:
  - pH: determines the extent of acidity or alkalinity, both of which are measured
  - $Paco_2$: reflects the adequacy of ventilation by the lungs
  - Bicarbonate level: reflects the activity of the kidneys in retaining or excreting bicarbonate.
- If hydrogen ion concentration increases, pH decreases (acidosis).
- If hydrogen ion concentration decreases, pH increases (alkalosis).

Respiratory acidosis

- Results from compromise in breathing
- Characterized by alveolar hypoventilation (body can't get rid of carbon dioxide)
- Leads to hypercapnia

Causes

- Hypoventilation from CNS trauma or tumor that depresses the respiratory center
- Neuromuscular disorders that affect respiratory drive
- Lung diseases that decrease amount of surface area available for gas exchange
- Airway obstruction
- Chest wall trauma
- Drugs that depress the respiratory center

Treatment

- Ventilation, bronchodilator, supplemental oxygen, and chest physiotherapy
- Antibiotics to treat infection
- Drug therapy to treat hyperkalemia
- Removal of foreign bodies from airway if needed
- Pain management

Respiratory alkalosis

- Occurs when carbon dioxide elimination increases

Causes

- Conditions that increase respiratory rate and depth
- Hyperventilation
- Hypercapnia
- Hypermetabolic states
- Liver failure
- Certain drugs
- Conditions that affect the brain's respiratory control center
- Acute hypoxia secondary to high altitude, pulmonary disease, severe anemia, pulmonary embolus, and hypotension

Treatment

- Removal of causative agent
- Fever reduction
- Sepsis treatment
- Oxygen therapy (if acute hypoxemia is the cause)
- Rebreathing exhaled carbon dioxide

(continued)

Acid-base imbalances review *(continued)*

Metabolic acidosis
- Occurs when hydrogen production increases
- Depresses the CNS and, if untreated, may lead to ventricular arrhythmias, coma, and cardiac arrest

Causes
- Loss of bicarbonate (base)
- Accumulation of metabolic acids (acid)
- Overproduction of ketone bodies
- Decreased ability of kidneys to excrete acids
- Excessive GI losses from diarrhea, intestinal malabsorption, or urinary diversion to ileum
- Hyperaldosteronism
- Use of potassium-sparing diuretics
- Poisoning or toxic drug reaction

Treatment
- Correction of acidosis as quickly as possible
- Respiratory compensation (mechanical ventilation if needed)
- Rapid-acting insulin (for diabetics)
- I.V. bicarbonate and I.V. fluids
- Dialysis (for patients with renal failure)

Metabolic alkalosis
- Commonly associated with hypokalemia
- Results from decrease in hydrogen production, a gain in bicarbonate, or both

Causes
- Excessive acid loss from the GI tract
- Diuretic therapy (kidney loss of hydrogen, potassium, and chloride)
- Cushing's disease (from sodium and chloride retention and potassium and hydrogen excretion)

Treatment
- I.V. fluids and acetazolamide to increase renal excretion
- Correction of underlying acid-base imbalance
- Discontinuation of thiazide diuretics and NG suctioning

For severe cases
- I.V. ammonia chloride

This chart shows pH, $Paco_2$, and bicarbonate values in respiratory and metabolic alkalosis and acidosis.

Acid-base imbalance	pH	$Paco_2$	Bicarbonate
Acute respiratory acidosis	Decreased	Increased	Normal
Chronic respiratory acidosis (with compensation)	Normal	Increased	Increased
Acute respiratory alkalosis	Increased	Decreased	Normal
Chronic respiratory alkalosis (with compensation)	Normal	Decreased	Decreased
Acute metabolic acidosis	Decreased	Normal	Decreased
Chronic metabolic acidosis (with compensation)	Normal	Decreased	Decreased
Acute metabolic alkalosis	Increased	Normal	Normal or increased
Chronic metabolic alkalosis	Normal	Increased	Normal or increased

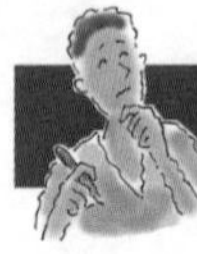

Quick quiz

1. The body compensates for chronic respiratory alkalosis by:
   A. increasing excretion of bicarbonate.
   B. decreasing excretion of bicarbonate.
   C. increasing $Paco_2$.
   D. decreasing $Paco_2$.

Answer: A. When hypocapnia lasts more than 6 hours, the body develops metabolic acidosis and the kidneys compensate by increasing excretion of bicarbonate and reducing excretion of hydrogen ions. Hydrogen ions return to the blood to decrease pH, causing chemoreceptors in the medulla to decrease the respiratory rate.

2. You're taking care of a patient with obesity-hypoventilation syndrome. You expect to see signs of chronic respiratory acidosis in the patient's ABG results. What do you look for?
   A. Increasing pH
   B. Increased $Paco_2$
   C. Increased bicarbonate
   D. Decreased bicarbonate

Answer: C. As respiratory mechanisms fail, the body compensates by using the increased $Paco_2$ to excrete hydrogen and to stimulate the kidneys to retain bicarbonate and sodium ions. As a result, more sodium bicarbonate (thus an increased bicarbonate) is available to buffer free hydrogen ions (metabolic alkalosis). Ammonium ions are also excreted to remove hydrogen.

3. If your patient's NG tube is attached to suction, you know the patient may develop metabolic alkalosis. You expect that his ABG results will show:
   A. decreased pH, increased $Paco_2$, and decreased bicarbonate.
   B. increased pH, increased $Paco_2$, and increased bicarbonate.
   C. decreased pH, decreased $Paco_2$, and decreased bicarbonate.
   D. increased pH, decreased $Paco_2$, and no change in bicarbonate.

Answer: B. Metabolic acidosis is caused by a loss in hydrogen ion production and a gain in bicarbonate, causing increased pH and bicarbonate levels. If respiratory compensation occurs, $Paco_2$ will increase above 45 mm Hg.

4. When assessing a patient with DKA, you detect Kussmaul's respirations. You realize the body is in:
   A. respiratory alkalosis with compensation.
   B. respiratory acidosis with compensation.
   C. metabolic alkalosis with compensation.
   D. metabolic acidosis with compensation.

Answer: D. A patient with DKA will develop metabolic acidosis. When excess hydrogen can't be buffered, the hydrogen reduces blood pH and stimulates chemoreceptors in the medulla, which in turn increases the respiratory rate (leading to respiratory alkalosis). This mechanism lowers carbon dioxide levels and allows more hydrogen to bind with bicarbonate.

5. In a patient with COPD, the primary imbalance is likely to be:
   A. respiratory alkalosis.
   B. respiratory acidosis.
   C. metabolic alkalosis.
   D. metabolic acidosis.

Answer: B. COPD results in destruction of the alveoli, thereby decreasing the surface area of the lungs available for gas exchange. With alveolar ventilation decreased, the $Paco_2$ increases. The carbon dioxide combines with water to form excessive amounts of carbonic acid. The carbonic acid dissociates to release free hydrogen and bicarbonate ions, thereby decreasing the pH (respiratory acidosis).

6. Your bedridden patient has these ABG results: pH, 7.5; $Paco_2$, 26 mm Hg; bicarbonate, 24 mEq/L. He's dyspneic and has a swollen right calf. The patient most likely is suffering from:
   A. a pulmonary embolus.
   B. heart failure.
   C. dehydration.
   D. hyperaldosteronism.

Answer: A. Unexplained respiratory alkalosis may mean a pulmonary embolus (in this case, most likely a thrombus in the leg as a result of immobility).

7. If administering dopamine to a patient with hypotension proves ineffective, how should you proceed?
   A. Change to dobutamine.
   B. Investigate the patient's pH.
   C. Check the patient's serum potassium level.
   D. Increase the rate of dopamine infusion.

Answer: B. If you're administering dopamine to a patient and it isn't elevating his blood pressure as you expected, you should investigate the patient's pH. A pH level below 7.1 causes resistance to vasopressor therapy.

8. Before and after you administer sodium bicarbonate, you should flush the I.V. line with:
   A. heparin.
   B. sterile water.
   C. normal saline solution.
   D. potassium.

Answer: C. You should flush the I.V. line with normal saline solution before and after giving bicarbonate.

Scoring

☆☆☆ If you answered all eight questions correctly, wow! Test the pH of the nearest pool, and jump in for a refreshing swim!

☆☆ If you answered five to seven correctly, excellent! You're just about ready to do your first solo balancing act!

☆ If you answered fewer than five correctly, take heart. You're still a boffo buffer in our book. (*Buffer*, get it? For chemical buffers? Oh well, can't win 'em all.)

References

Bronfenbrenner, R. (2013). *Acid-base interpretation*. Retrieved from http://emedicine.medscape.com/article/2058760-overview

Lippincott's visual nursing: A guide to disease skills and treatment (2nd ed.). (2012). Philadelphia, PA: Lippincott Williams & Wilkins.

Williamson, M. A., & Snyder, L. M. (2009). *Wallach's interpretation of diagnostic tests* (9th ed.). Philadelphia, PA: Lippincott Williams & Wilkins.

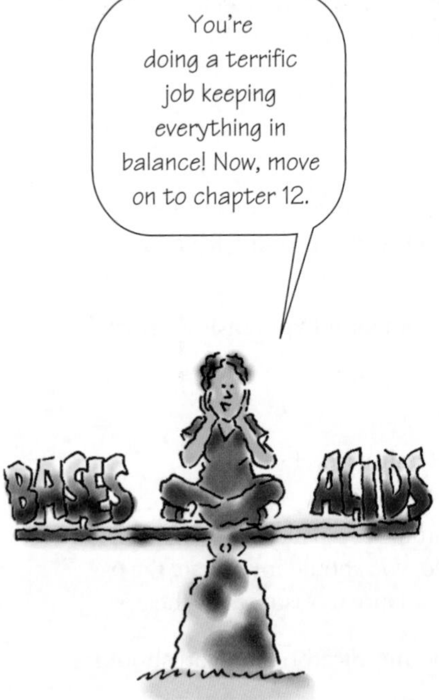
You're doing a terrific job keeping everything in balance! Now, move on to chapter 12.
BASES
ACIDS

Part III

Disorders that cause imbalances

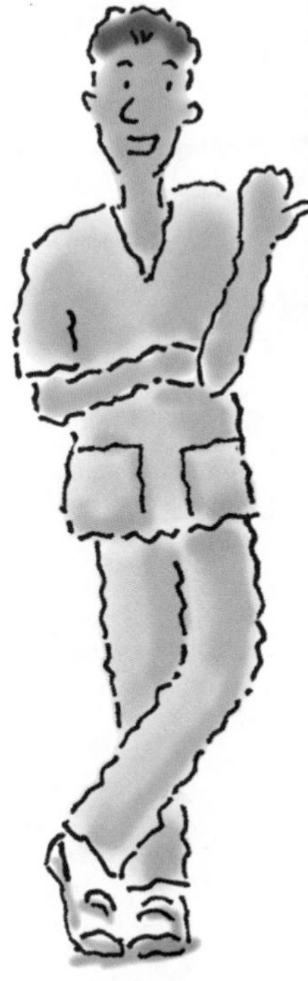

Chapter 12

Heat-related health alterations

Just the facts

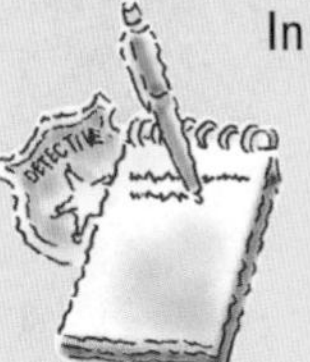

In this chapter, you'll learn:

- the differences among the five types of heat-related health alterations
- signs and symptoms of heat-related health alterations
- proper ways to manage heat-related health alterations.

A look at heat-related health alterations

Heat-related health alterations are a major cause of preventable deaths worldwide, especially in regions with high temperatures. Heat-related health alterations develop when the body can't offset its rising temperature, thus retaining too much heat (hyperthermia). When the body gets too hot too quickly (temperature above 99° F [37.2° C]), heat-related health alterations occur.

Just cool it!

Although the body initially tries to cool itself down when it's exposed to too much heat, the mechanisms that regulate body heat can fail if the stress becomes too great. Normally, the body adjusts to excessive temperatures through complex cardiovascular and neurologic changes coordinated by the hypothalamus. Heat loss offsets heat production to regulate body temperature.

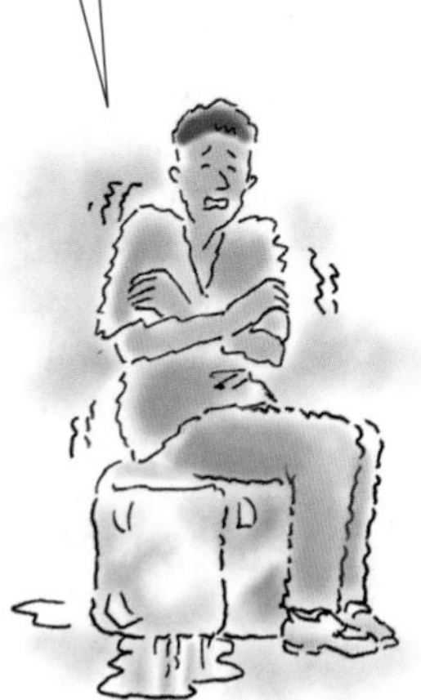

If the body can't cool itself quickly enough, a heat-related health alteration may occur. This may not have been the best way to cool down . . .

To and fro

Heat transfer to and from the body occurs in four ways:

1. *Conduction* is the transfer of heat through direct physical contact and accounts for less than 2% of the body's heat loss.
2. In *convection,* heat is transferred from the body to the air and water vapor surrounding the body. It accounts for less than 10% of the body's heat loss. When air temperature is higher than body temperature, the body gains heat energy.
3. *Radiation* is the transfer of heat via electromagnetic waves and accounts for most heat loss. As long as the air temperature is less

than the body temperature, about 65% of the body's heat is lost by radiation.

4. In *evaporation*, heat is transferred when a liquid changes into a vapor. It accounts for about 30% of the body's heat loss.

If you can't take the heat . . .

In hot temperatures, the body loses heat mainly by radiation and evaporation. However, when air temperature is higher than 95° F (35° C), radiation of heat from the body stops and evaporation becomes the only means of heat loss.

When air temperatures increase and a person is exercising, he can sweat 1 to 2 L every hour. However, if humidity reaches 100%, evaporation of sweat is no longer possible and the body loses its ability to lose heat.

How they happen

Sweat is the body's main way to get rid of extra heat. When a person sweats, water evaporates from the skin. The heat that makes this evaporation possible comes from the heat created by blood flowing through the skin. As long as blood is flowing properly, extra heat from the core of the body is "pumped" to the skin and removed by sweat evaporation.

Weather forecast

The effectiveness of sweat sometimes depends on the weather. If the air is humid, it's harder for sweat to evaporate. This means it's easier to sweat (and for the body to rid itself of excess heat) when it's relatively dry than when it's humid.

Don't sweat the small stuff

Because the evaporation that occurs during sweating causes water loss, it's important for a person to drink water when sweating. If the body doesn't have enough water, dehydration can occur. This condition makes it harder for the body to cool itself because less water is available for the body to use during evaporation.

Heat-related health alterations are easy to prevent with adequate hydration. Discuss with your patients the importance of drinking water, especially when exerting themselves in hot weather (U.S. Department of Labor, n.d.).

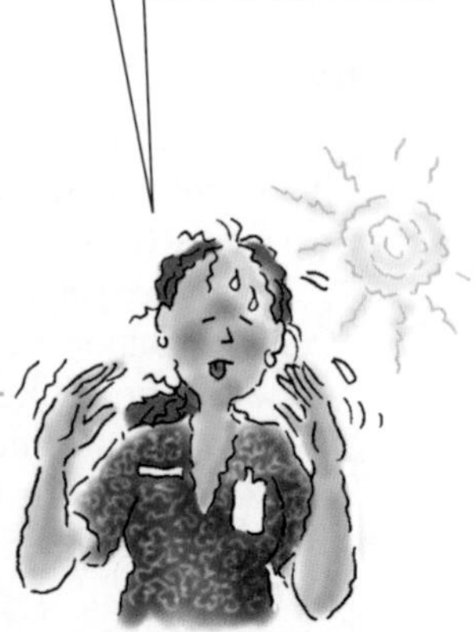

It's important to drink water and other nonalcoholic fluids when you're sweating this much! It could be the key to preventing heat-related health alterations.

What causes them

Heat-related health alterations result when the body's production of heat increases at a faster rate than the body's ability to dissipate it (heat loss). Heat production increases with exercise, fever, infection, and the use of certain drugs, such as amphetamines. Heat loss decreases with high temperatures or humidity, lack of acclimatization, lack of air conditioning or proper ventilation, excess clothing, obesity, decreased fluid intake, dehydration, extensive burns, cardiovascular disease, skin diseases, sweat gland dysfunction, endocrine disorders (such as hyperthyroidism, diabetes, and pheochromocytoma), ingestion of alcohol, and use of certain medications. (See *Drugs that can cause heat-related health alterations*.)

When the body uses all its tricks and still can't keep its temperature down, the excess heat is retained and heat-related health alterations can develop.

Drugs that can cause heat-related health alterations

Drugs that may cause decreased heat loss include:

- anticholinergics
- antihistamines
- beta-adrenergic blockers
- cyclic antidepressants
- diuretics
- ethanol
- lithium
- phenothiazines
- salicylates
- sympathomimetics (e.g., cocaine and amphetamines) that cause vasodilation.

Types of heat-related health alterations

Heat-related health alterations fall into five categories: heat rash, heat cramps, heat exhaustion, heat syncope, and heatstroke.

Heat rash

Heat rash is a skin irritation that can develop from excessive sweating during hot weather. It is usually found on the neck or upper torso, or in skin folds such as the axillae, groin, or breast creases, and looks like red pimples or tiny blisters.

Heat cramps

Heat cramps are muscle contractions that typically occur in the gastrocnemius or hamstring muscles. These painful contractions are caused by a deficiency of water and sodium and are generally attributed to dehydration and poor muscle conditioning. Cramps usually occur after exertion in high temperatures (> 100° F [37.8° C]) with profuse sweating and water intake without adequate electrolyte replacement. Heat cramps are common in manual laborers, athletes, and skiers who overdress for the cold as well as in those who aren't used to hot, dry climates in which excessive sweating is almost undetected because of rapid evaporation. Symptoms usually improve with rest, water consumption, and a cool environment.

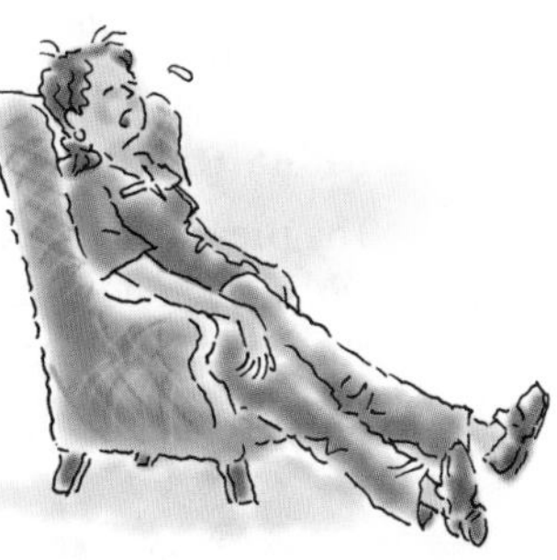

Heat exhaustion can really make a person feel exhausted!

Heat exhaustion

Heat exhaustion is caused by heat and fluid loss from excessive sweating without fluid replacement. Rest, water, ice packs, and a cool environment may help in mild heat exhaustion. More severely exhausted patients may need I.V. fluids, especially if vomiting keeps them from drinking enough. Circulatory collapse may occur if this condition isn't promptly treated.

Heat syncope

Heat syncope (fainting or dizziness) occurs when a patient stands up quickly or has been standing for a prolonged period of time. Dehydration is often to blame for heat syncope.

Heatstroke

Heatstroke, also known as *sunstroke,* is the most severe form of heat-related health alteration. It commonly occurs in patients who exercise in hot weather.

Elderly patients and patients taking certain medications are also at risk for heatstroke in hot weather, even in the absence of exercise. Signs to look for include warm, flushed skin and lack of sweating. Some patients may have symptoms that resemble a regular stroke, such as slurred speech, bizarre behavior, confusion, or dizziness. (Athletes who have heatstroke after vigorous exercise in hot weather may still sweat considerably.)

Whether exercise-related or not, a person with heatstroke usually has a very high temperature (104° F [40° C] or higher) and may be delirious or unconscious or having seizures.

Cool moves

Patients suffering from heatstroke need to have their temperature reduced quickly (often with ice packs) and must also be given I.V. fluids for rehydration. Because many body organs can fail in heatstroke, patients are typically hospitalized for observation. The body's attempt to regulate its temperature during heat-related health alterations causes a loss of excessive amounts of water and electrolytes. These must be replaced to counteract the hyperthermia. Extremely high body temperature may damage tissues, including muscle and brain tissues, and may lead to permanent disability and even death.

What to look for

Signs and symptoms of heat-related health alterations vary depending on the severity of the syndrome. (See *Signs and symptoms of heat-related health alterations.*)

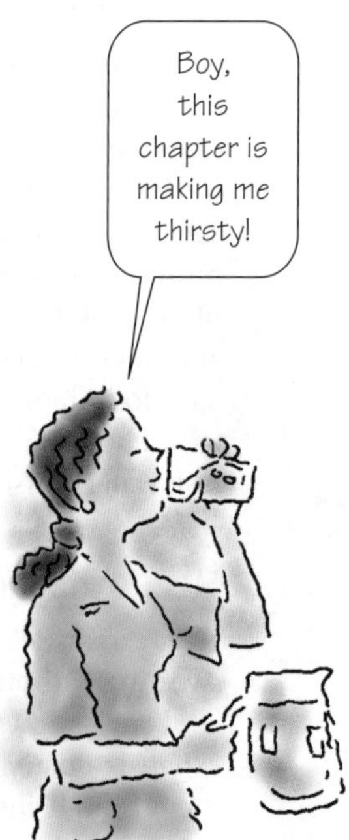
Boy, this chapter is making me thirsty!

Risks of heat-related health alterations

The presence of certain fluid and electrolyte imbalances is associated with increased risk of heat-related health alterations. These imbalances include dehydration, hyponatremia, and hypokalemia.

Signs and symptoms of heat-related health alterations

Heat-related health alterations may be classified as mild (heat cramps or heat rash), moderate (heat exhaustion or heat syncope), or critical (heatstroke). This table highlights the major assessment findings associated with each classification.

Classification	Assessment findings
Mild hyperthermia Heat rash Heat cramps	• Red pimples or tiny blisters on upper torso or in skin folds (*heat rash only*) • Mild agitation (central nervous system findings otherwise normal) • Mild hypertension • Moist, cool skin and muscle tenderness; involved muscle groups possibly hard and lumpy • Muscle twitching and spasms • Nausea and abdominal cramps • Report of prolonged activity in a very warm or hot environment without adequate salt intake • Tachycardia • Temperature ranging from 99° to 102° F (37.2° to 38.9° C)
Moderate hyperthermia Heat exhaustion Heat syncope	• Dizziness • Headache • Hypotension • Muscle cramping • Nausea and vomiting • Oliguria • Pale, moist skin • Rapid, thready pulse • Syncope or confusion • Temperature elevated up to 104° F (40° C) • Thirst • Weakness
Critical hyperthermia Heatstroke	• Atrial or ventricular tachycardia • Confusion, combativeness, and delirium • Bizarre behavior • Fixed, dilated pupils • Hot, dry, reddened skin • Loss of consciousness • Seizures • Tachypnea • Temperature greater than 104° F (40° C)

Dry idea

Signs and symptoms of dehydration include thirst; dry mucous membranes; hot, dry skin; decreased urine output; confusion; dizziness; postural hypotension; tachycardia; and eventually anhidrosis (absence of sweating).

Pass the salt, please

Signs and symptoms of hyponatremia (decreased serum sodium levels) include lethargy, nausea and vomiting, muscle cramps and weakness, muscle twitching, and seizures.

Special K

Signs and symptoms of hypokalemia (decreased serum potassium levels) include fatigue, paresthesia, hypoactive reflexes, ileus, cardiac arrhythmias, and electrocardiogram changes (flattened T waves, the development of U waves, ST-segment depression, and prolonged PR intervals).

Who's at risk?

Patients who are most at risk for fluid and electrolyte loss with heat-related illness include elderly people, young children, people with chronic and debilitating diseases, those not acclimated to heat, alcoholics, and people taking certain medications (such as anticholinergics, diuretics, and beta-adrenergic blockers). (See *Age-related heat-related health alteration risk.*) Fluid and electrolyte loss also occurs in healthy people who work or exercise in extreme heat and humidity and in those who don't increase their fluid intake accordingly. Football players are prone to heat-related health alterations because their uniforms cover nearly all of the body and practice usually begins in late summer, when the temperature outside is highest. Athletes should pay careful attention to the fluids they drink and lose and should wear lightweight clothing when possible.

What tests show

These test results can help diagnose heat-related health alterations and determine their severity:

- Serum sodium and potassium levels will be decreased.
- Urine specific gravity will be increased.
- Alanine transaminase levels will be elevated (almost universal in heatstroke).

Other laboratory tests are used to detect end-organ damage (especially in patients with heatstroke) or to rule out other disorders.

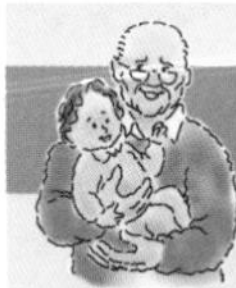

Ages and stages

Age-related heat-related health alteration risk

With aging, an individual's thirst mechanism and ability to sweat decrease. These factors put elderly patients at risk for heat-related health alterations, especially during hot summer days.

Heatstroke is a medical emergency and must be treated rapidly to prevent serious complications or death. To help prevent heatstroke, teach your older patient to follow these instructions:

- Reduce activity in hot weather, especially outdoor activity.
- Wear lightweight, loose-fitting clothing during hot weather; when outdoors, wear a hat and sunglasses and avoid wearing dark colors that absorb sunlight.
- Drink plenty of fluids, especially water, and avoid tea, coffee, and alcohol because they can cause dehydration.
- Stay inside when possible, and use air conditioning or open windows (making sure that a secure screen is in place). Teach the patient to use a fan to help circulate air. (If the patient doesn't have air conditioning at home, suggest that he or she goes to community resources that have air conditioning during periods of excessive heat, such as senior centers, libraries, and churches. Some community centers may even provide transportation for the patient.)

Little ones, too

Neonates are also at increased risk for heat-related health alterations. In part, this is due to their bodies' poorly developed heat-regulating abilities.

How they're treated

The goal of treatment for heat-related health alterations is to lower the patient's body temperature as quickly as possible. Elderly patients may require more aggressive treatment and should be evaluated for even the mildest cases of heat-related health alterations.

For heat rash

Patients can avoid heat rash by staying in cool environments with low humidity whenever possible. Treatment of heat rash includes keeping the affected area dry and powdering with corn starch to decrease discomfort.

For heat cramps

Hospitalization for heat cramps is rare, and the signs and symptoms are usually self-limiting. Treatment includes rest, intake of electrolyte-rich fluids (sports drinks), and ingestion of salty foods. Clothing can be removed or loosened, and stretching or direct pressure on the muscles may decrease cramping. If the patient can't eat or drink, he may need an I.V. infusion of normal saline solution (U.S. Department of Labor, n.d.).

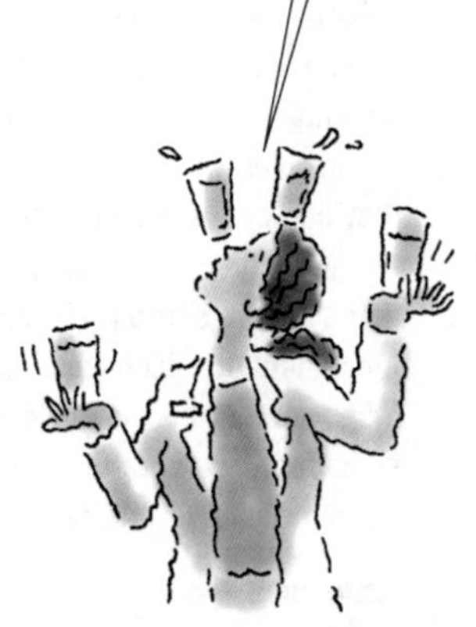
Treatment of heat-related health alterations involves more than just balancing fluids.

For heat exhaustion

Hospitalization usually isn't necessary for heat exhaustion. It's typically treated by having the patient rest in a cool location and drink water, slightly salty fluids, or electrolyte-rich sports drinks every few minutes. Clothing can be removed or loosened and the feet can be elevated 12″ (30.5 cm). For severe cases, isotonic I.V. fluids may be given if available and if necessary. Rarely, cardiac stimulants and plasma volume expanders (such as albumin and dextran) are given; these should be used cautiously to avoid volume overload. Untreated heat exhaustion may lead to heatstroke (Centers for Disease Control and Prevention, 2014; U.S. Department of Labor, n.d.).

For heat syncope

Teach your patients to avoid heat syncope by staying hydrated, remaining in cooler environments when possible, and to immediately sit or lie down if they begin to feel light-headed.

Depending on the circumstances, patients who experience heat syncope may need hospitalization or medical attention, particularly if they have sustained an injury during the syncopal episode (U.S. Department of Labor, n.d.).

For heatstroke

Hospitalization or immediate medical attention is required for patients with heatstroke. Treatment focuses on cooling the body as quickly as possible. Ice packs should be placed on the patient's neck, armpits, and groin. He should remain undressed and should be sponged with water, sprayed with tepid water, or dabbed with wet towels. A fan may also be used to blow cool air over the patient. This causes evaporative cooling—the best cooling method for patients with heatstroke. He'll also need cool I.V. fluids. Other ways to support the cooling process may include oxygen therapy and, in severe cases, endotracheal intubation. If the patient has uncontrollable seizures, he'll need I.V. diazepam and barbiturates (Centers for Disease Control and Prevention, 2014; U.S. Department of Labor, n.d.).

Beating the heat—carefully

Other options for cooling the patient include covering him with ice and immersing him in an ice bath. Although effective at rapidly lowering body temperature, these methods can create complications such as peripheral vasoconstriction, which can lead to less heat dissipation. These techniques also are uncomfortable for the patient, limit the ability to monitor the patient's vital signs and cardiac status, may result in hypothermia, and eventually may cause the patient to shiver. Shivering slows the cooling process because it increases core body temperature.

Say no to (these) drugs

For all types of heat-related health alterations, patients shouldn't take salicylates to decrease body temperature because salicylates increase the risk of coagulopathy. Patients shouldn't also take acetaminophen because it doesn't reduce body temperature during heat-related health alterations. Taking acetaminophen may actually worsen existing hepatic damage because the liver metabolizes acetaminophen.

How you intervene

Treatment of heat-related health alterations requires frequent monitoring of laboratory values (central venous and pulmonary wedge pressures), instituting rehydration measures, replacing sodium and potassium, and starting cooling measures to decrease body temperature. Also institute the interventions discussed here.

For heat-related health alterations

- Replace fluid and electrolytes by encouraging fluid intake with a balanced electrolyte drink; give salt tablets.
- Loosen the patient's clothing.
- Ask the patient to lie down in a cool place.
- Massage his muscles.
- If heat cramps are severe, start an I.V. infusion with normal saline solution.
- If the patient has heat exhaustion, he may require oxygen administration.

For heatstroke

- Initiate the ABCs (airway, breathing, and circulation) of life support.
- Quickly lower the patient's body temperature using hypothermia blankets and ice packs on arterial pressure points.
- Monitor the patient's temperature continuously. Temperatures shouldn't be allowed to fall below 101° F (38.3° C) or the patient may develop hypothermia.
- Replace fluids and electrolytes I.V.
- When necessary, give diazepam to control seizures, chlorpromazine I.V. to reduce shivering, or mannitol I.V. to maintain urine output as ordered.

- Insert a nasogastric tube to prevent aspiration as ordered.
- Monitor temperature, intake, output, and cardiac status. Assist with the insertion of a central venous catheter or a pulmonary artery catheter. Give dobutamine I.V. to correct cardiogenic shock. Vasoconstrictors shouldn't be used. (See *Documenting heat-related health alterations.*)
- Avoid stimulants and sedatives.
- Encourage bed rest for a few days.
- Warn the patient that his temperature may fluctuate for weeks.

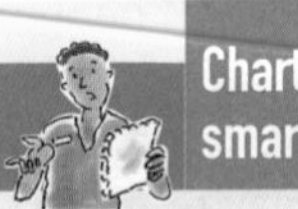

Chart smart

Documenting heat-related health alterations

If your patient has a heat-related health alteration, make sure you document the following information:

- prescribed medications
- cooling procedures and their effect
- intake and output
- level of consciousness
- cardiac output
- vital signs
- heart sounds
- lung sounds
- central venous pressure and pulmonary artery wedge pressure if central line in place
- oxygen administration
- patient teaching.

Preventing heat-related health alterations

Prevention of heat-related health alterations is possible. By encouraging your patient to keep well hydrated and be sensible about exertion in hot, humid weather, you're helping him to stay on the right track. Remember to tell him that water is the best fluid to drink when he's sweating, not an electrolyte drink. (See *Teaching about heat-related health alterations.*)

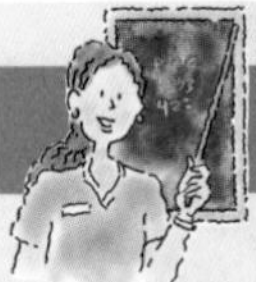

Teaching points

Teaching about heat-related health alterations

Heat-related health alterations are easily preventable, so it's important to educate individuals about the various factors that cause them. This information is especially vital for athletes, laborers, and soldiers in field training. Be sure to follow these guidelines when performing patient teaching:

- Advise patients to take these precautions in hot weather: rest frequently, avoid hot places, drink adequate fluids, and wear loose-fitting, lightweight clothing.
- Advise patients who are obese, elderly, or taking drugs that impair heat regulation to avoid overheating.
- Tell patients who have had heat cramps or heat exhaustion to increase their salt and water intake. They should also refrain from exercising until signs and symptoms resolve and resume exercises gradually, making sure to drink plenty of electrolyte-containing fluids. Advise them to take precautions to prevent overheating.
- Warn patients with heatstroke that residual hypersensitivity to high temperatures may persist for several months.
- Teach parents how to take steps to prevent young children and infants from overheating in hot weather.

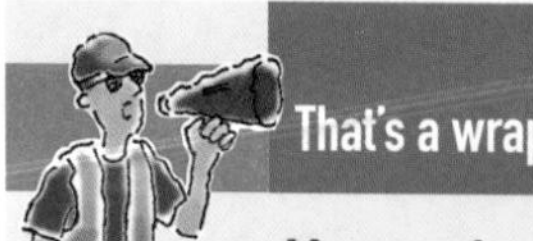

Heat-related health alterations review

Heat-related health alterations basics
- Develop when the body can't offset rising temperature and retains too much heat
- Result from failure of the mechanisms that regulate body temperature
- Are easily prevented with adequate hydration

Heat transfer
- Four methods: conduction, convection, radiation, and evaporation
- Body heat lost mainly through radiation and evaporation; if air temperature > 95° F (35° C), evaporation is only means of heat loss

Sweat
- Body's main way to get rid of extra heat
- Heat created by blood flowing through the skin evaporates water from the skin's surface.
- Weather and dehydration influence the effectiveness of sweating.

Types of heat-related health alterations
- Heat rash (mild)
- Heat cramps (mild)
- Heat exhaustion (moderate)
- Heat syncope (moderate)
- Heatstroke (critical)

Heat rash
- Develops from excessive sweating during hot weather
- Usually found on the neck or upper torso or in skin folds
- Looks like red pimples or tiny blisters

Heat cramps
- Caused by deficiency of water and sodium
- Generally attributed to dehydration and poor muscle conditioning

Heat exhaustion
- Caused by heat and fluid loss from excessive sweating without fluid replacement
- Can result in circulatory collapse if not treated promptly

Heat syncope (fainting)
- Occurs when a patient stands up quickly or has been standing for a prolonged period of time
- Dehydration is often to blame for heat syncope!

Heatstroke
- Caused by rising body temperature
- Leads to damage of internal organs
- Considered a medical emergency

Causes
- Fever
- Infection
- Dehydration
- Burns
- Cardiovascular disease
- Skin diseases
- Sweat gland dysfunction
- Diabetes
- Hyperthyroidism
- Pheochromocytoma
- Obesity
- High temperatures or humidity
- Lack of acclimatization
- Drugs (such as amphetamines) and alcohol

(continued)

Heat-related health alterations review *(continued)*

Treatment

- Institute cooling measures to lower body temperature.
- Remove or loosen clothing.
- Institute rehydration measures and replace sodium and potassium losses.
- Treat heatstroke as a medical emergency by initiating the ABCs of life support if needed.
- For heatstroke, monitor temperature, intake, output, and cardiac status.
- Patients experiencing heatstroke may require administration of benzodiazepines to control seizures, dobutamine I.V. to correct cardiogenic shock, chlorpromazine I.V. to reduce shivering, or mannitol I.V. to maintain urine output (Centers for Disease Control and Prevention, 2014; U.S. Department of Labor, n.d.).

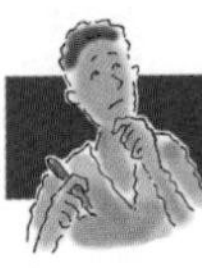

Quick quiz

1. Which mechanism accounts for most of the body's heat loss under typical environmental conditions?
   A. Convection
   B. Conduction
   C. Radiation
   D. Evaporation

Answer: C. Radiation accounts for approximately 65% of the body's heat loss when the outside temperature is less than the body's temperature.

2. After cooling a patient with heatstroke, he begins to shiver. You expect to administer:
   A. aspirin.
   B. acetaminophen.
   C. diazepam.
   D. chlorpromazine.

Answer: D. Chlorpromazine should be used when a patient is shivering to prevent significant heat production.

3. Which feature can help you determine whether a patient has heat exhaustion or heatstroke?
   A. Temperature higher than 102° F (38.9° C)
   B. Altered CNS function
   C. Dehydration
   D. Elevated liver transaminase levels

Answer: B. Altered CNS function (including seizures, coma, delirium, bizarre behavior, and dilated pupils) is the hallmark of heatstroke. Heat exhaustion causes fatigue and weakness; however, the patient is usually aware. Heat exhaustion, if it is severe and left untreated, may progress to heatstroke.

4. When treating a patient with heatstroke, you need to monitor temperature continuously to make sure that it doesn't fall below:
   - A. 101° F (38.3° C).
   - B. 98.6° F (37° C).
   - C. 104° F (40° C).
   - D. 99° F (37.2° C).

Answer: A. For patients with heatstroke, a rapid decrease in body temperature below 101° F (38.3° C) can cause hypothermia.

5. The best cooling method for heatstroke is:
   - A. water immersion.
   - B. iced peritoneal lavage.
   - C. evaporative cooling.
   - D. I.V. fluids.

Answer: C. Evaporative cooling, which includes undressing the patient, spraying tepid water on him, and using cool fans to maximize evaporation, is the best cooling method for a patient with heatstroke.

Scoring

☆☆☆ If you answered all five questions correctly, grab a bottle of water! You're hot, hot, hot!

☆☆ If you answered four questions correctly, good job! You've worked up a sweat in this chapter. Now move onto the next one.

☆ If you answered fewer than four questions correctly, don't worry! You're sure to hit a hot stroke—err, streak—soon.

References

Centers for Disease Control and Prevention. (2014). *Heat stress.* Retrieved from http://www.cdc.gov/niosh/topics/heatstress/

U.S. Department of Labor. (n.d.). *Heat related illnesses and first aid.* Retrieved from https://www.osha.gov/SLTC/heatstress/heat_illnesses.html

Chapter 13

Heart failure

Just the facts

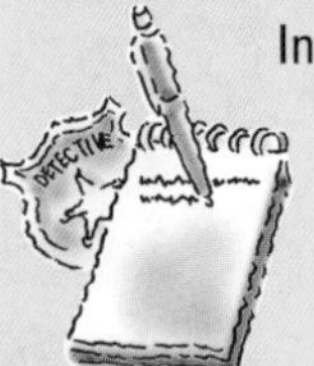

In this chapter, you'll learn:

- conditions that lead to heart failure
- signs and symptoms of heart failure
- imbalances that can occur as a result of heart failure or its treatment and ways to manage them.

A look at heart failure

Heart failure is a complex clinical syndrome that results from any structural or functional impairment of ventricular filling or ejection that causes diminished cardiac output. From the subtle loss of normal ventricular function to the presence of signs and symptoms that no longer respond to medical therapy, heart failure occurs when the heart can't pump enough blood to meet the body's metabolic needs. There is no single diagnostic test for heart failure because it is clinically diagnosed based on symptoms and physical exam.

How the ventricles function depends on the interaction among the four factors that regulate the cardiac output:

- preload (volume)
- afterload (pressure)
- contractility (squeeze)
- heart rate.

(Woods, 2010)

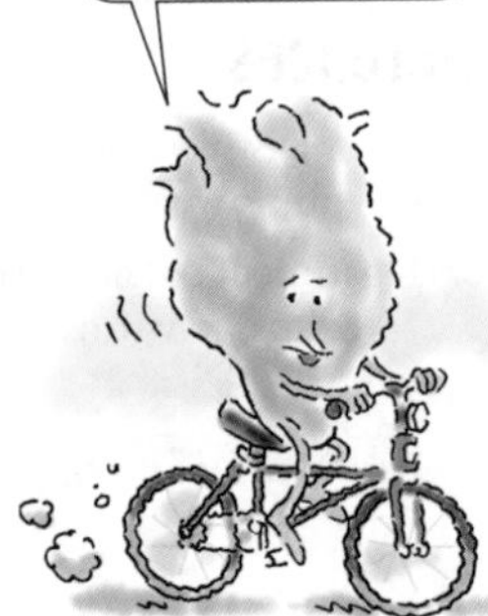

Remember, diastole and systole are the two phases of the cardiac cycle.

Cycle survey

It's important to remember that two periods—diastole and systole—make up the normal cardiac cycle. Diastole is the portion of the cycle when the heart is at rest, filling the ventricles with blood. Systole is the portion of the cycle when the ventricles contract, ejecting their volume of blood.

Chain reaction

When any of the four interrelated factors are altered, cardiac output may be affected. For example, when the preload (volume) delivered to the ventricles during diastole is inadequate, cardiac output may be compromised, and heart failure may result. Furthermore, when the afterload (pressure) against which the ventricles must contract is elevated during systole, cardiac output may be compromised, leading to heart failure.

Heart failure may result when the balance of these four interrelated factors is altered during either diastole or systole. When heart failure stems from inadequate filling of the ventricles, the syndrome is described as diastolic heart failure. When heart failure stems from inadequate contraction, the syndrome is described as systolic heart failure. This ventricular dysfunction may occur in either the left or right ventricle (Woods, 2010; Yancy et al., 2013).

How it happens

Normally, the pumping actions of the right and left sides of the heart complement each other, producing a synchronized and continuous blood flow. However, when an underlying disorder is present, one side may fail while the other continues to function normally for some time. Because of the prolonged strain, the functioning side eventually fails, resulting in total heart failure (Eckman, 2011).

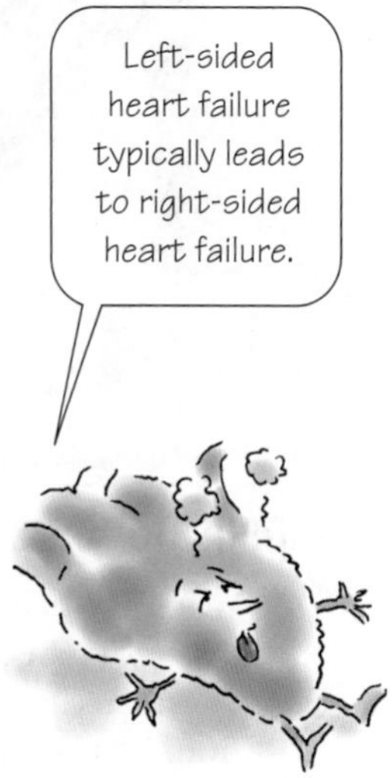

Left-sided heart failure typically leads to right-sided heart failure.

The left leads off

Usually, the heart's left side fails first. Left-sided heart failure typically leads to and is the main cause of right-sided heart failure.

Here's what happens: Diminished left ventricular function allows blood to pool in the ventricle and atrium and eventually back up into the pulmonary veins and capillaries. (See *Left-sided heart failure,* page 250.)

As the pulmonary circulation becomes engorged, rising capillary pressure pushes sodium and water into the interstitial space, causing pulmonary edema. The right ventricle becomes stressed because it's pumping against greater pulmonary vascular resistance and left ventricular pressure, leading to pulmonary congestion, dyspnea, and cardiomegaly (Eckman, 2011; Woods, 2010).

The right responds

As the right ventricle starts to fail, signs and symptoms worsen. Blood pools in the right ventricle and right atrium. The backed-up blood causes pressure and congestion in the venae cavae and systemic circulation. (See *Right-sided heart failure,* page 251.)

Blood also distends the visceral veins, especially the hepatic vein. As the liver and spleen become engorged, their function is impaired. Rising capillary pressure forces excess fluid from the capillaries into the interstitial space. This causes tissue edema, especially in the lower extremities and abdomen.

Left-sided heart failure

This illustration shows what happens when left-sided heart failure develops. The left side of the heart normally receives oxygenated blood returning from the lungs and then pumps blood through the aorta to all tissues. Left-sided heart failure causes blood to back up into the lungs, which results in such respiratory symptoms as tachypnea and shortness of breath.

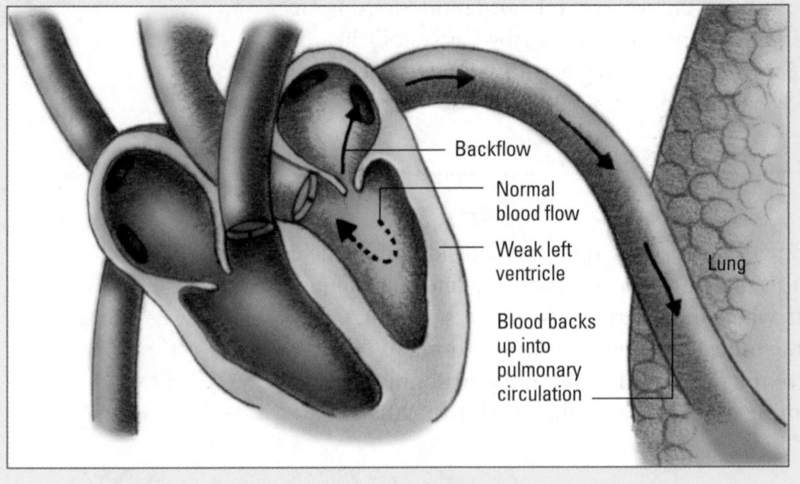

Compensatory responses

When the heart begins to fail, the body responds with three compensatory mechanisms to maintain blood flow to the tissues. These mechanisms include sympathetic nervous system activation, increased preload, and hypertrophy of the cardiac cells. Initially, the compensatory mechanisms increase the cardiac output. However, these mechanisms eventually contribute to heart failure.

The sympathetic nervous system

Diminished cardiac output activates the sympathetic nervous system, which increases heart rate and contractility. This initially increases cardiac output. However, this increased heart rate and contractility cause the heart's demand for oxygen to rise, thereby increasing the work that the heart must do to meet this demand. (Over time, this demand contributes to heart failure rather than compensating for it.) (Eckman, 2011; Woods, 2010)

Right-sided heart failure

This illustration shows what happens when right-sided heart failure develops. The right side of the heart normally receives deoxygenated blood returning from the tissues and then pumps that blood through the pulmonary artery into the lungs. Right-sided heart failure causes blood to back up past the vena cava and into the systemic circulation. This, in turn, causes enlargement of the abdominal organs and tissue edema.

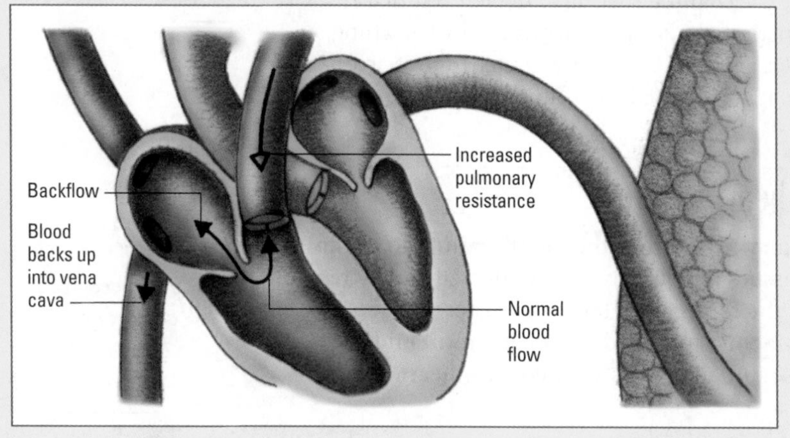

With increased demand, blood then shunts away from areas of low priority (such as the skin and kidneys) to areas of high priority (such as the heart and brain).

Pulmonary congestion, a complication of heart failure, can lead to pulmonary edema, a life-threatening condition. Decreased perfusion to major organs, particularly the brain and kidneys, may cause these organs to fail, necessitating dialysis for kidney failure. The patient's level of consciousness (LOC) may decrease, possibly leading to coma. Myocardial infarction (MI) may occur because myocardial oxygen demands can't be sufficiently met.

Increased preload

When blood is shunted away from areas of low priority, the kidneys, sensing a reduced renal blood flow, activate the renin-angiotensin-aldosterone system. This results in sodium and water retention, which increases blood volume (preload). Again, initially, this serves to increase cardiac output. However, over time, the heart can't pump this increased volume effectively, making heart failure worse, not better.

Cardiac hypertrophy

When the heart is under strain, it responds by increasing its muscle mass, a condition called *cardiac hypertrophy*. As the cardiac wall thickens, the heart's demand for blood and oxygen grows. The patient's heart may be unable to meet this demand, further compromising the patient's condition.

All stretched out

When pressure inside the chambers (usually the left ventricle) rises for a sustained period, the heart compensates by stretching, a condition called *cardiac dilation*. Eventually, stretched muscle fibers become overstrained, reducing the heart's ability to pump.

Imbalances caused by heart failure

Several imbalances may result from the heart's failure to pump blood and perfuse tissues adequately. Imbalances also may result from stimulation of the renin-angiotensin-aldosterone system or from certain treatments, such as diuretic therapy. Fluid, electrolyte, and acid-base imbalances associated with heart failure include:

- hypervolemia and hypovolemia
- hyperkalemia and hypokalemia
- hypochloremia, hypomagnesemia, and hyponatremia
- metabolic acidosis and alkalosis
- respiratory acidosis and alkalosis.

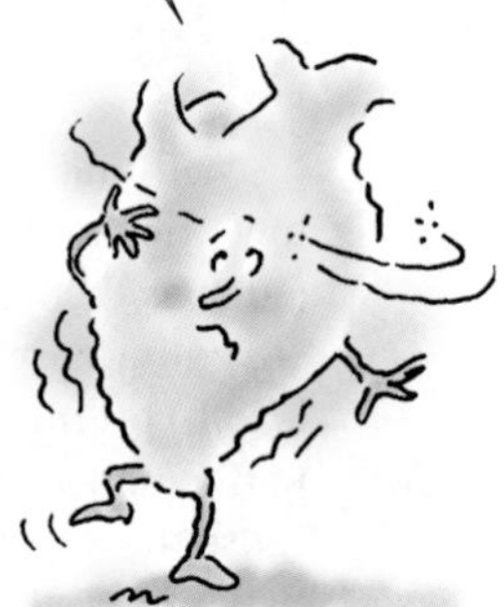

As my ability to pump becomes compromised, imbalances can occur.

A flood of fluid

Hypervolemia—the most common fluid imbalance associated with heart failure—results from the heart's failure to propel blood forward, consequent vascular pooling, and sodium and water reabsorption triggered by the renin-angiotensin-aldosterone system. Excess extracellular fluid volume commonly causes peripheral edema.

Hypovolemia is usually associated with overly aggressive diuretic therapy and can be especially dangerous in elderly patients because it causes confusion and hypotension.

Lowdown on low sodium

Hyponatremia may result from sodium loss due to diuretic abuse. In some cases, it may result from a dilutional effect that occurs when water reabsorption is greater than sodium reabsorption.

Other electrolyte highs and lows

In patients with heart failure, prolonged use of a diuretic without adequate potassium replacement can cause hypokalemia. Likewise, use of a potassium-sparing diuretic can cause hyperkalemia. Both hypokalemia and hyperkalemia can lead to life-threatening arrhythmias. Therefore, potassium levels require careful monitoring whenever a patient receives any kind of diuretic, oral or I.V.

Hypomagnesemia may accompany hypokalemia, particularly if the patient is receiving a diuretic (many diuretics cause the kidneys to excrete magnesium). Hypochloremia may also result from excessive diuretic therapy.

Lactic acid on the rise

When cells don't receive enough oxygen, they produce more lactic acid. Poor tissue perfusion in a patient with heart failure allows lactic acid to accumulate, which in turn leads to metabolic acidosis. Metabolic alkalosis may be caused by excessive diuretic use, which causes bicarbonate retention.

In the early stages of heart failure, as respiratory rate increases, more carbon dioxide is blown off from the lungs, which raises pH and leads to respiratory alkalosis. As heart failure progresses, gas exchange is further impaired. Carbon dioxide accumulates, resulting in respiratory acidosis.

What causes heart failure

A wide range of pathophysiologic processes can cause heart failure, including conditions that directly damage the heart, such as MI, myocarditis, myocardial fibrosis, and ventricular aneurysm. The damage from these disorders causes a subsequent decrease in the contractility of the heart.

Ventricular overload can also cause heart failure. This overload may be caused by increased blood volume in the heart (called *increased preload*) as a result of aortic insufficiency or a ventricular septal defect. Systemic or pulmonary hypertension or an elevation in pressure against which the heart must pump (called *increased afterload*) as a result of aortic or pulmonic stenosis can also cause this overload.

Restricted ventricular diastolic filling, characterized by the presence of so little blood that the ventricle can't pump it effectively, can also cause heart failure. Such diastolic filling is triggered by constrictive pericarditis or cardiomyopathy, tachyarrhythmias, cardiac tamponade, or mitral or aortic stenosis and usually occurs in older patients.

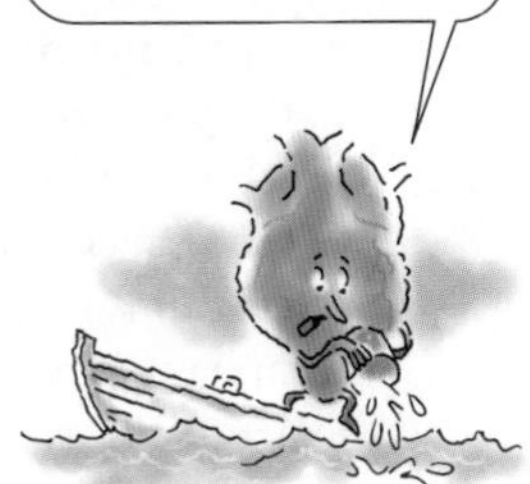

Too much blood volume in the heart can cause ventricular overload, which can lead to heart failure. I've got a sinking feeling about this whole situation!

Risk raisers

Certain conditions can predispose a person to heart failure, especially if there is an underlying disease. They include:

- anemia, which causes the heart rate to speed up to maintain tissue oxygenation
- pregnancy and thyrotoxicosis, which increase the demand for cardiac output
- infections, which increase metabolic demands and further burden the heart
- increased physical activity, emotional stress, greater sodium or water intake, or failure to comply with the prescribed treatment regimen for underlying heart disease
- pulmonary embolism, which elevates pulmonary arterial pressures and can cause right-sided heart failure
- connective tissue disorders (sarcoidosis).

What to look for

Signs and symptoms of heart failure vary according to the site of failure and stage of the disease. Expect to encounter a combination of the findings discussed here.

Left-sided heart failure

If your patient has left-sided heart failure and tissue hypoxia, they will probably complain of fatigue, weakness, orthopnea, and exertional dyspnea. The patient may also report paroxysmal nocturnal dyspnea.

The patient may use two or three pillows to elevate his head to sleep or may have to sleep sitting up in a chair. Shortness of breath may awaken the patient shortly after they fall asleep, forcing them to quickly sit upright to catch his breath. The patient may have dyspnea, coughing, and wheezing even when sitting up. Tachypnea may occur, and you may note crackles on inspiration. Coughing may progress to the point where the patient produces pink, frothy sputum as he develops pulmonary edema.

The patient may be tachycardic. Auscultation of heart sounds may reveal third and fourth heart sounds as the myocardium becomes less compliant. Hypoxia and hypercapnia can affect the central nervous system, causing restlessness, confusion, and a progressive decrease in the patient's LOC. Later, with continued decrease in cardiac output, the kidneys may be affected, and oliguria may develop as a result of hypoperfusion.

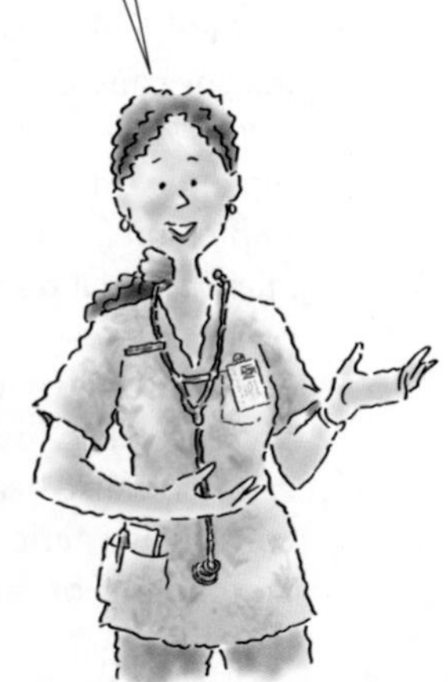
Signs and symptoms of heart failure vary according to the site of failure and stage of the disease.

Right-sided heart failure

Inspection of a patient with right-sided heart failure may reveal venous engorgement. When the patient sits upright, neck veins may appear distended, feel rigid, and exhibit exaggerated pulsations. Edema may develop, and the patient may report a weight gain. Nail beds may appear cyanotic. Anorexia and nausea may occur. The liver may be enlarged and slightly tender. This condition may progress to congestive hepatomegaly, ascites, and jaundice.

Advanced heart failure

In a patient with advanced heart failure, pulse pressure may be diminished, reflecting reduced stroke volume. Occasionally, diastolic pressure rises from generalized vasoconstriction. The patient's skin feels cool and clammy. Progression of heart failure may lead to palpitations, chest tightness, and arrhythmias. Cardiac arrest may occur. (See *Recognizing advanced heart failure*.)

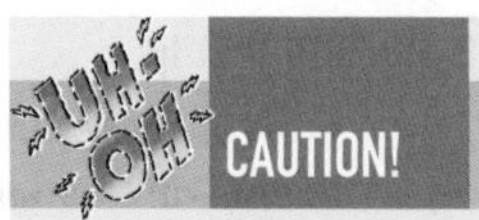

Recognizing advanced heart failure

The following assessment findings commonly occur in patients with heart failure:

- cool, clammy skin
- diminished pulse pressure
- elevated diastolic pressure
- chest tightness
- arrhythmias.

What tests show

Several tests may help confirm the diagnosis of heart failure:

- Electrocardiograms can detect arrhythmias, MI, or the presence of coronary artery disease.
- Chest X-rays show cardiomegaly, alveolar edema, pleural effusion, and pulmonary edema.
- A two-dimensional echocardiogram with Doppler should be performed during initial evaluation to assess ventricular function, size, wall thickness, wall motion, and valve function.
- Cardiac catheterizations and echocardiograms reveal enlarged heart chambers, changes in ventricular function, and the presence of valvular disease. Echocardiogram, the gold standard for detecting heart failure, shows left ventricular dysfunction.
- Hemodynamic pressure readings reveal increased central venous and pulmonary artery wedge pressures.
- Measurement of B-type natriuretic peptide (BNP) or N-terminal prohormone of brain natriuretic peptide (NT-proBNP) to support diagnosis of acutely decompensated heart failure.
- Measurement of cardiac troponin to determine disease severity in acutely decompensated cases (Yancy et al., 2013).

How it's treated

Heart failure is a medical emergency. Relieving dyspnea and improving arterial oxygenation are the immediate therapeutic goals. Secondary goals include minimizing or eliminating the underlying cause, reducing sodium and water retention, optimizing cardiac preload and afterload, and enhancing myocardial contractility.

The starting lineup

One or more drugs—such as a diuretic, a vasodilator, or an inotropic agent—are usually needed to manage heart failure. Diuretic therapy, the starting point of this treatment, increases sodium and water elimination by the kidneys. By reducing fluid overload, diuretics decrease total blood volume and relieve circulatory congestion. For most diuretics to work effectively, the patient must control his sodium intake.

Types of diuretics include thiazide and loop diuretics, such as furosemide, torsemide, and bumetanide. Because thiazide and loop diuretics work at different sites in the nephron, they produce a synergistic effect when given in combination. Potassium-sparing diuretics, such as amiloride, spironolactone, and triamterene, may also be used.

Any patient who takes a diuretic needs careful monitoring because these drugs can disturb the electrolyte balance and lead to metabolic alkalosis, metabolic acidosis, or other complications.

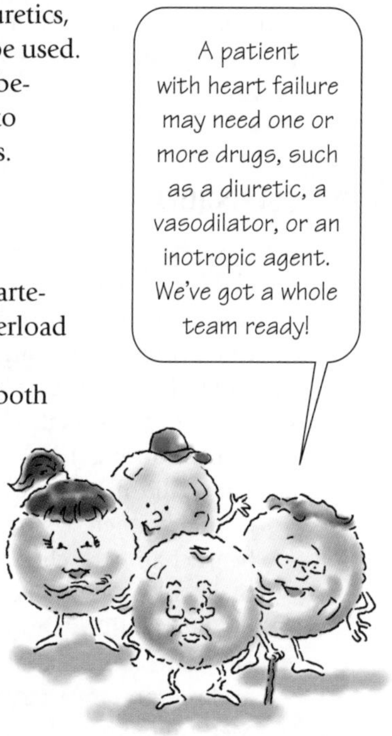

A patient with heart failure may need one or more drugs, such as a diuretic, a vasodilator, or an inotropic agent. We've got a whole team ready!

The other players

Other drugs also help manage heart failure:

- Vasodilators can reduce preload or afterload by decreasing arterial and venous vasoconstriction. Reducing preload and afterload helps increase stroke volume and cardiac output.
- Angiotensin-converting enzyme (ACE) inhibitors decrease both afterload and preload. Because ACE inhibitors prevent potassium loss, hyperkalemia may develop in patients who are also taking a potassium-sparing diuretic, so these patients need close monitoring.
- Angiotensin-receptor blocker (ARB) is recommended for patients who are ACE inhibitor intolerant. It decreases both afterload and preload.
- Nitrates, primarily vasodilators, also dilate arterial smooth muscle at higher doses. Most patients with heart failure tolerate nitrates well. Nitrates come in several forms, as I.V., oral, and topical ointments.
- Beta-adrenergic blockers such as carvedilol decrease afterload through their vasodilating action. Specifically, they cause peripheral vasodilation, decreasing systemic pressure directly and cardiac workload indirectly. Beta-adrenergic blocker therapy also enhances longevity.
- Inotropic drugs such as digoxin increase contractility in the failing heart muscle and slow conduction through the atrioventricular node. However, there's a narrow margin of safety between therapeutic and toxic levels. A concurrent electrolyte imbalance, such as hypokalemia, may contribute to digoxin toxicity because it decreases digoxin excretion from the body. This toxicity may lead to fatal cardiac arrhythmias, muscle weakness, and respiratory distress.

- Other drugs—such as dopamine, dobutamine, milrinone, and inamrinone—may be indicated for patients with acute heart failure to increase myocardial contractility and cardiac output. Hydralazine and nitroprusside may also be used to treat heart failure.
- Morphine is commonly used in patients with heart failure who also have acute pulmonary edema. Besides reducing anxiety, it decreases preload and afterload by dilating veins (Eckman, 2011; Nettina, 2010; Woods, 2010; Yancy et al., 2013).

Urgency may call for surgery

Patients with severe heart failure may require surgery. In cardiomyoplasty, a muscle is wrapped around the failing heart to boost its pumping action. In left ventriculectomy, a section of nonviable myocardium is removed to reduce ventricular size, which allows the heart to pump more effectively. To help the ventricles propel blood through the vascular system, an intra-aortic balloon counterpulsation or other ventricular assist device, such as a biventricular pacemaker or an implantable cardioverter defibrillator (sometimes necessary because a patient with heart failure may have a concurrent life-threatening arrhythmia), may be implanted. Heart transplant is used only as a last resort.

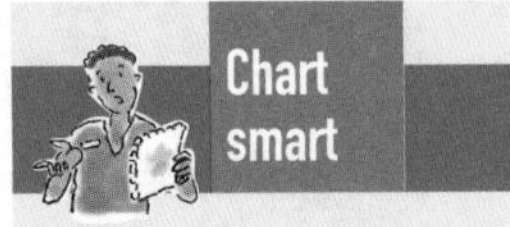

Documenting heart failure

If your patient has heart failure, make sure you document the following information:
- prescribed medications
- daily weight, intake, and output (any weight gain over 2 lb [0.9 kg] in less than 24 hours puts the patient at risk for fluid overload)
- edema
- diet restrictions
- vital signs
- lung sounds
- heart sounds
- skin conditions
- patient positioning and response
- mental status
- tolerance of activity
- safety measures implemented
- notification of practitioner
- patient teaching.

How you intervene

To properly care for a patient with heart failure, you'll need to investigate the patient's signs and symptoms and perform a number of specific interventions:

- Assess the patient's vital signs and mental status and immediately report any changes.
- Assess the patient for signs and symptoms of impending cardiac failure, such as fatigue; restlessness; hypotension; rapid respiratory rate; shortness of breath; orthopnea; dyspnea; coughing; decreased urine output; liver enlargement; and a rapid, thready pulse.
- Assess the patient for edema. Note the amount and location of edema and the degree of pitting, if present. (See *Documenting heart failure*.)
- Monitor sodium and fluid intake as prescribed. Hyponatremia and fluid volume deficit can stimulate the renin-angiotensin-aldosterone system and exacerbate heart failure. Usually, mild sodium restriction (no added salt allowed) is prescribed.
- Check the patient's weight and fluid intake and output daily for significant changes to determine if the patient is in a state of fluid overload. If the patient has gained 2 lb (0.9 kg) or more over 24 hours, he'll need further diuretic therapy. (See *Teaching about heart failure*, page 258.)
- Monitor vital signs, including blood pressure, pulse, respirations, and heart and breath sounds, for abnormalities that might indicate a fluid excess or deficit.

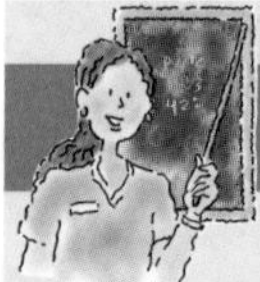

Teaching points

Teaching about heart failure

When teaching a patient with heart failure, be sure to cover the following topics and then evaluate your patient's learning:

- basics of the condition and its treatment
- need for adequate rest
- proper skin care
- prescribed medications
- dietary restrictions
- need to reduce stress and anxiety level
- need for regular exercise
- need for daily weights
- warning signs and symptoms and when to report them
- importance of follow-up.

- Monitor serum electrolyte levels—especially sodium and potassium—for changes that may indicate an imbalance. Remember that hypokalemia can lead to digoxin toxicity. Monitor arterial blood gas results to assess adequacy of ventilation.
- Maintain continuous cardiac monitoring during acute and advanced stages of the disease to identify arrhythmias promptly.
- Administer prescribed medications—such as digoxin, diuretics, ACE inhibitors, ARB, and potassium supplements—to support cardiac function and minimize symptoms.
- Administer oral potassium supplements in orange juice or with meals to promote absorption and prevent gastric irritation.
- Place the patient in semi-Fowler's or Fowler's position as tolerated, and give supplemental oxygen as ordered to help him breathe more easily.
- Encourage independent activities of daily living as tolerated, although some patients may require bed rest. Reposition the patient as needed every 1 to 2 hours. Edematous skin is prone to breakdown.
- Instruct the patient and his family to notify the staff of any changes in the patient's condition, such as increased shortness of breath, chest pain, or dizziness.
- Instruct the patient to call the practitioner if his pulse rate is irregular; if it measures fewer than 60 beats/minute; or if he experiences dizziness, blurred vision, shortness of breath, a persistent dry cough, palpitations, increased fatigue, nocturnal dyspnea that comes and goes, swollen ankles, or decreased urine output (Eckman, 2011; Nettina, 2010; Woods, 2010; Yancy et al., 2013).

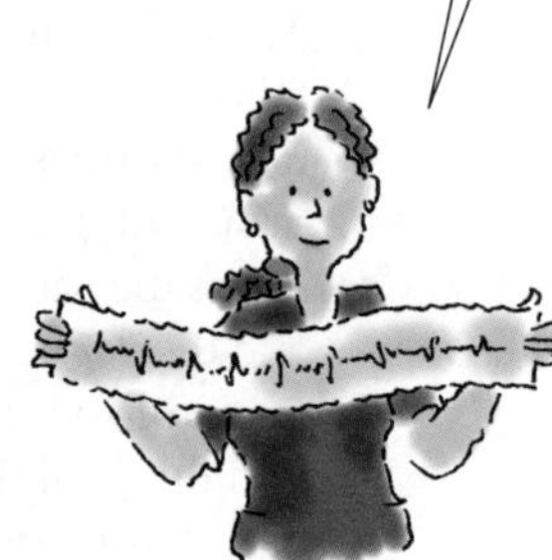
The patient needs continuous cardiac monitoring during acute and advanced stages of heart failure.

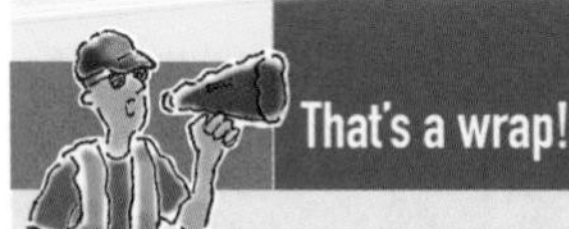

That's a wrap!

Heart failure review

Heart failure
- Clinical syndrome of myocardial dysfunction that causes diminished cardiac output
- Occurs when the heart can't pump enough blood to meet the body's metabolic needs

Left-sided heart failure
- Typically leads to and is the main cause of right-sided heart failure
- Causes pulmonary edema, hypoxia, and hypercapnia
- Clinical symptoms: fatigue; weakness; orthopnea; exertional dyspnea; pulmonary edema; paroxysmal nocturnal dyspnea; tachycardia; third and fourth heart sounds; tachypnea; shortness of breath; oliguria; and coughing with pink, frothy sputum

Right-sided heart failure
- Causes enlargement of the abdominal organs and tissue edema
- Clinical signs and symptoms: venous engorgement, edema, weight gain, anorexia, nausea, cyanosis of nail beds, cool and clammy skin, chest tightness, palpitations, neck vein distention and rigidity, cardiac arrest, and hepatomegaly

Causes
- MI
- Myocarditis
- Myocardial fibrosis
- Ventricular aneurysm
- Ventricular overload as a result of aortic insufficiency or ventricular septal defect
- Systemic or pulmonary hypertension as a result of aortic or pulmonic stenosis
- Restricted ventricular diastolic filling triggered by constrictive pericarditis or cardiomyopathy, tachyarrhythmias, cardiac tamponade, or mitral or aortic stenosis

Imbalances caused by heart failure
- Hypervolemia or hypovolemia
- Hyperkalemia or hypokalemia
- Hypochloremia, hypomagnesemia, and hyponatremia
- Metabolic acidosis or alkalosis
- Respiratory acidosis or alkalosis

Hypervolemia
- Most common fluid imbalance associated with heart failure
- Results from heart's failure to propel blood forward, resulting in vascular pooling and sodium and water reabsorption
- Commonly causes peripheral edema

Hypovolemia
- Associated with overuse of diuretics
- Causes confusion and hypotension in elderly patients
- May cause electrolyte imbalances

Hyponatremia
- May result from sodium loss due to diuretic abuse
- May result from a dilutional effect when water reabsorption is greater than sodium reabsorption
- May cause confusion

Other electrolyte imbalances
- Hypokalemia—results from prolonged use of a diuretic without adequate potassium replacement

(continued)

Heart failure review *(continued)*

- Hyperkalemia—occurs with use of potassium-sparing diuretics
- Hypokalemia and hyperkalemia—lead to life-threatening arrhythmias
- Hypomagnesemia—occurs with hypokalemia, especially with diuretic use
- Hypochloremia—results from excessive diuretic therapy

Metabolic and respiratory acidosis and alkalosis

- Metabolic acidosis—occurs when poor tissue perfusion allows lactic acid to accumulate
- Metabolic alkalosis—occurs with excessive diuretic use, which causes bicarbonate retention
- Respiratory alkalosis—occurs early in heart failure when increased respirations cause more carbon dioxide to be blown off and pH to rise
- Respiratory acidosis—occurs as heart failure progresses, gas exchange is impaired, and carbon dioxide accumulates

Treatment

- Medical emergency
- Relief of dyspnea
- Improved arterial oxygenation
- Diuretics to relieve fluid overload, vasodilators to reduce preload and afterload, or inotropics to increase heart contractility
- Possibly surgery for severe heart failure (heart transplant as last resort)
- Patient and family education about the disease and its management

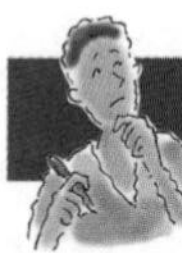

Quick quiz

1. When assessing a patient with left-sided heart failure, you would expect to detect:
   A. distended neck veins.
   B. edema of the lower extremities.
   C. dyspnea on exertion.
   D. hepatomegaly.

Answer: C. Diminished left ventricular function allows blood to pool in the ventricle and atrium and eventually back up into the pulmonary veins and capillaries. As the pulmonary circulation becomes engorged, rising capillary pressure pushes sodium and water into the interstitial space, causing pulmonary edema. Reasons for seeking care include fatigue, exertional dyspnea, orthopnea, weakness, and paroxysmal nocturnal dyspnea.

2. The most common fluid imbalance associated with heart failure is:
   A. hypervolemia.
   B. hypovolemia.
   C. hyperkalemia.
   D. hypokalemia.

Answer: A. Extracellular fluid volume excess results from the heart's failure to propel blood forward, which causes vascular pooling, and from the sodium and water reabsorption triggered by the renin-angiotensin-aldosterone system.

3. A patient with heart failure is more likely to develop a toxic reaction to digoxin if he has concurrent:
   A. hyponatremia.
   B. hyperkalemia.
   C. hypernatremia.
   D. hypokalemia.

Answer: D. Hypokalemia, which can occur with diuretic therapy, may lead to digoxin toxicity.

4. Which drug class given to treat heart failure has been shown to increase longevity?
   A. ACE inhibitors
   B. Nitrates
   C. Beta-adrenergic blockers
   D. Digoxin

Answer: C. Beta-adrenergic blocker therapy enhances longevity.

Scoring

☆☆☆ If you answered all four questions correctly, we salute your heartfelt effort!

☆☆ If you answered three questions correctly, great! We applaud your boisterous bravado!

☆ If you answered fewer than three questions correctly, relax. We still commend your veritable valor!

References

Woods, S. (Ed.). (2010). *Cardiac nursing* (6th ed.). Philadelphia, PA: Lippincott Williams & Wilkins.

Eckman, M. (Ed.). (2011). *Professional guide to pathophysiology* (3rd ed.). Philadelphia, PA: Lippincott Williams & Wilkins.

Nettina, S. M. (2010). *Lippincott manual of nursing practice* (9th ed.). Philadelphia, PA: Lippincott Williams & Wilkins.

Yancy, C. W., Jessup, M., Bozkurt, B., Butler, J., Casey, D. E., Jr., Drazner, M. H., . . . Wilkoff, B. L. (2013). ACCF/AHA guidelines for the management of heart failure. *Journal of the American College of Cardiology, 62*(16), e147–e239.

Chapter 14

Respiratory failure

Just the facts

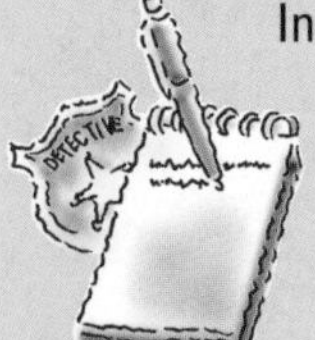

In this chapter, you'll learn:

- conditions that lead to respiratory failure
- signs and symptoms of respiratory failure
- imbalances that occur with respiratory failure and ways to manage them.

A look at respiratory failure

When the lungs can't sufficiently maintain arterial oxygenation or eliminate carbon dioxide, acute respiratory failure results. Unchecked and untreated, this condition can lead to decreased oxygenation of the body tissues and metabolic acidosis.

In patients with essentially normal lung tissue, respiratory failure usually produces hypercapnia (an above-normal amount of carbon dioxide in the arterial blood) and hypoxemia (a deficiency of oxygen in the arterial blood). In patients with chronic obstructive pulmonary disease (COPD), respiratory failure may be signaled only by an acute drop in arterial blood gas (ABG) levels and clinical deterioration. This is because some patients with COPD consistently have high partial pressure of arterial carbon dioxide ($Paco_2$) levels and low partial pressure of arterial oxygen (Pao_2) levels but are able to compensate and maintain a normal, or near-normal, pH level.

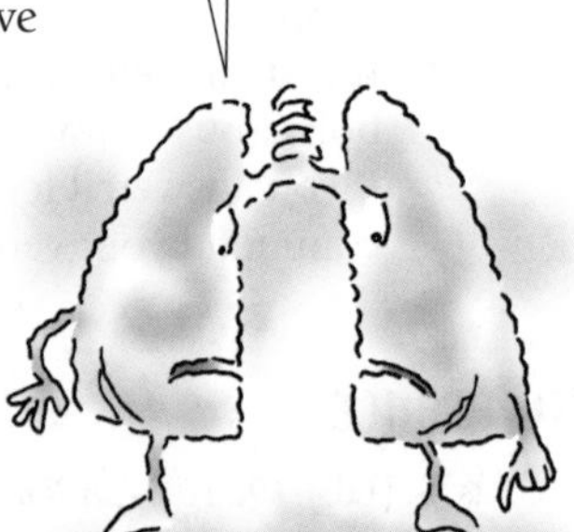
When the lungs can't maintain arterial oxygenation or eliminate carbon dioxide, acute respiratory failure results.

How it happens

In patients with acute respiratory failure, gas exchange is diminished by any combination of these malfunctions:

- alveolar hypoventilation
- ventilation-perfusion ($\dot{V}/\dot{Q}$) mismatch
- intrapulmonary shunting.

Imbalances associated with respiratory failure include hypervolemia, hypovolemia, hypokalemia, hyperkalemia, respiratory acidosis, respiratory alkalosis, and metabolic acidosis. Let's look at each one individually. (See *What happens in acute respiratory failure*.)

What happens in acute respiratory failure

Three major malfunctions account for impaired gas exchange and subsequent acute respiratory failure: alveolar hypoventilation, ventilation-perfusion ($\dot{V}/\dot{Q}$) mismatch, and intrapulmonary (right to left) shunting.

Alveolar hypoventilation
In alveolar hypoventilation (shown below as the result of airway obstruction), the amount of oxygen brought to the alveoli is diminished, which causes a drop in the partial pressure of arterial oxygen and an increase in alveolar carbon dioxide (CO_2). The accumulation of CO_2 in the alveoli prevents diffusion of adequate amounts of CO_2 from the capillaries, which increases the partial pressure of arterial CO_2.

($\dot{V}/\dot{Q}$) mismatch
($\dot{V}/\dot{Q}$) mismatch, the leading cause of hypoxemia, occurs when insufficient ventilation exists with a normal flow of blood or when, as shown below, normal ventilation exists with an insufficient flow of blood.

Intrapulmonary shunting
Intrapulmonary shunting occurs when blood passes from the right side of the heart to the left side without being oxygenated, as shown below. Shunting can result from untreated ventilation or perfusion mismatches.

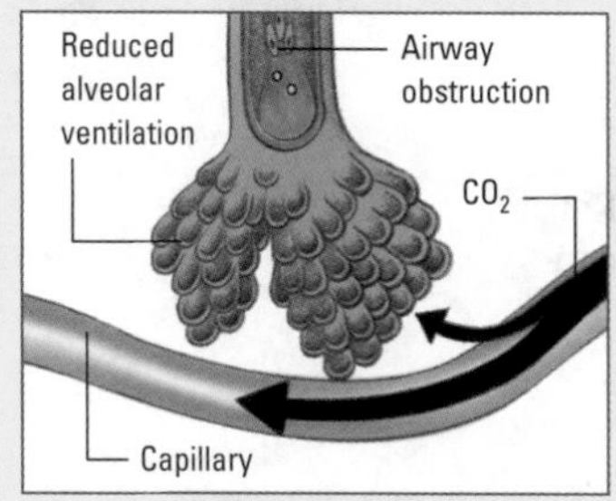

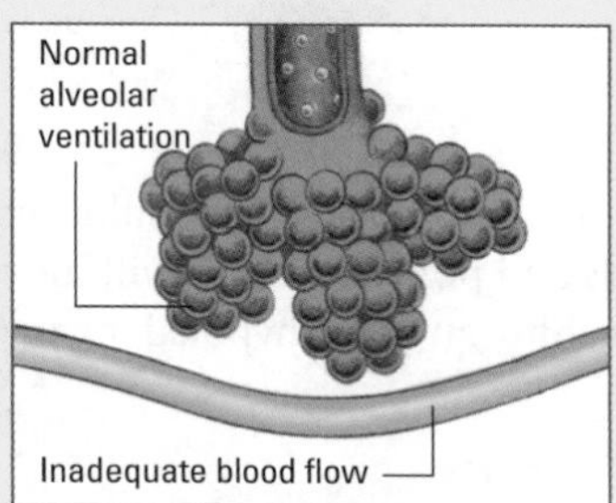

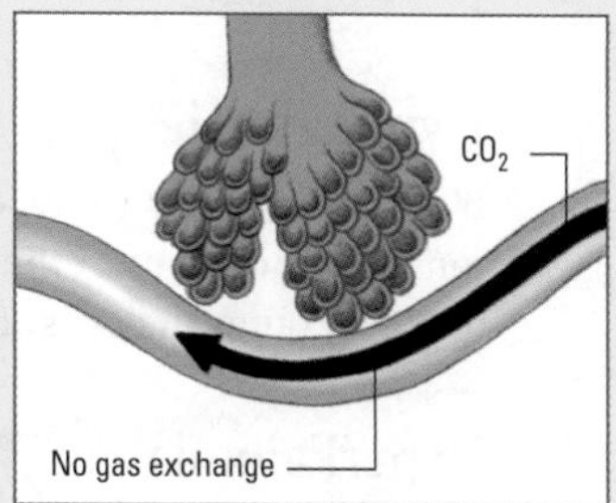

Hypervolemia

Prolonged respiratory treatments, such as nebulizer use, can lead to inhalation and absorption of water vapor. Excessive fluid absorption may also result from increased lung capillary pressure or permeability, which typically occurs in acute respiratory distress syndrome (ARDS). The excessive fluid absorption may precipitate pulmonary edema.

Hypovolemia

Because the lungs remove water daily through exhalation, an increased respiratory rate can promote excessive loss of water. Excessive loss can also occur with fever or any other condition that increases the metabolic rate and thus the respiratory rate. (See *Causes of respiratory failure,* page 264.)

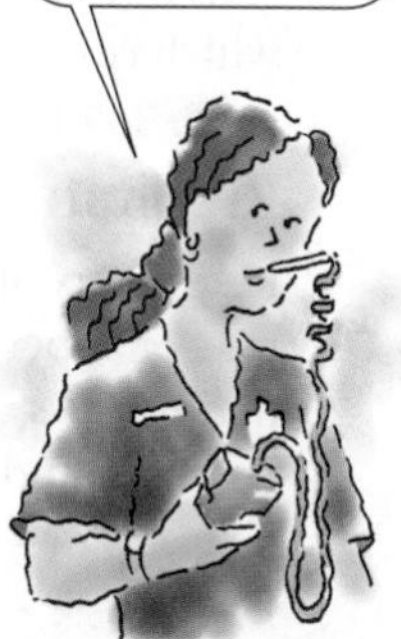

Fever increases metabolic rate, which increases respiratory rate and can lead to hypovolemia.

Causes of respiratory failure

Problems with the brain, lungs, muscles, and nerves or with pulmonary circulation can impair gas exchange and cause respiratory failure. Here's a list of conditions that can cause respiratory failure.

Brain
- Anesthesia or certain medications (opioids)
- Cerebral hemorrhage
- Cerebral tumor
- Drug overdose
- Head trauma
- Skull fracture

Lungs
- Acute respiratory distress syndrome (ARDS)
- Asthma
- Chronic obstructive pulmonary disease (COPD)
- Cystic fibrosis
- Flail chest
- Massive bilateral pneumonia
- Sleep apnea
- Tracheal obstruction

Muscles and nerves
- Amyotrophic lateral sclerosis
- Guillain-Barré syndrome
- Multiple sclerosis
- Muscular dystrophy
- Myasthenia gravis
- Polio
- Spinal cord trauma

Pulmonary circulation
- Heart failure
- Pulmonary edema
- Pulmonary embolism

Hypokalemia

If a patient begins to hyperventilate and alkalosis results, hydrogen ions will move out of the cells and potassium ions will move from the blood into the cells. That shift can cause hypokalemia.

Hyperkalemia

In acidosis, excess hydrogen ions move into the cell. Potassium ions then move out of the cell and into the blood to balance the positive charges between the two fluid compartments. Hyperkalemia may result.

Respiratory acidosis

Respiratory acidosis, which is due to hypoventilation, results from the inability of the lungs to eliminate sufficient quantities of carbon dioxide. The excess carbon dioxide combines with water to form carbonic acid. Increased carbonic acid levels result in decreased pH, which contributes to respiratory acidosis.

Respiratory alkalosis

Respiratory alkalosis develops from an excessively rapid respiratory rate, or hyperventilation, and causes excessive carbon dioxide elimination. Loss of carbon dioxide decreases the blood's acid-forming potential and results in respiratory alkalosis.

Metabolic acidosis

Conditions that cause hypoxia cause cells to use anaerobic metabolism. That metabolism creates an increase in the production of lactic acid, which can lead to metabolic acidosis.

What to look for

Hypoxemia and hypercapnia, which are characteristic of acute respiratory failure, stimulate strong compensatory responses from all body systems, especially the respiratory, cardiovascular, and central nervous systems (CNS).

Labored breathing may signify respiratory failure.

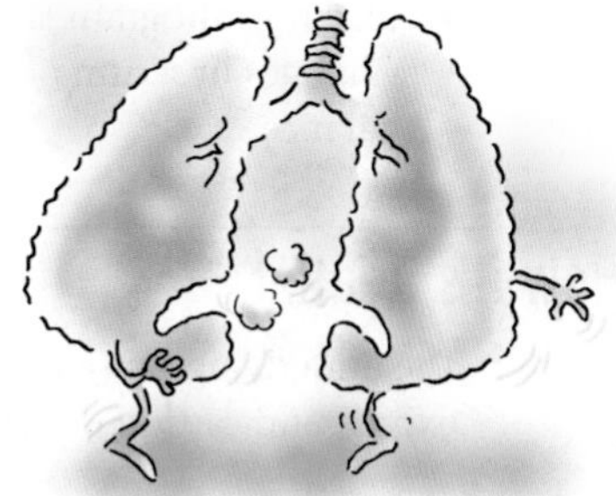

Leading with the lungs

When the body senses hypoxemia or hypercapnia, the respiratory center responds by increasing respiratory depth and then respiratory rate. Signs of labored breathing—flared nostrils, pursed-lip exhalation, and the use of accessory breathing muscles, among others—may signify respiratory failure.

As respiratory failure worsens, muscle retractions between the ribs, above the clavicle, and above the sternum may also occur. The patient is dyspneic and may become cyanotic. Auscultation of the chest reveals diminished or absent breath sounds over the affected area. You may also hear wheezes, crackles, or rhonchi. Respiratory arrest may occur.

The heart heats up

The sympathetic nervous system usually compensates by increasing the heart rate and constricting blood vessels in an effort to improve cardiac output. The patient's skin may become cool, pale, and clammy. Eventually, as myocardial oxygenation diminishes, cardiac output, blood pressure, and heart rate drop. Arrhythmias develop, and cardiac arrest may occur.

S.O.S. from the CNS

Even a slight disruption in oxygen supply and carbon dioxide elimination can affect brain function and behavior. Hypoxia initially causes early signs of anxiety and restlessness, which can progress to marked confusion, agitation, and lethargy. The primary indicator of hypercapnia, headache, occurs as cerebral vessels dilate in an effort to increase the brain's blood supply. If the carbon dioxide level continues to rise, the patient will display fatigue and be at risk for seizures and coma. (See *Recognizing worsening respiratory failure,* page 266.)

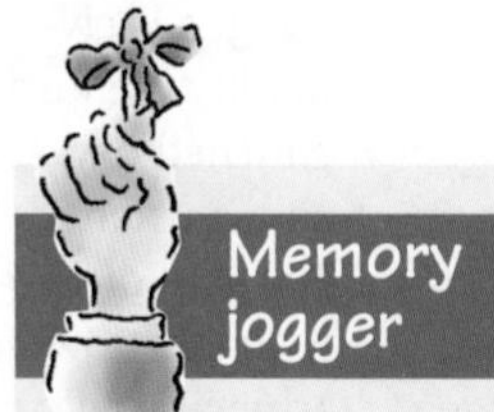

Memory jogger

When you auscultate a patient with worsening respiratory failure, certain signs may stick in your **CRAW:**

Crackles

Rhonchi

Absent breath sounds

Wheezes.

What tests show

The following diagnostic test results can help diagnose respiratory failure and guide its treatment:

- ABG changes indicate respiratory failure. (Always compare ABG results with your patient's baseline values. For a patient with previously normal lungs, the ABG changes may reveal the pH usually less than 7.35, the PaO_2 less than 50 mm Hg, and the $PaCO_2$ greater than 50 mm Hg. In a patient with COPD, an acute drop in the PaO_2 level of 10 mm Hg or more indicates respiratory failure. Keep in mind that patients with COPD have a chronically low PaO_2, increased $PaCO_2$, increased bicarbonate levels, but a normal pH.)
- Chest X-rays may identify an underlying pulmonary condition.
- Electrocardiogram (ECG) changes may show arrhythmias.
- Changes in serum potassium levels may be related to acid-base balance.

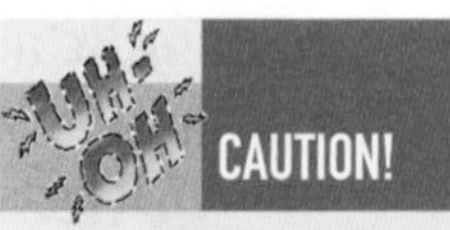

Recognizing worsening respiratory failure

The following assessment findings commonly occur in patients with worsening respiratory failure:

- arrhythmias
- bradycardia
- cyanosis
- diminished or absent breath sounds over affected area and, possibly, wheezes, crackles, or rhonchi
- dyspnea
- air hunger
- hypotension
- muscle retractions.

How it's treated

The underlying cause of respiratory failure must be addressed and oxygen and carbon dioxide levels improved.

Up the oxygen—but not too much

Oxygen is given in controlled concentrations, often using a Venturi mask. A Venturi mask mixes oxygen with room air, creating high-flow enriched oxygen of a settable concentration. It provides an accurate and constant delivery of oxygen (American Thoracic Society, 2014). The goal of oxygen therapy is to prevent oxygen toxicity by administering the lowest dose of oxygen for the shortest period of time while achieving an oxygen saturation of 90% or more or a PaO_2 level of at least 60 mm Hg. Oxygen therapy must be used cautiously in patients with chronic lung disease.

Intubate, ventilate, saturate

Intubation and mechanical ventilation are indicated if conservative treatment fails to raise oxygen saturation above 90%. The patient may also be intubated and ventilated if acidemia continues, if he becomes exhausted, or if respiratory arrest occurs. Intubation provides a patent airway. Mechanical ventilation decreases the work of breathing, ventilates the lungs, and improves oxygenation.

Positive end-expiratory pressure (PEEP) therapy may be ordered during mechanical ventilation or with a bilevel positive airway pressure (BiPAP) mask to improve gas exchange. PEEP maintains positive pressure at the end of expiration, thus preventing the airways and alveoli from collapsing between breaths. BiPAP is a pressure-controlled ventilation system with two cycles that supports spontaneous breathing.

Keep the airways open for business

Bronchodilators, especially inhalants, are used to open the airways. If the patient can't inhale effectively or is on a mechanical ventilator, he may receive a bronchodilator via a nebulizer. A corticosteroid, theophylline, and an antibiotic may also be ordered. The patient may also need chest physiotherapy, including postural drainage, chest percussion, and chest vibration and possibly suctioning to clear the airways. I.V. fluids may be ordered to correct dehydration and to help thin secretions. A diuretic may help if the patient is experiencing fluid overload.

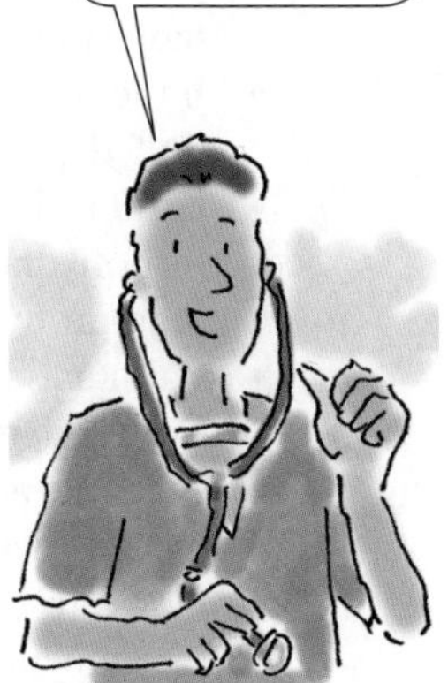

Keep a close eye on your patient's respiratory status, including breath sounds.

How you intervene

To care effectively for a patient with respiratory failure, follow these guidelines:

- Assess respiratory status; monitor rate, depth, and character of respirations, checking breath sounds for abnormalities.
- Monitor vital signs frequently.
- Monitor the patient's neurologic status; it may become depressed as respiratory failure worsens.
- Make sure your ongoing respiratory assessment includes skin and mucous membrane color; accessory muscle use; changes in breath sounds; ABG analysis; secretion production and clearance; and respiratory rate, depth, and pattern. Notify the practitioner if interventions don't improve the patient's condition.
- Monitor fluid status by maintaining accurate fluid intake and output records. Obtain daily weights.
- Evaluate serum electrolyte levels for abnormalities that can occur with acid-base imbalances.
- Evaluate ECG results for arrhythmias.
- Monitor oxygen saturation values with a pulse oximeter.
- Intervene as needed to correct underlying respiratory problems and associated alterations in acid-base status.
- Keep a handheld resuscitation bag at the bedside.
- Maintain patent I.V. access as ordered for medication and I.V. fluid administration.

- Administer oxygen as ordered to help maintain adequate oxygenation and restore normal respiratory rate.
- Use caution when administering oxygen to a patient with COPD. Increased oxygen levels can depress the breathing stimulus.
- Make sure the ventilator settings are at the ordered parameters.
- Perform chest physiotherapy and postural drainage as needed to promote adequate ventilation.
- If the patient is retaining carbon dioxide, encourage slow deep breaths with pursed lips to prevent alveolar collapse. Urge to the coughing up of secretions. If the patient can't mobilize secretions, suction when necessary.
- Unless the patient is retaining fluid or has heart failure, increase his fluid intake to 2 qt (2 L)/day to help liquefy secretions.
- Reposition the immobilized patient every 1 to 2 hours.
- Position the patient for optimum lung expansion. Sit the conscious patient upright as tolerated in a supported, forward-leaning position to promote diaphragm movement. Supply an overbed table and pillows for support.
- If the patient isn't on a ventilator, avoid giving narcotics or another CNS depressant because either may further suppress respirations.
- Limit carbohydrate intake and increase protein intake because carbohydrate metabolism causes more carbon dioxide production than protein metabolism.
- Calm and reassure the patient while giving care. Anxiety can raise oxygen demands.
- Pace care activities to maximize the patient's energy level and to provide needed rest. Limit the need to respond verbally. Talking may cause shortness of breath.
- Implement safety measures as needed to protect the patient. Reorient the confused patient.
- Stress the importance of returning for routine follow-up appointments with the doctor.
- Explain how to recognize signs and symptoms of overexertion, fluid retention, and heart failure. These may include a weight gain of 2 to 3 lb (0.9 to 1.4 kg)/day, edema of the feet or ankles, nausea, loss of appetite, shortness of breath, or abdominal tenderness. (See *Teaching about respiratory failure*.)
- Help the patient develop the knowledge and skills he needs to perform pulmonary hygiene. Encourage adequate hydration to thin secretions—but instruct the patient to notify the doctor of any signs or symptoms of fluid retention or heart failure.
- Document all instructions given and care provided. (See *Documenting respiratory failure*.)

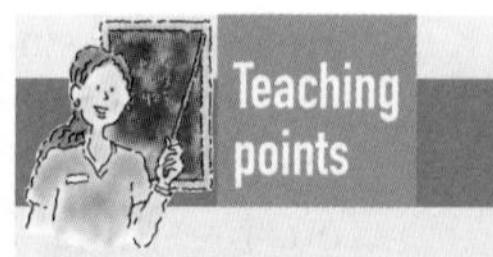

Teaching about respiratory failure

When teaching a patient with respiratory failure, be sure to cover the following topics and then evaluate your patient's learning:

- basics of respiratory failure and its treatment
- proper pulmonary hygiene and coughing techniques
- need for proper rest
- need to quit smoking, if appropriate
- prescribed medications
- warning signs and symptoms and when to report them
- importance of follow-up appointments
- diet restrictions, if appropriate.

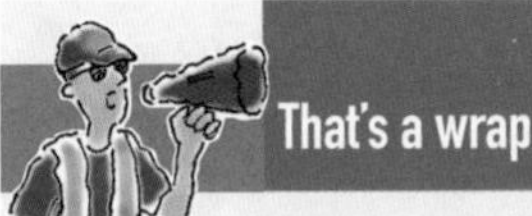

Respiratory failure review

Respiratory failure basics
- Occurs when the lungs can't sufficiently maintain arterial oxygenation or eliminate carbon dioxide
- Usually produces hypercapnia and hypoxemia in patients with normal lung tissue
- May be signaled only by an acute drop in ABG levels and clinical deterioration in patients with COPD
- Gas exchange diminished by three major malfunctions: alveolar hypoventilation, ($\dot{V}/\dot{Q}$) mismatch, and intrapulmonary shunting

Imbalances associated with respiratory failure

Hypervolemia
- May be caused by excessive fluid absorption as a result of prolonged respiratory treatments or increased lung capillary pressure or permeability
- May precipitate pulmonary edema

Hypovolemia
- May be caused by increased respiratory rate, which can promote excessive water loss
- May also occur with fever or any other condition that increases the metabolic rate and thus the respiratory rate

Hypokalemia
- May be caused by hyperventilation and resulting alkalosis, which causes hydrogen ions to move out of the cells and potassium ions to shift from the blood and into the cells

Hyperkalemia
- May be caused by acidosis, in which excess hydrogen ions move into the cells while potassium ions shift from the cells and into the blood

Respiratory acidosis
- Results from hypoventilation (lungs can't eliminate carbon dioxide; carbon dioxide combines with water to form carbonic acid)
- Contributed to by decreased pH levels that result from increased carbonic acid

Respiratory alkalosis
- Results from hyperventilation (rapid respiration causes excessive carbon dioxide elimination, which decreases the blood's acid-forming potential, resulting in alkalosis)

Metabolic acidosis
- Results from hypoxia, which causes cells to use anaerobic metabolism
- Produces an increase in lactic acid, leading to metabolic acidosis

Signs and symptoms
- Increased respiratory depth and rate
- Muscle retraction between the ribs, above the clavicle, and above the sternum
- Increased heart rate and arrhythmias
- Constriction of blood vessels
- Anxiety and restlessness, progressing to fatigue, confusion, agitation, and lethargy
- Headaches
- Changes in serum potassium levels

(continued)

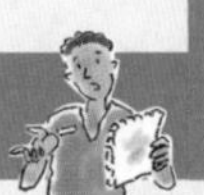

Documenting respiratory failure

If your patient has respiratory failure, make sure you document the following information:
- breath sounds
- lung secretions
- laboratory results
- breathing exercises and the patient's response
- color and temperature of skin
- daily weight
- intake and output
- measures taken to promote ventilation and the patient's response
- neurologic status
- notification of doctor
- oxygen therapy
- safety measures
- patient teaching.

Respiratory failure review *(continued)*

Treatment
- Lowest possible dose of oxygen for the shortest amount of time to prevent oxygen toxicity
- Intubation and ventilation if unable to achieve oxygen saturation above 90%
- Bronchodilators as ordered to open airways
- Corticosteroids, theophylline, antibiotics, chest physiotherapy, and suctioning as ordered
- I.V. fluids for dehydration or diuretics for a fluid overload as ordered

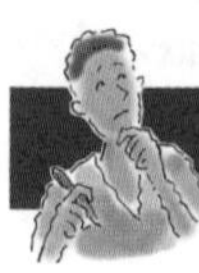

Quick quiz

1. When the body senses hypoxemia or hypercapnia, the brain's respiratory center responds by:
   A. slowing down the respiratory rate.
   B. decreasing the heart rate.
   C. increasing the depth and rate of respirations.
   D. increasing the heart rate.

Answer: C. The brain's respiratory center initially causes an increase in respiratory rate. It then causes an increase in respiratory depth in an effort to blow off excess carbon dioxide.

2. Respiratory alkalosis can develop from:
   A. hyperventilation.
   B. excessive vomiting.
   C. prolonged use of antacids.
   D. decreased respiratory rate.

Answer: A. Respiratory alkalosis develops from an excessively rapid respiratory rate—hyperventilation—which causes excessive carbon dioxide elimination.

3. Prolonged respiratory treatment, such as nebulizer use, can lead to which of the following conditions?
   A. Hypovolemia
   B. Respiratory alkalosis
   C. Respiratory acidosis
   D. Hypervolemia

Answer: D. Prolonged respiratory treatments, such as nebulizer use, can lead to the inhalation and absorption of water vapor, which can lead to hypervolemia.

4. You're concerned about possible respiratory failure in your newly admitted patient. When administering drug therapy, you should avoid giving him which of the following agents?
   A. Anticholinergics
   B. Corticosteroids
   C. Opioids
   D. Antihypertensives

Answer: C. Opioids depress the respiratory center of the brain and may hasten the development of respiratory failure.

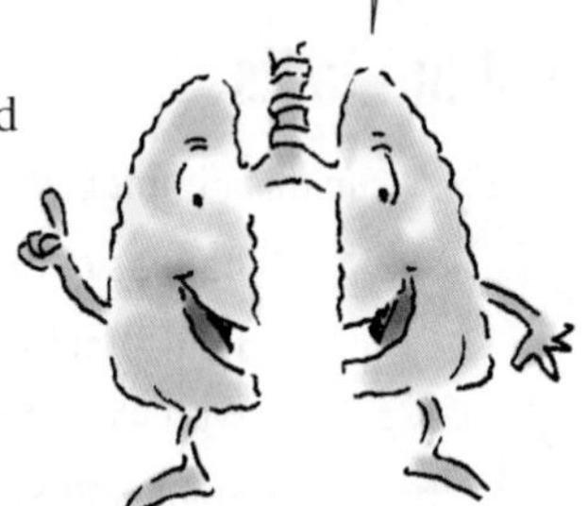
I'm
feeling better
already!

5. A patient with respiratory failure should limit his intake of:
   A. protein.
   B. carbohydrates.
   C. water.
   D. sodium.

Answer: B. A patient with respiratory failure should limit carbohydrate intake and increase protein intake because carbohydrate metabolism causes more carbon dioxide production than protein metabolism.

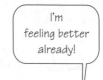

Scoring

☆☆☆ If you answered all five questions correctly, outstanding! You're an inspiration when it comes to respiration!

☆☆ If you answered four questions correctly, great! Breathe deeply and appreciate your accomplishment!

☆ If you answered fewer than four questions correctly, don't worry. Keep your head up and catch your breath; you have more chapters to run through!

References

American Thoracic Society. (2014). *Oxygen delivery methods*. Retrieved from https://www.thoracic.org/clinical/copd-guidelines/for-health-professionals/exacerbation/inpatient-oxygen-therapy/oxygen-delivery-methods.php

Chapter 15

Excessive GI fluid loss

Just the facts

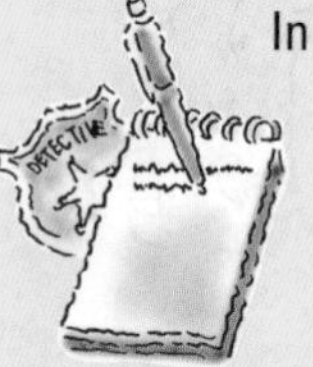

In this chapter, you'll learn:

- causes of excessive gastrointestinal (GI) fluid loss
- fluid, electrolyte, and acid-base imbalances that occur with excessive GI fluid loss and ways to treat them
- signs and symptoms of excessive GI fluid loss
- teaching points for patients with excessive GI fluid loss.

A look at excessive GI fluid loss

Normally, very little fluid is lost from the GI system. Most fluid is reabsorbed in the intestines. However, the potential for significant loss exists because large amounts of fluids—isotonic and hypotonic—pass through the GI system in the course of a day.

Isotonic fluids that may be lost from the GI tract include gastric juices, bile, pancreatic juices, and intestinal secretions. The only hypotonic fluid that may be lost is saliva, which has a lower solute concentration than other GI fluids.

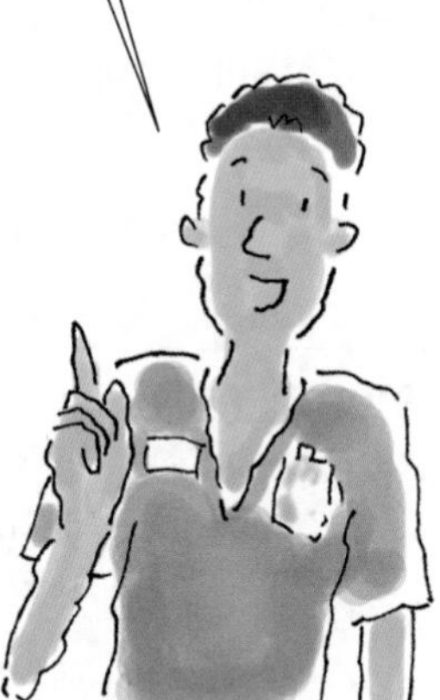
Normally, the body loses very little fluid from the GI system.

How it happens

Excessive GI fluid loss may come from physical removal of secretions as a result of vomiting, suctioning, or increased or decreased GI tract motility. Excessive fluids can be excreted as waste products or secreted from the intestinal wall into the intestinal lumen, both of which lead to fluid and electrolyte imbalances. (See *Imbalances caused by excessive GI fluid loss.*)

Osmotic diarrhea may occur in the intestines when a high solute load in the intestinal lumen attracts water into the cavity. Both acids and bases can be lost from the GI tract.

Imbalances caused by excessive GI fluid loss

Excessive GI fluid loss can lead to a number of fluid, electrolyte, and acid-base imbalances. Here's a breakdown of those imbalances.

Fluid imbalances

- *Hypovolemia and dehydration*—Large amounts of fluid can be lost during prolonged, uncorrected vomiting and diarrhea. Hypovolemia can also result if gastric and intestinal suctioning occur without proper monitoring of intake and output to make sure lost fluid and electrolytes are adequately replaced.

Electrolyte imbalances

- *Hypokalemia*—The excessive loss of gastric fluids rich in potassium can lead to hypokalemia.
- *Hypomagnesemia*—Although gastric secretions contain little magnesium, several weeks of vomiting, diarrhea, or gastric suctioning can result in hypomagnesemia. Because hypomagnesemia itself can cause vomiting, the patient's condition may be self-perpetuating.
- *Hyponatremia*—Prolonged vomiting, diarrhea, or gastric or intestinal suctioning can deplete the body's supply of sodium and lead to hyponatremia.
- *Hypochloremia*—Any loss of gastric contents causes the loss of chloride. Prolonged gastric fluid loss can lead to hypochloremia.

Acid-base imbalances

- *Metabolic acidosis*—Any condition that promotes intestinal fluid loss can result in metabolic acidosis. Intestinal fluid contains large amounts of bicarbonate. With the loss of bicarbonate, pH falls, creating an acidic condition.
- *Metabolic alkalosis*—Loss of gastric fluids from vomiting or the use of drainage tubes in the upper GI tract can lead to metabolic alkalosis. Gastric fluids contain large amounts of acids that, when lost, lead to an increase in pH and alkalosis. Excessive use of antacids can also worsen the imbalance by adding to the alkalotic state.

Vomiting and suctioning

Vomiting or mechanical suctioning of stomach contents, as with a nasogastric tube, causes the loss of hydrogen ions and electrolytes, such as chloride, potassium, and sodium. Vomiting also depletes the body's fluid volume supply and causes hypovolemia. Dehydration occurs when more water than electrolytes is lost. When assessing acid-base balance, remember that the pH of the upper GI tract is low and that vomiting causes the loss of those acids and raises the risk of alkalosis. (See *Characteristics and causes of vomiting,* page 274.)

Characteristics and causes of vomiting

Vomiting may lead to serious fluid, electrolyte, and acid-base disturbances and can occur for a variety of reasons. By carefully observing the characteristics of the vomitus and, as needed, questioning the patient, you may gain clues as to the underlying disorder. Here's what the vomitus may indicate.

Bile-stained (greenish)
Obstruction below the pylorus, as from a duodenal lesion

Bloody
Upper GI bleeding, as from gastritis or peptic ulcer (if bright red) or from gastric or esophageal varices (if dark red)

Brown with a fecal odor
Intestinal obstruction or infarction

Burning, bitter-tasting
Excessive hydrochloric acid in gastric contents

Coffee-ground consistency
Digested blood from slowly bleeding gastric or duodenal lesions

Undigested food
Gastric outlet obstruction, as from gastric tumor or ulcer

Bowel movements

An increase in the frequency and amount of bowel movements and a change in the stool toward a watery consistency can cause excessive fluid loss, resulting in hypovolemia and dehydration. In addition to fluid loss, diarrhea can cause a loss of potassium, magnesium, and sodium. Fluids lost from the lower GI tract carry a large amount of bicarbonate with them, which lowers the amount of bicarbonate available to counter the effects of acids in the body.

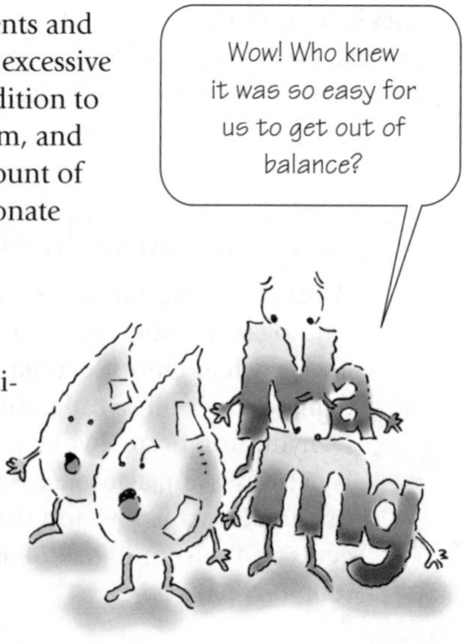

Wow! Who knew it was so easy for us to get out of balance?

Laxatives and enemas

Laxatives and enemas may be used by patients to treat constipation, or they may be given to patients before abdominal surgery or diagnostic studies to clean the bowel. Excessive use of laxatives—such as magnesium sulfate, milk of magnesia, and Fleet Phospho-soda—can cause high magnesium (hypermagnesemia) and phosphorus (hyperphosphatemia) levels.

Excessive use of commercially prepared enemas containing sodium and phosphate, such as Fleet enemas, can cause high phosphorus and sodium (hypernatremia) levels if the enemas are absorbed before they can be eliminated. Excessive use of tap water enemas can cause a decrease in sodium levels because water absorbed by the colon can have a dilutional effect on sodium.

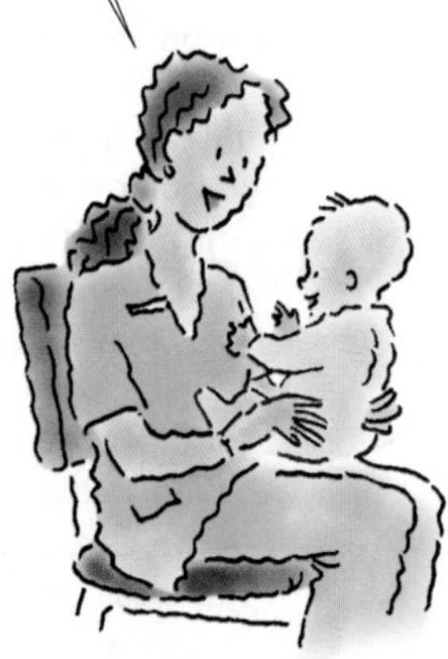

I had better keep an eye on you. Young children are particularly vulnerable to fluid loss from diarrhea.

Factor in fluid loss

Excessive GI fluid loss can result from several other factors, too. Bacterial infections of the GI tract typically cause vomiting and diarrhea. Antibiotic administration removes the normal flora and promotes diarrhea. Age can also play a role; infants and young children are especially vulnerable to diarrhea. Pregnancy, pancreatitis, hepatitis and, in young children, pyloric stenosis can all be accompanied by vomiting.

An abundance of imbalances

Imbalances can also result from fecal impaction, poor absorption of foods, poor digestion, anorexia nervosa, or bulimia as well as excessive intake of alcoholic substances and some illicit drugs. Such disorders as anorexia nervosa and bulimia, which primarily affect young women, typically involve the use of laxatives and vomiting as a means of controlling weight. This can lead to numerous fluid, electrolyte, and acid-base imbalances. (See *Adolescents and excessive GI fluid loss*.) Other disorders that can cause disturbances in fluid, electrolyte, or acid-base balance include the presence of fistulas involving the GI tract, GI bleeding, intestinal obstruction, and paralytic ileus.

The use of enteral tube feedings and ostomies (especially ileostomies) may also lead to imbalances. Enteral tube feedings may cause diarrhea or vomiting, depending on their composition, concentration,

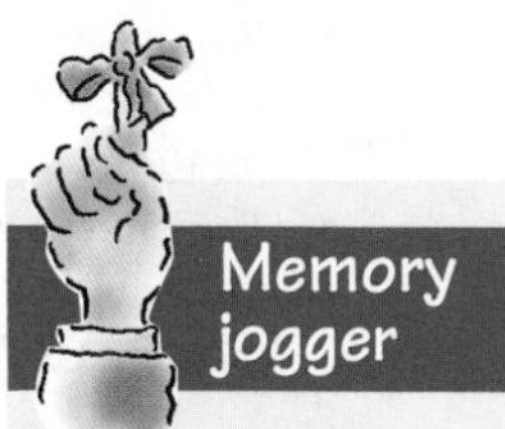

Memory jogger

Remember, laxatives and enemas can make a patient HYPER:

Excessive laxative use can cause **hyper**magnesemia and **hyper**phosphatemia.

Excessive use of enemas that contain sodium and phosphate can cause **hyper**natremia and **hyper**phosphatemia.

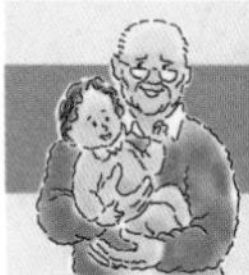

Ages and stages

Adolescents and excessive GI fluid loss

When treating an adolescent, especially a female, for excessive GI fluid loss, assess for signs and symptoms of anorexia and bulimia. Teeth that appear yellow and worn away and a history of laxative or diet pill use are two obvious signs.

Also, assess the patient for use of alternative diet therapies, particularly pills containing ma huang or ephedrine, which speed the metabolism by mimicking the effects of adrenaline on the GI system. Other agents such as orlistat (Xenical) bind to gastric and pancreatic enzymes to prevent digestion of fats and may produce GI fluid loss as well as decreased absorption of vitamins.

and the patient's condition. Suctioning of gastric secretions through tubes may deplete the body of vital fluids, electrolytes, and acids. Dysphagia related to extensive head and neck cancer and other conditions that interfere with swallowing may result in saliva loss.

What to look for

With excessive GI fluid loss, the patient may show signs of hypovolemia. Look for these signs and symptoms:

- Tachycardia occurs as the body tries to compensate for hypovolemia by increasing the heart rate. Blood pressure also falls as intravascular volume is lost.
- The patient's skin may be cool and dry as the body shunts blood flow to major organs. Skin turgor may be decreased or the eyeballs may appear to be sunken, as occurs with dehydration. Urine output decreases as kidneys try to conserve fluid and electrolytes.
- Cardiac arrhythmias may occur from electrolyte imbalances, such as those related to potassium and magnesium. The patient may become weak and confused. Mental status may deteriorate as fluid, electrolyte, and acid-base imbalances progress.

Taking a deep breath

- Respirations may change according to the type of acid-base imbalance the patient develops. For instance, acidosis will cause respirations to be deeper as the patient tries to blow off acid.
- The patient will also have signs and symptoms related to the underlying disorder—for instance, pancreatitis. (See *Recognizing excessive GI fluid loss*.)

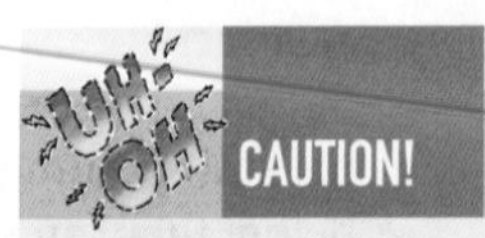

Recognizing excessive GI fluid loss

In addition to the signs and symptoms related to the underlying disorder, a patient with excessive GI fluid loss may show these signs and symptoms of hypovolemia:

- changes in respiration
- weight loss
- confusion or deteriorated mental status
- cool, dry, pale skin
- muscle cramps
- decreased blood pressure
- decreased/tenting skin turgor or sunken eyeballs
- decreased output with concentrated urine
- possible arrhythmias
- tachycardia
- weakness.

What tests show

Diagnostic tests, such as endoscopy, ultrasound, computerized tomography, or magnetic resonance imaging, may reveal the cause and extent of the disorder. In addition, diagnostic test results related to the fluid, electrolyte, and acid-base imbalances associated with excessive GI fluid loss can help direct your nursing interventions. Such results include:

- changes in arterial blood gas levels related to metabolic acidosis or metabolic alkalosis
- alterations in the levels of certain electrolytes, such as potassium, magnesium, and/or sodium
- hematocrit that may be falsely elevated in a volume-depleted patient
- cultures of body fluid samples that may help to identify bacteria responsible for the underlying disorder.

How they're treated

Treatment is aimed at the underlying cause of the imbalance to prevent further fluid and electrolyte loss. For instance, an antiemetic and an antidiarrheal may be given for vomiting and diarrhea, respectively. In another instance, GI drainage tubes and the suction applied to them should be discontinued as soon as possible.

The patient should also receive I.V. or oral fluid replacement, depending on his tolerance and the cause of the fluid loss. He may also need electrolytes replaced if his serum levels are decreased. Long-term parenteral nutrition may be needed. If infection is the underlying cause of fluid loss, the patient may need antibiotics.

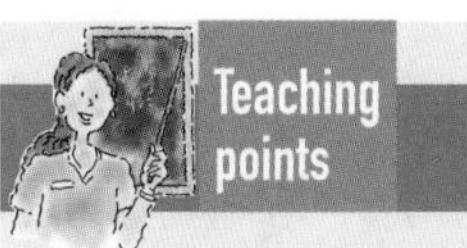

Teaching about excessive GI fluid loss

When teaching a patient with excessive GI fluid loss, be sure to cover the following topics and then evaluate your patient's learning:

- basics of the condition and its treatment
- need to report prolonged vomiting or diarrhea
- importance of avoiding repeated use of enemas and laxatives
- proper technique for irrigating a gastric tube, if appropriate
- proper technique for monitoring I.V. infusion, if appropriate.

How you intervene

A patient with a condition that alters fluid and electrolyte balance through GI losses requires close monitoring. You'll need to report any increase in the amount of drainage or change in drainage characteristics from GI tubes or increase in the frequency of vomiting or diarrhea. Follow these interventions when caring for a patient with GI fluid losses:

- Measure and record the amount of fluid lost through vomiting, diarrhea, or gastric or intestinal suctioning. Remember to include GI losses as part of the patient's total output. Significant increases in GI loss places the patient at increased risk for fluid and electrolyte imbalances and metabolic alkalosis or acidosis.
- Assess the patient's fluid status by monitoring intake and output, daily weight, and skin turgor.
- Assess vital signs and report any changes that may indicate fluid deficits, such as a decreased blood pressure or increased heart rate.
- Report vomiting to keep imbalances from becoming severe and to initiate prompt treatment.
- Administer oral fluids containing water and electrolytes, such as Gatorade or Pedialyte, if the patient can tolerate fluids. (See *Teaching about excessive GI fluid loss*.)
- Perform oral care and provide lip balm because the mucous membranes and lips may be dry and cracked.

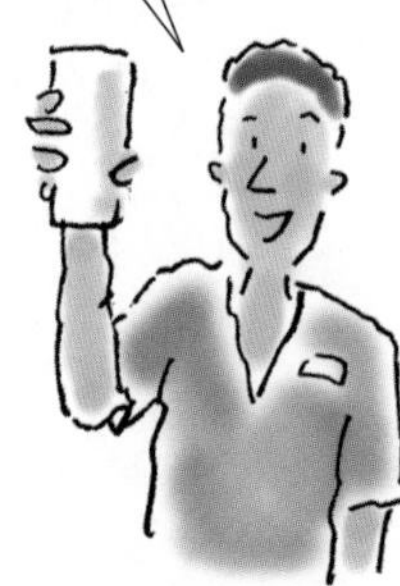
If your patient can tolerate fluids, give him oral fluids that contain water and electrolytes.

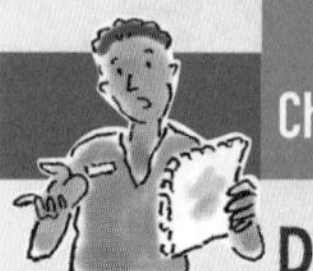

Chart smart

Documenting excessive GI fluid loss

If your patient has excessive GI fluid loss, make sure you document the following information:

- vital signs
- intake and output
- daily weight
- presence and characteristics of vomitus, diarrhea, and/or GI fluid drainage
- skin turgor
- correct placement of GI tube, if present, plus care related to the tube
- interventions used to decrease GI fluid loss
- I.V. or oral fluid and electrolyte replacement therapy and the patient's response.

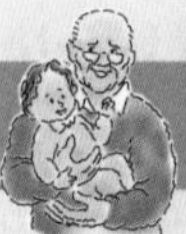

Ages and stages

Don't go too fast with fluids

Elderly patients can develop heart failure if I.V. fluids are infused too rapidly. Therefore, use caution when administering I.V. fluids to replace fluid losses in these patients.

- Maintain patent I.V. access as ordered. Administer I.V. replacement fluids as prescribed. Monitor the infusion rate and volume to prevent hypervolemia. (See *Don't go too fast with fluids.*)
- If the patient is undergoing gastric suctioning, monitor GI tube placement often to prevent fluid aspiration or tube migration.
- Irrigate the suction tube with isotonic normal saline solution as ordered. Remember, never use plain water for irrigation. It draws more gastric secretions into the stomach in an attempt to make the fluid isotonic for absorption. Also, the fluid is suctioned out of the stomach, causing further depletion of fluids and electrolytes.
- When the patient is connected to gastric suction, restrict the amount of ice chips given by mouth and explain the reason for the restriction. Gastric suctioning of ice chips can deplete fluid and electrolytes from the stomach.
- Administer medications, such as an antiemetic or antidiarrheal, as prescribed to control the patient's underlying condition.
- Evaluate serum electrolyte levels and pH to detect abnormalities and to monitor the effectiveness of therapy.
- Chart all instructions given and care provided. (See *Documenting excessive GI fluid loss.*)

Have you got all that?
The quiz is coming shortly!

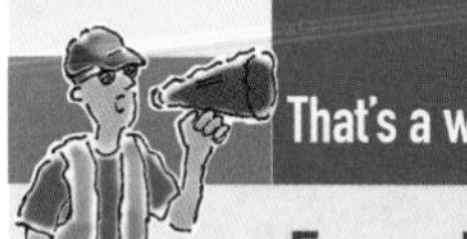

Excessive GI fluid loss review

Excessive GI fluid loss

- May result from vomiting, suctioning, or increased or decreased GI tract motility
- May be excreted as waste products or secreted from the intestinal wall into the intestinal lumen, leading to fluid and electrolyte imbalances

Causes

- Anorexia nervosa
- Antibiotic use
- Bacterial GI infections
- Bulimia
- Enteral tube feedings and ostomies
- Excessive intake of alcohol and illicit drugs
- Excessive use of enemas and laxatives
- Fecal impaction
- GI bleeding
- GI fistulas
- Intestinal obstruction
- Pancreatitis or hepatitis
- Paralytic ileus
- Poor absorption of foods
- Poor digestion
- Pyloric stenosis in young children

Signs and symptoms

- Altered respirations
- Arrhythmias
- Cool, dry skin or decreased skin turgor
- Decreased, concentrated urine output
- Falsely elevated hemoglobin level and hematocrit
- Increased heart rate and decreased blood pressure
- Sunken eyeballs
- Muscle cramps
- Weakness and confusion

Imbalances associated with excessive GI fluid loss

Hypovolemia and dehydration

- Can occur with prolonged vomiting and diarrhea or if gastric and intestinal suctioning occur without proper monitoring of intake and output

Hypokalemia

- Can occur with excessive loss of gastric fluids rich in potassium

Hypomagnesemia

- Can occur with prolonged (lasting several weeks) vomiting, diarrhea, or gastric suctioning

Hyponatremia

- Can occur with prolonged vomiting, diarrhea, or gastric suctioning
- Can also occur with excessive use of tap water enemas because water absorbed by the colon can have a dilutional effect on sodium

Hypochloremia

- Can be caused by any loss of gastric contents

Metabolic acidosis

- Caused by a loss of intestinal fluid, which causes loss of bicarbonate, leading to decreased pH and an acidic state

Metabolic alkalosis

- Caused by a loss of gastric fluids, including acid, which increases pH and creates an alkalotic state

(continued)

Excessive GI fluid loss review *(continued)*

Hypermagnesemia and hyperphosphatemia
- May be caused by excessive use of laxatives, such as magnesium sulfate, milk of magnesia, and Fleet Phospho-soda

Hypernatremia and hyperphosphatemia
- May be caused by excessive use of enemas containing sodium and phosphorus, such as Fleet enemas

Treatment
- Prevention of further fluid and electrolyte loss
- Antiemetics for nausea and vomiting if indicated
- Antidiarrheals if diarrhea is the cause
- I.V. or oral fluid replacement, depending on the severity
- Electrolyte replacement
- Long-term parenteral nutrition if needed
- Antibiotics if infection is the underlying cause

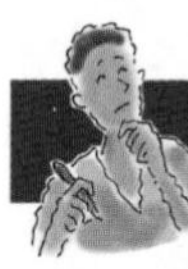

Quick quiz

1. Which of the following fluid and electrolyte imbalances can occur with excessive GI fluid loss?
   A. Hypomagnesemia, hypermagnesemia, and hyponatremia
   B. Hypomagnesemia, hypernatremia, and hyperchloremia
   C. Hypervolemia, hyponatremia, and hypernatremia
   D. Hypervolemia, hypomagnesemia, and hyperkalemia

Answer: A. Hypomagnesemia, hypermagnesemia, and hyponatremia—and others—may occur with varying types of GI fluid loss.

2. A patient with fluid losses from the upper GI tract is likely to suffer from which of the following imbalances?
   A. Metabolic alkalosis
   B. Metabolic acidosis
   C. Respiratory acidosis
   D. Metabolic acidosis

Answer: A. Fluid losses from the upper GI tract can result in metabolic alkalosis; losses from the lower GI tract can result in metabolic acidosis.

3. Warning signs of hypovolemia associated with GI losses include:
   A. bradycardia, decreased blood pressure, and decreased urine output.
   B. tachycardia, increased blood pressure, and increased urine output.
   C. decreased blood pressure; increased urine output; and warm, flushed skin.
   D. tachycardia, decreased blood pressure, and decreased urine output.

Answer: D. Tachycardia, decreased blood pressure, and decreased urine output indicate that the patient is experiencing hypovolemia from GI losses.

4. You carefully observe the characteristics of the patient's vomitus and document your finding as brown with fecal odor. This type of vomitus may indicate:
   A. excessive hydrochloric acid in gastric contents.
   B. intestinal obstruction.
   C. obstruction below the pylorus.
   D. gastric outlet obstruction.

Answer: B. Brown vomitus that has a fecal odor may indicate intestinal obstruction or infarction.

Scoring

☆☆☆ If you answered all four questions correctly, here's a high five! You're a GI genius!

☆☆ If you answered three questions correctly, we want to shake your hand! You're certainly not at a loss for the right answers!

☆ If you answered fewer than three correctly, don't fret! With a little (certainly not excessive!) review, you'll get this down just fine.

Reference

Hinkle, J., & Cheever, K. (2014). *Brunner & Suddarth's textbook of medical-surgical nursing* (13th ed.). Philadelphia, PA: Lippincott Williams & Wilkins.

Chapter 16

Acute pancreatitis

Just the facts

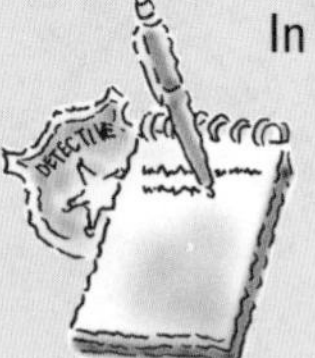

In this chapter you'll learn:

- types and causes of acute pancreatitis
- signs and symptoms of acute pancreatitis
- fluid and electrolyte imbalances that can occur with acute pancreatitis
- treatments for acute pancreatitis
- nursing interventions for patients with acute pancreatitis.

A look at acute pancreatitis

Pancreatitis is an inflammation of the pancreas. An accessory organ of the gastrointestinal (GI) tract, the pancreas lies in the left upper abdomen behind the stomach and between the spleen and duodenum. It functions as both an exocrine and endocrine gland, producing enzymes that promote digestion and hormones that aid in glucose balance. (See *Functions of the pancreas*.)

Adults of any age can develop acute pancreatitis; however, children rarely develop the disorder. It can occur in either edematous (interstitial) or necrotizing form. Both types cause inflammation that begins in the acinar cells. (See *Edematous vs. necrotizing*, page 284.) Most cases of acute pancreatitis are mild; however, about 15% of patients experience a severe form of the disease that can cause life-threatening complications, including fluid and electrolyte disturbances.

Acute pancreatitis that occurs on two or more occasions is classified as acute recurrent pancreatitis. When progressive recurring episodes of inflammation cause structural damage and loss of glandular function, pancreatitis becomes chronic. (See *Chronic pancreatitis*, page 285.)

About 15% of patients with acute pancreatitis have a severe form of the disease that can cause life-threatening complications. That doesn't make me happy!

Functions of the pancreas

The pancreas works in two ways. As an exocrine gland, it secretes its products through ducts—in this case, enzymes and bicarbonate that promote digestion. As an endocrine gland, the pancreas secretes hormones directly into the bloodstream. These hormones help maintain glucose balance.

Exocrine function

Within the pancreas, groups of acinar cells produce precursor digestive enzymes that the pancreas secretes into the intestine through the main pancreatic duct. These enzymes play a crucial role in breaking down and metabolizing carbohydrates, proteins, and fats.

When these enzymes first come from the acinar cells, they aren't active; that doesn't happen until they combine with enzymes in the intestinal mucosa of the duodenum. The combined enzymes then convert partially digested food into substances the body can use for energy. The pancreas produces three main types of enzymes: amylase, which digests carbohydrates; trypsinogen and chymotrypsinogen, which digest protein; and pancreatic lipase, which combines with bile acids to digest triglycerides, a major component of dietary fats.

Pancreatic secretions also contain bicarbonate, which comes from the epithelial cells lining the smaller pancreatic ducts. The bicarbonate helps in digestion by neutralizing the acidic chyme that the stomach releases into the small intestine.

Endocrine function

The pancreas also secretes hormones directly into the bloodstream, where they're carried to different cells in the body. It produces these hormones in the islets of Langerhans, a specialized group of cells. Islet cells are dispersed throughout the pancreas, although the tail of the pancreas has the highest concentration.

Four different types of cells in the islets of Langerhans produce hormones. Beta cells, which compose 65% to 80% of islet cells, produce insulin, amylin, and C-peptide. Insulin regulates the use and storage of glucose. It acts by forcing many body cells to absorb and use glucose, which decreases blood glucose levels. When blood glucose levels rise again, the pancreas secretes more insulin. Amylin supplements insulin's actions by reducing blood glucose levels. It also inhibits the secretion of glucagon, slows the emptying of the stomach, and sends a satiety signal to the brain. C-peptide is a byproduct of insulin production. Levels of this hormone help to identify viable beta cell mass.

Alpha cells—15% to 20% of islet cells—produce glucagon. This hormone helps maintain a steady blood glucose level. It does this by forcing many body cells to release or produce glucose. Low blood glucose levels stimulate its secretion; high glucose and amylin levels inhibit its secretion.

Delta cells, which make up 3% to 10% of islet cells, produce somatostatin. This hormone decreases the rate of nutrient absorption, inhibits the secretion of many other hormones—including growth hormone, insulin, glucagon, and other GI hormones—and suppresses pancreatic exocrine secretions. It also has various complex effects on the nervous system.

Gamma or pancreatic polypeptide cells make up a mere 1% of islet cells. These cells produce pancreatic polypeptide. Although its function is unknown, it's thought to inhibit appetite. Secretion of this hormone increases after a protein meal, fasting, exercise, and acute hypoglycemia. Somatostatin and I.V. glucose decrease its production.

Edematous vs. necrotizing

Acute pancreatitis occurs in two forms: edematous (or interstitial) and necrotizing. Both forms begin in the acinar cells, causing inflammation. The severity of the disease depends on the degree of the inflammatory response and resulting cell damage.

Edematous pancreatitis

- Usually mild
- Eighty-five percent of cases
- Self-limiting, typically resolving in 5 to 7 days
- Triggers an inflammatory response
- Causes fluid accumulation and swelling
- Results in minimal organ damage
- May cause scattered areas of fat necrosis

Necrotizing pancreatitis

- Severe
- Fifteen percent of cases
- Progressive
- Triggers a hyperinflammatory response
- Causes tissue damage and cell death
- Results in organ failure
- May cause life-threatening complications

How it happens

Gallstones are the most common cause of acute pancreatitis, accounting for 45% of all cases in the United States (Fernandez & Kerman, 2013). They pass into the bile duct and temporarily block the opening into the duodenum at the point where it's joined by the pancreatic duct. This obstructs pancreatic juices from flowing out of the pancreas into the duodenum. The backflow of these digestive juices causes lysis (dissolving) of pancreatic cells and subsequent pancreatitis. This typically mild type of pancreatitis resolves with the passage or removal of the gallstones.

Evil spirits

It's believed that ethyl alcohol, the second most common cause of acute pancreatitis, can cause the disease in several ways. Ethyl alcohol is implicated as the causative factor in 35% of all pancreatitis cases and is the most common cause of pancreatitis in males worldwide (Fernandez & Kerman, 2013). Alcohol can affect the motility of the

Chronic pancreatitis

In chronic pancreatitis, widespread scarring and destruction of pancreatic tissue occurs. In about 80% of cases, the disorder results from prolonged and excessive alcohol intake.

Chronic pancreatitis typically affects the exocrine functions of the pancreas first and results in weight loss because of the intestines' inability to digest food and absorb nutrition. Patients with chronic pancreatitis are at risk for developing:

- calculi that can block or cause stenosis of bile ducts
- diabetes mellitus
- gastric bleeding
- pancreatic cancer
- portal hypertension
- pseudocysts
- severe, chronic pain.

sphincter of Oddi, have direct toxic and metabolic effects on the pancreas, and form protein plugs that obstruct small ducts in the pancreas. It's also believed that alcohol produces a temporary but significant reduction in blood flow to the pancreas. When these episodes occur repeatedly, they result in ischemic damage to the cells.

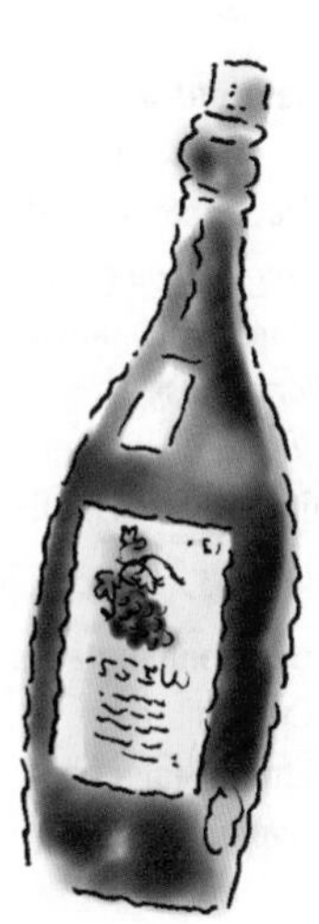

These effects can occur from long-term abuse or from a single episode of binge drinking. A person sensitive to the effects of alcohol may have an attack of acute pancreatitis a few hours to a day or two after drinking; such a person may not need to drink very much alcohol to precipitate an attack. Alcohol typically results in a more severe type of pancreatitis because of the cell necrosis that occurs. With repeated attacks, pancreatitis becomes chronic.

Cause and exocrine effect

Acute pancreatitis can result from several other, less common, causes. (See *Causes of acute pancreatitis*, page 286.) But no matter what the cause, it's the exocrine functions that fail during acute pancreatitis. The enzymes that the pancreas normally excretes into the duodenum are instead activated within the pancreas or its ducts and begin to digest the pancreatic tissue itself. The inflammation that results causes intense pain, third-space shift of large volumes of fluids (which results in hypovolemia), pancreatic fat necrosis (with accompanying consumption of serum calcium), and, occasionally, hemorrhage.

Causes of acute pancreatitis

Although gallstones and alcohol consumption are the most common causes of acute pancreatitis, many factors can lead to the disorder. Here's a list of possible causes.

Biliary tract disease
- Gallstones
- Spasm or obstruction of the sphincter of Oddi

Drugs
- Glucocorticoids
- Hormonal contraceptives
- Immunosuppressant regimens
- Nonsteroidal anti-inflammatory drugs
- Sulfonamides
- Tetracycline
- Thiazide diuretics

Infectious agents
- Bacteria (such as *Legionella, Mycobacterium tuberculosis,* and *Mycoplasma pneumoniae*)
- Parasites (such as *Ascaris* and *Clonorchis*)
- Viruses (such as cytomegalovirus, hepatitis viruses, HIV [Fernandez & Kerman, 2013], measles, mumps, and rubella)

Toxins and metabolic processes
- Cystic fibrosis
- Ethanol (alcohol)
- Hypercalcemia
- Hyperthyroidism
- Hypertriglyceridemia
- Methanol (Fernandez & Kerman, 2013)
- Organophosphorus insecticides (Fernandez & Kerman, 2013)
- Renal failure
- Scorpion venom

Trauma
- Blunt trauma
- Injury during endoscopic retrograde cholangiopancreatography
- Injury during upper abdominal, renal, or cardiovascular surgery
- Organ transplantation

Other
- Abnormal pancreatic structure
- Atherosclerosis
- Autoimmune disease
- Cysts or tumors
- Emotional or neurogenic factors
- Heredity
- Hypothermia
- Inflammatory bowel disease
- Penetrating peptic ulcer
- Pregnancy (third trimester)
- Shock

Imbalances caused by acute pancreatitis

Acute pancreatitis—whether mild or severe—can cause fluid and electrolyte imbalances, including hypovolemia, hyponatremia, hypocalcemia, hypomagnesemia, and hypokalemia.

Turn up the (blood) volume!

Hypovolemia is a major cause of death in patients with acute pancreatitis. Severe pancreatic damage triggers the release of systemic inflammatory mediators that produce increased capillary permeability and vasodilation. This, in turn, produces massive fluid shifts from the intravascular spaces to the interstitial spaces and the retroperitoneum, resulting in hypovolemia. Vomiting, diarrhea, excessive sweating, and, possibly, hemorrhage also contribute to hypovolemia.

The case of the lost electrolytes

Acute pancreatitis can also result in the loss of calcium, magnesium, and potassium. Vomiting and diarrhea can result in hyponatremia, hypokalemia, and (when severe) hypomagnesemia. Hyponatremia can also result from excessive sweating and increased antidiuretic hormone secretion caused by hypovolemia.

Hypocalcemia in acute pancreatitis usually results from concomitant hypoalbuminemia. Fat necrosis—caused by lipase necrosing the fat tissue in pancreatic interstitium and peripancreatic spaces—may result in the release of free fatty acids and intraperitoneal saponification, further decreasing serum calcium levels. Fat necrosis can also lead to hypomagnesemia because magnesium is deposited in areas of fat necrosis, which reduces serum levels. Because hypomagnesemia can contribute to hypocalcemia, hypomagnesemia should be corrected first.

What to look for

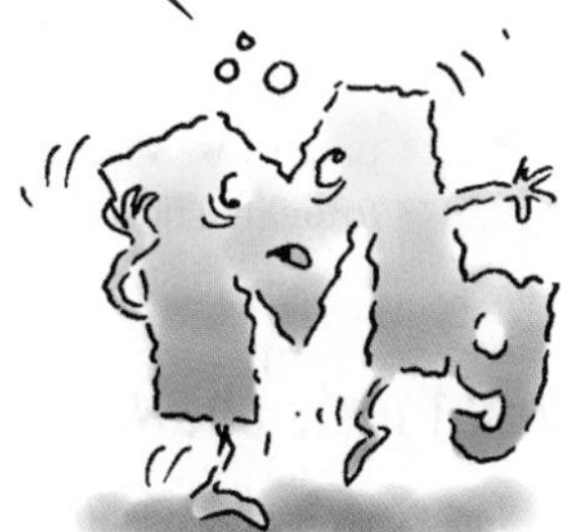

I'm stretched so thin, it's making me dizzy!

Often, the only symptom of mild pancreatitis is steady epigastric pain centered near the navel that's unrelieved by vomiting. In severe pancreatitis, the patient will likely report severe, persistent, piercing abdominal pain, usually in the midepigastric region, although the pain may generalize or occur in the left upper quadrant and radiate to the back or other areas. The patient typically describes the pain as boring or penetrating and may report recent consumption of a large meal or alcohol. His pain may ease when he leans forward or when he lies on his side with his knees drawn toward his chest.

Sign language

Other possible signs and symptoms include nausea; vomiting; fever; mild jaundice; tachycardia; tachypnea; muscle spasms; and fatty, foul-smelling stools. Depending on the severity of the illness and degree of fluid loss and hemorrhage, the patient may also be hypotensive. Assessment may reveal Grey Turner's sign (flank ecchymosis); Cullen's sign (periumbilical ecchymosis); Chvostek's and Trousseau's signs (hypocalcemia); and abdominal distention, rigidity, and tenderness with hypoactive bowel sounds.

Complications of acute pancreatitis

The patient with acute pancreatitis can rapidly develop complications, especially if he has pancreatic necrosis. Monitor closely for signs and symptoms of these complications:

- acute renal failure
- acute respiratory distress syndrome
- acute tubular necrosis
- atelectasis
- chronic pancreatitis
- diabetes mellitus
- disseminated intravascular coagulation
- duodenal or common bile duct obstruction
- GI bleeding
- hemorrhage from ruptured necrotic pancreatic blood vessels
- hypocalcemia
- hypotension
- infectious pancreatic necrosis
- intravascular fluid volume deficit
- multiple organ dysfunction syndrome
- pancreatic abscess
- pancreatic pseudocyst (and possible rupture)
- paralytic ileus
- pleural effusion
- pneumonia
- pulmonary edema
- reduced cardiac contractility, output, and perfusion pressure
- respiratory failure
- shock
- splenic artery pseudoaneurysms
- systemic inflammatory response syndrome
- tetany
- thrombosis of the splenic vein, superior mesenteric vein, and portal veins.

Pancreatitis can lead to severe, life-threatening complications. The patient will need close monitoring for signs and symptoms that may indicate such complications. (See *Complications of acute pancreatitis*.)

What tests show

Several types of diagnostic tests can help identify acute pancreatitis, including imaging and blood studies. Severity scoring can help predict the severity of the disease and the patient's prognosis.

Imaging studies

- Chest X-rays show such pulmonary complications as atelectasis, pleural effusions (most commonly on the left side), or infiltrates that suggest adult respiratory distress syndrome.
- Abdominal X-rays exclude other causes of acute abdominal pain and show bowel dilation and ileus.
- Contrast-enhanced computed tomography (CT) scanning and ultrasonography show an enlarged pancreas with fluid

collection, gallstones, cysts, abscess, masses, and pseudocysts. CT scanning also shows areas of necrosis. This is the most useful of all imaging techniques for diagnosis, detection of a pseudocyst, and recognition of pancreatic necrosis (Fernandez & Kerman, 2013).

- Endoscopic retrograde cholangiopancreatography (ERCP) shows swelling and ductal system abnormalities.
- Magnetic resonance cholangiopancreatography may show stones in the common bile duct and necrosis; the test doesn't require an I.V. contrast medium.

Abdominal X-rays may shine some light on whether the patient's abdominal pain comes from pancreatitis or another cause.

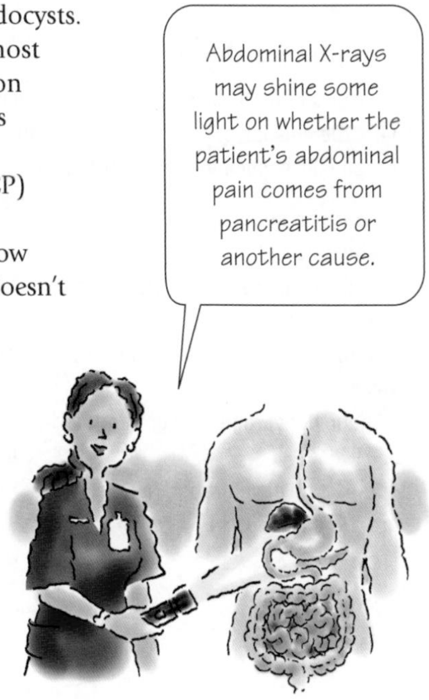

Blood studies

- Elevated serum amylase levels (more than three times normal) almost always indicate pancreatitis. Levels normally peak in 12 to 24 hours and return to normal within 1 week.
- Serum lipase levels usually rise within 4 to 8 hours of the onset of symptoms and peak in about 24 hours. They typically return to normal in 8 to 14 days.
- Several other levels also rise, including glucose, triglyceride, bilirubin, aspartate aminotransferase, alanine aminotransferase, lactate dehydrogenase, alkaline phosphatase, and blood urea nitrogen. Tests also show a prolonged prothrombin time and increased white blood cell count.
- Hematocrit; partial pressure of arterial oxygen; and calcium, magnesium, potassium, and albumin levels all decrease.

Severity scoring

Several tools help predict the severity of acute pancreatitis and the patient's prognosis. It's crucial to use these tools early on because early recognition of severe pancreatitis can significantly improve the outcome. Tools include Ranson's criteria, the acute physiologic assessment and chronic health evaluation (APACHE II) score, the multiorgan system failure (MOSF) score, the modified Glasgow prognostic criteria, and the Balthazar score.

Ranson's criteria look at several factors on admission (the local inflammatory effects of pancreatic enzymes) and then again 48 hours later (the systemic effects). If the patient meets three or more criteria, the criteria predict a severe course and an increased mortality risk. (See *Ranson's criteria*, page 290.)

The APACHE II score uses a point score calculated from routine physiologic measurements to provide a statistical prediction of mortality. However, the scoring system is time-consuming—a minus for assessing severe acute pancreatitis.

Ranson's criteria

Ranson's criteria allow early diagnosis of severe acute pancreatitis. The more criteria the patient meets, the more severe the episode of pancreatitis—and the greater the risk of mortality. The lists below detail the criteria used and the prognostic implications. Assign 1 point for each criterion met.

Criteria on admission
- Age greater than 55 years
- White blood cell count greater than 16,000/mm^3
- Serum glucose greater than 200 mg/dl
- Lactic dehydrogenase greater than 350 IU/L
- Aspartate aminotransferase greater than 250 IU/L

Criteria 48 hours after admission
- Greater than 10% decrease in hematocrit
- Blood urea nitrogen increase greater than 5 mg/dl
- Serum calcium less than 8 mg/dl
- Partial pressure of arterial oxygen less than 60 mm Hg
- Base deficit greater than 4 mEq/L
- Estimated fluid sequestration greater than 6 L

Prognostic implications
- Score 0 to 2: 2% mortality
- Score 3 to 4: 15% mortality
- Score 5 to 6: 40% mortality
- Score 7 to 11: 100% mortality

Extra sensitive

More sensitive than Ranson's criteria and the APACHE II, the MOSF score predicts the severity of the disease at admission and can be recalculated daily. It's typically used on intensive care units. The scoring system evaluates seven organ systems, with a higher score indicating more severe disease. All patients with a MOSF score greater than three have severe disease.

Similar to Ranson's criteria but with fewer criteria, the modified Glasgow criteria allows for daily scoring. The Balthazar score uses CT scan results to arrive at a prognosis. (See *The Balthazar score: A CT scan severity index.*)

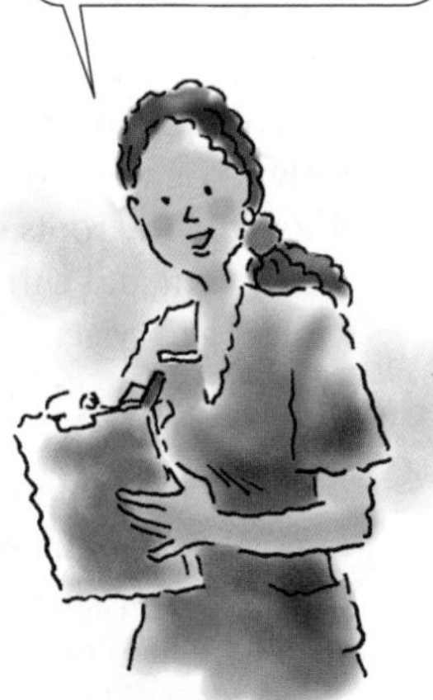

Aggressive fluid replacement may be necessary in patients with acute pancreatitis.

How it's treated

Treatment for acute pancreatitis aims to maintain circulation and fluid volume, relieve pain, decrease pancreatic secretions, maintain nutrition, and prevent infection and complications, as well as correcting contributing factors, such as removal of gallstones in acute pancreatitis caused by gallstones (Fernandez & Kerman, 2013).

The Balthazar score: A CT scan severity index

The Balthazar scoring system uses CT scanning to stage the severity of disease. Patients with severe acute pancreatitis should undergo a contrast-enhanced CT scan after the first 3 days to distinguish interstitial from necrotizing pancreatitis.

The first table shows grades for acute pancreatitis and the degree of pancreatic necrosis. The second table gives the risk for mortality and complications for each score. The score itself is a combination of the points for the grade of acute pancreatitis combined with the points for the degree of pancreatic necrosis.

Finding	Points
Grade of acute pancreatitis	
Normal pancreas	0
Pancreatic enlargement	1
Inflammation involving pancreas and peripancreatic fat	2
Single fluid collection or phlegmon	3
Two or more fluid collections or phlegmons	4
Degree of pancreatic necrosis	
No necrosis	0
Necrosis of one-third of the pancreas	2
Necrosis of one-half of the pancreas	4
Necrosis of more than one-half of the pancreas	6

Severity index	Mortality	Complications
0 to 1	0%	0%
2 to 3	3%	8%
4 to 6	6%	35%
7 to 10	17%	92%

Keep those fluids flowing

Patients with evidence of significant third-space fluid shift and those who have a large amount of fluid in the retroperitoneal space need aggressive fluid replacement. These fluid shifts deplete intravascular volume and may lead to tachycardia, hypotension, renal failure, hemoconcentration, and generalized circulatory collapse. Patients who develop hemoconcentration are also at increased risk for pancreatic necrosis and organ failure.

Most cases of pancreatitis respond well to colloids or lactated Ringer's solution to treat hypovolemia and shock. Patients require close monitoring for electrolyte abnormalities, particularly hypocalcemia, hypokalemia, and hypomagnesemia. Fluid replacement aims to correct these imbalances and replace volume. If a patient develops necrotizing pancreatitis or experiences a sudden, severe attack with hemorrhaging, he may also need packed red blood cells to maintain hemodynamic stability.

Pushing back at pancreatic pain

The severe pain that typically accompanies pancreatitis calls for pain relief. Meperidine was long thought to be the best choice for pain management because it seemed to have less spasmodic effects on the sphincter of Oddi compared with such opiates as morphine and fentanyl. However, more recent studies show that opiates may provide more pain relief, and patients tolerate them well. Due to the depressing effects on the respiratory system with opioids, careful observation of patients must be maintained with the administration of any opioid (Fernandez & Kerman, 2013). Positioning patients in the knee-to-chest position may also help relieve pain.

No food, please—just rest

Part of treatment includes letting the pancreas rest—and that means giving the pancreas a break from food, which stimulates enzyme secretion. Initially, the patient with pancreatitis should receive nothing by mouth. As pain subsides and the patient's condition improves, he can begin oral intake, with careful monitoring. The patient should at first receive small amounts of high-carbohydrate foods because they don't stimulate the pancreas as much as fat and protein.

If needed, antacids can help neutralize gastric secretions, and histamine antagonists can decrease hydrochloric acid production. Anticholinergic drugs can reduce vagal stimulation, decrease GI motility, and inhibit pancreatic enzyme secretion. If the patient has severe pancreatitis with significant pancreatic necrosis, he may need insulin to correct hyperglycemia.

A patient with recurrent vomiting, gastric distention, or intestinal ileus may need a nasogastric (NG) tube inserted. An NG tube with suctioning also suppresses pancreatic secretions by decreasing gastric fluids.

Although controversial, antibiotic therapy for acute pancreatitis is indicated if secondary infection or necrotizing pancreatitis is present (Fernandez & Kerman, 2013).

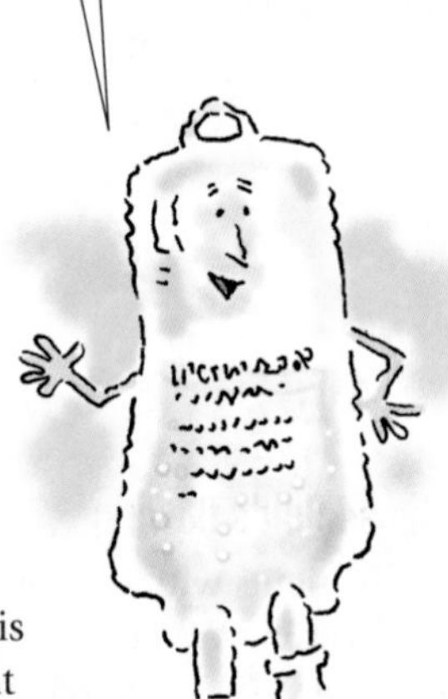

A patient with severe pancreatitis may need total parenteral nutrition to help him cope with the high stress and hypercatabolism of the disease.

The oral route is out

Until a patient with pancreatitis can tolerate oral intake, he must receive nutrition by an alternate method. In milder cases, food should be withheld for no more than 7 days. A patient with severe pancreatitis requires nutritional support because of the inherently high level of stress and hypercatabolism. Such a patient may receive total parenteral nutrition (without lipids if triglycerides are increased) or enteric feedings to maintain nutrition.

Eradicating infections

An inactive bowel allows intestinal flora to cross the colonic wall and infect the pancreas, particularly necrotic areas, which are the most vulnerable to infection. When necrotic pancreatic tissue becomes infected, the mortality rate increases to 40% to 70%.

Antibiotics can help prevent infection or treat one that's already present. If infected pancreatic necrosis arises, the patient may need surgical debridement and drainage. The doctor may also use a CT scan to guide aspiration of necrotic areas. This allows identification of the infecting organism, leading to more effective treatment.

Coping with complications

To prevent the disease from progressing, the patient may need surgery or ERCP to remove gallstones or other biliary tract obstructions. A patient with a pancreatic abscess or pseudocyst may need surgical drainage. If a patient develops complications in the cardiovascular, renal, pulmonary, GI, or neurologic system, he'll need treatment for the specific complication.

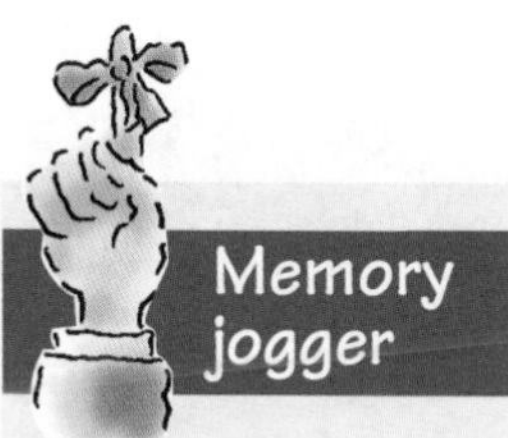

To remember some of the key treatments for acute pancreatitis, just think of the word **PANCREAS**:

Pain control

Arresting shock with I.V. fluids

Nasogastric intubation

Calcium monitoring

Renal evaluation

Ensuring pulmonary function

Antibiotic administration

Surgery or special procedures as needed.

How you intervene

Patients with acute pancreatitis need careful monitoring, thorough assessments, and diligent nursing care. Follow these guidelines:

- Teach the patient and his family about acute pancreatitis, and include them whenever possible in care planning. (See *Teaching about acute pancreatitis*, page 294.)
- Ensure a patent airway, and assess the patient's respiratory status at least every hour or as ordered. Assess for adventitious or diminished breath sounds. Check oxygen saturation levels and arterial blood gas results as ordered.
- Closely monitor the patient's cardiac and hemodynamic status at least every hour or as ordered.
- Monitor the patient's vital signs at least every hour or as ordered.
- Place the patient in a comfortable position that minimizes pain such as sitting and leaning forward, lying on his side with his knees bent, or sitting with his knees flexed toward his chest.

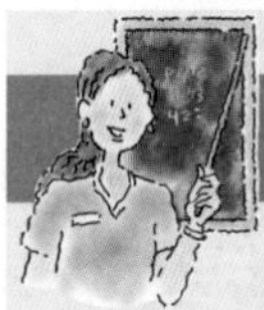

Teaching points

Teaching about acute pancreatitis

When teaching a patient with acute pancreatitis, be sure to cover these topics and then evaluate your patient's learning:

- explanation about acute pancreatitis, including its causes, signs and symptoms, treatment, possible complications, and risk for recurrence
- role of alcohol in the development of acute pancreatitis
- importance of avoiding factors that may precipitate an attack, especially alcohol and products containing alcohol, such as certain cough and cold medications, and high-fat foods
- dietary counseling and, if necessary, the role of lipid-lowering drugs if pancreatitis resulted from high triglyceride levels
- prescribed medications and possible adverse effects
- dietary modifications as indicated, including the need for a diet high in carbohydrates and low in fats and proteins as well as recommendations to avoid caffeine and irritating foods
- need to stop smoking, if applicable
- signs and symptoms to report to the practitioner
- importance of follow-up appointments
- referral to an appropriate support group such as Alcoholics Anonymous, if indicated.

- Allow for periods of rest to reduce metabolic stress.
- If the patient develops acute respiratory syndrome, anticipate the need for additional therapies such as prone positioning.
- Provide supplemental oxygen as ordered.
- Initiate I.V. fluid replacement therapy as ordered. Assess for signs of fluid overload, including dyspnea, edema, and crackles.
- Monitor serum laboratory values (hematology, coagulation, and chemistry) for changes.

Dangerous drop-offs

- Watch closely for signs and symptoms of hypokalemia (hypotension, muscle weakness, apathy, confusion, and cardiac arrhythmias), hypomagnesemia (hypotension, tachycardia, confusion, tremors, twitching, hypoactive deep tendon reflexes, and confusion), and hypocalcemia (positive Chvostek's and Trousseau's signs, tetany, seizures, and prolonged QT intervals on an electrocardiogram). Have emergency equipment readily available.
- Assess for Cullen's and Grey Turner's signs, which indicate hemorrhagic pancreatitis.

- Monitor the patient's intake and output closely, and notify the practitioner if the patient has a urine output of less than 0.5 ml/kg/hour. Weigh the patient daily.
- Monitor the patient's neurologic status, noting confusion or lethargy.
- Maintain the patient in a normothermic state to reduce the body's demand for oxygen.
- Assess the patient's pain level and administer medications as ordered.
- Administer antibiotics as ordered, and monitor serum peak and trough levels as appropriate.
- Withhold all oral fluids and food as ordered to prevent stimulation of pancreatic enzymes.
- Insert an NG tube as ordered. Check placement at least every 4 hours. Irrigate with normal saline solution to maintain patency. Monitor drainage for frank bleeding, and watch for bleeding in vomitus and stool.
- Assess the patient's abdomen for distention and for diminished or absent bowel sounds; measure his abdominal girth.
- As ordered, administer stool softeners to relieve constipation caused by immobility and opioid use.
- Administer parenteral nutrition therapy or enteral feedings as ordered. Monitor blood glucose levels. Administer insulin as ordered.
- When bowel sounds become active and the patient's condition improves, anticipate switching to high-carbohydrate, low-protein, low-fat oral feedings after 1 or 2 days on clear liquids.
- Perform range-of-motion exercises to maintain joint mobility.
- Perform meticulous skin care.
- Provide emotional support to the patient and his family, and encourage them to express their feelings.
- Prepare the patient for surgery as indicated.
- Document your assessments and interventions. (See *Documenting acute pancreatitis*, page 296.)

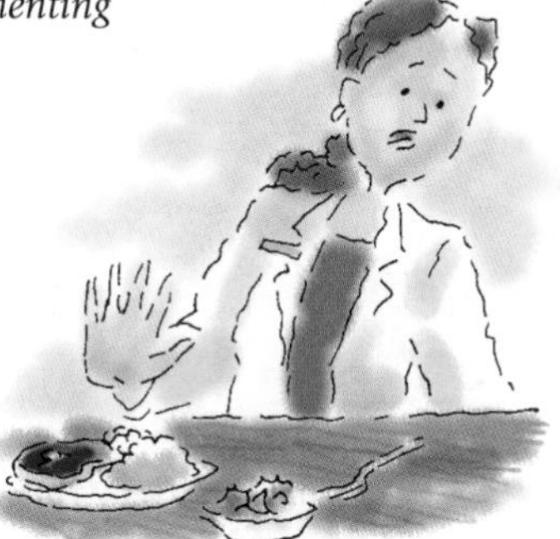
Withhold all oral fluids and food to prevent the stimulation of pancreatic enzymes. Nothing at all for me, thanks!

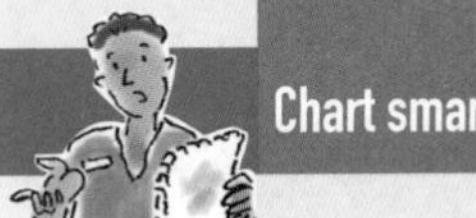

Chart smart

Documenting acute pancreatitis

If your patient has acute pancreatitis, make sure you document the following information:

- vital signs
- intake and output
- laboratory and imaging test results
- tolerance of testing procedures
- respiratory status
- daily weight
- I.V. fluid therapy
- patency and appearance of I.V. site
- nutrition supplementation
- diet, when applicable
- medications administered
- oxygen administered, if indicated
- pain level and response to medications
- positioning and response
- mental status
- presence and characteristics of vomitus and diarrhea
- correct placement of NG tube and care provided, if present
- signs and symptoms of improving or worsening condition
- safety measures
- notification of practitioner
- all nursing assessments, observations, and interventions and the patient's response
- patient and family teaching and their understanding.

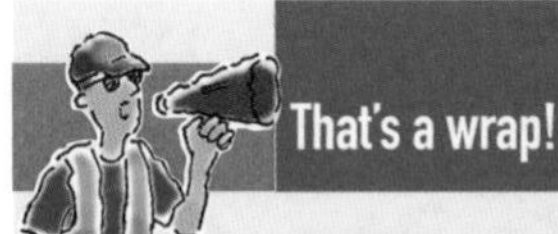

Acute pancreatitis review

Acute pancreatitis basics

- Inflammation of the pancreas
- Two types: edematous, which is usually mild, accounts for about 85% of cases, is self-limiting, and resolves in 5 to 7 days; and necrotizing, which is severe, accounts for about 15% of cases, is progressive, and causes tissue damage and cell death
- May progress to chronic pancreatitis with progressive recurrent episodes

Causes

- Gallstones most common cause
- Alcohol consumption second most common cause
- Other biliary tract disease, drugs, infection, toxins and metabolic processes, trauma, and other factors less common causes

Effects on pancreas

- Exocrine functions fail
- Activated enzymes in pancreas digest pancreatic tissue

Imbalances caused by acute pancreatitis

Hypovolemia

- Major cause of death in acute pancreatitis
- Occurs when severe pancreatic damage triggers release of systemic inflammatory mediators that produce increased capillary permeability and vasodilation, leading to massive fluid shifts from intravascular to interstitial spaces and retroperitoneum
- Can also result from vomiting, diarrhea, excessive sweating, and, possibly, hemorrhage

Hyponatremia

- Can result from vomiting, diarrhea, and excessive sweating
- Also occurs when hypovolemia causes an increase in antidiuretic hormone secretion

Hypocalcemia

- Usually results from concomitant hypoalbuminemia
- Can be worsened by fat necrosis (caused by lipase necrosing fat tissue in pancreatic interstitium and peripancreatic spaces) that may result in the release of free fatty acids and intraperitoneal saponification
- Can also stem from hypomagnesemia (hypomagnesemia should be addressed before hypocalcemia)

Hypomagnesemia

- Can result from vomiting and diarrhea
- Can occur when magnesium is deposited in areas of fat necrosis, decreasing serum levels

Hypokalemia

- May be caused by severe vomiting and diarrhea

Signs and symptoms

- Mild pancreatitis: steady epigastric pain centered near the navel and unrelieved by vomiting

(continued)

Acute pancreatitis review *(continued)*

- Severe pancreatitis: severe, persistent, piercing abdominal pain, usually in the midepigastric region; may generalize or occur in left upper quadrant and radiate to the back or other areas; typically precipitated by a large meal or alcohol consumption; may improve when patient leans forward or lies on side with knees drawn toward chest
- Nausea
- Vomiting
- Fever
- Mild jaundice
- Tachycardia
- Tachypnea
- Muscle spasms
- Fatty, foul-smelling stools
- Possible hypotension
- Grey Turner's sign (flank ecchymosis)
- Cullen's sign (periumbilical ecchymosis)
- Chvostek's and Trousseau's signs (hypocalcemia)
- Abdominal distention, rigidity, and tenderness with hypoactive bowel sounds

Treatment

- Maintenance of circulation and fluid volume (typically requires aggressive fluid replacement)
- Pain relief (using medications, such as morphine and fentanyl, and positioning)
- Reduction of pancreatic secretions to allow pancreas to rest (no oral intake, medications to rest pancreas, and possibly NG tube insertion)
- Maintenance of nutrition (nutritional support, such as total parenteral nutrition and enteric feedings)
- Prevention or treatment of infection and complications (antibiotic therapy or surgery as needed)

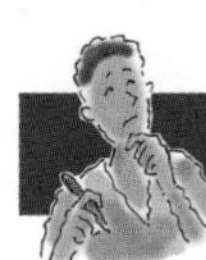

Quick quiz

1. The pancreas functions as both an exocrine and endocrine gland. Which of these is an example of its exocrine function?
   A. The pancreas produces hydrochloric acid.
   B. Amylase is produced in the acinar cells.
   C. Insulin is produced in the islets of Langerhans.
   D. The pancreas secretes its enzymes into the stomach.

Answer: B. The production of amylase in the acinar cells is an example of exocrine function.

2. The most common cause of acute pancreatitis is:
   A. alcohol.
   B. eating low-fat foods.
   C. gallstones.
   D. pregnancy.

Answer: C. Gallstones are the most common cause of acute pancreatitis.

3. Which of these imbalances typically occurs in acute pancreatitis?
   A. Hypovolemia
   B. Hypercalcemia
   C. Hypernatremia
   D. Hypermagnesemia

Answer: A. In acute pancreatitis, fluid shifting from the intravascular space into the interstitial spaces and retroperitoneum causes hypovolemia.

4. The patient with acute pancreatitis may report that his pain decreases:
   A. when he lies on his stomach.
   B. after vomiting.
   C. after eating a large meal.
   D. when he lies on his side with his knees drawn toward his chest.

Answer: D. Pain caused by acute pancreatitis is commonly relieved when the patient lies on his side with his knees drawn toward his chest.

5. Patients recovering from acute pancreatitis should eat foods that are:
   A. low in carbohydrates and high in fats and proteins.
   B. low in carbohydrates, proteins, and fats.
   C. high in carbohydrates and fats and low in proteins.
   D. high in carbohydrates and low in fats and proteins.

Answer: D. The patient recovering from acute pancreatitis should eat foods that are high in carbohydrates and low in fats and proteins.

Scoring

☆☆☆ If you answered all five questions correctly, bravo! You're not only acute, you're pancreatitis proficient.

☆☆ If you answered four questions correctly, that's cool! You're on your way to glandular glory.

☆ If you answered fewer than four questions correctly, that's okay! Just review the chapter until you can fully digest the information.

Reference

Fernandez, H., & Kerman, D. (2013). Pancreatitis. In R. Buttaro, J. Trybulski, P. Bailey, & J. Sandberg-Cook (Eds.), *Primary care: A collaborative practice* (4th ed.). St. Louis, MO: Elsevier Mosby.

Chapter 17

Renal failure

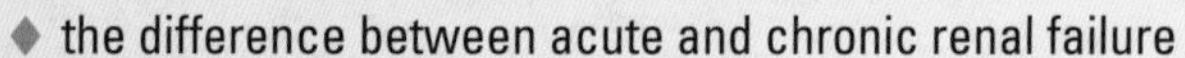

Just the facts

In this chapter, you'll learn:

- the difference between acute and chronic renal failure
- fluid, electrolyte, and acid-base imbalances that can occur with renal failure
- signs and symptoms of renal failure
- appropriate nursing interventions for patients with renal failure.

A look at renal failure

Renal failure involves a disruption of normal kidney function. The kidneys play a major role in regulating fluids, electrolytes, acids, and bases. Acute renal failure occurs suddenly and is usually reversible. In contrast, chronic renal failure occurs slowly and is irreversible.

Both acute and chronic renal failure affect the kidneys' functional unit, the nephron, which forms urine. Imbalances occur as the kidneys lose the ability to excrete water, electrolytes, wastes, and acid-base products through the urine. Patients may also develop hypertension, anemia, and uremia, as well as renal osteodystrophy, which includes increased bone resorption and a reduction of bone mass. Let's look at how acute and chronic renal failure develop.

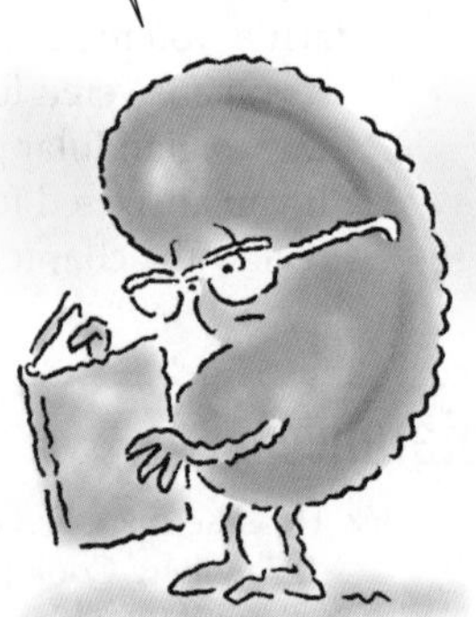

All this business about renal failure is getting me worried!

How acute renal failure happens

Acute renal failure can stem from prerenal conditions such as heart failure, which causes a diminished blood flow to the kidneys; from intrarenal conditions, which damage the kidneys themselves; or from obstructive postrenal conditions such as prostatitis, which can cause urine to back up into the kidneys. (See *Causes of acute renal failure*.)

Causes of acute renal failure

The causes of acute renal failure can be broken down into three categories: prerenal, intrarenal, and postrenal. Prerenal causes include conditions that diminish blood flow to the kidneys. Intrarenal causes include conditions that damage the kidneys themselves. Postrenal causes include conditions that obstruct urine outflow, which causes urine to back up into the kidneys. For each type, the affected structures are highlighted in the illustrations below.

Prerenal causes

- Serious cardiovascular disorders
- Peripheral vasodilation
- Severe vasoconstriction
- Renal vascular obstruction
- Trauma
- Shock (septic, hypovolemic, cardiogenic)

Intrarenal causes

- Acute tubular necrosis
- Nephrotoxins
- Exposure to heavy metals
- Aminoglycosides, nonsteroidal anti-inflammatory drugs, or cephalosporins
- Ischemic damage from poorly treated renal failure
- Eclampsia, postpartum renal failure, or uterine hemorrhage
- Myopathy, sepsis, or transfusion reaction
- Trauma (crush injury, etc.)

Postrenal causes

- Bladder obstruction
- Ureteral or urethral obstruction
- Trauma

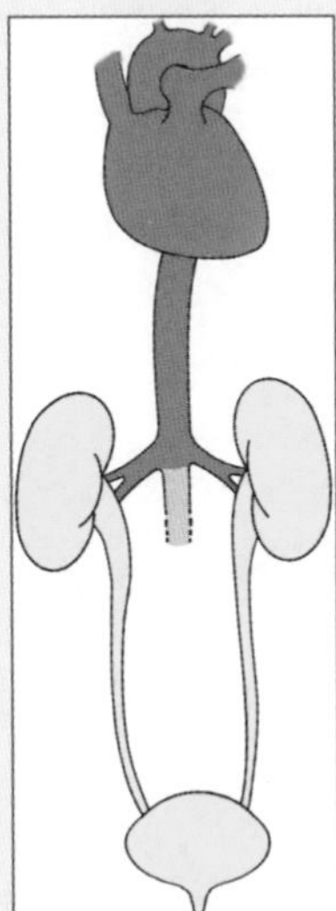

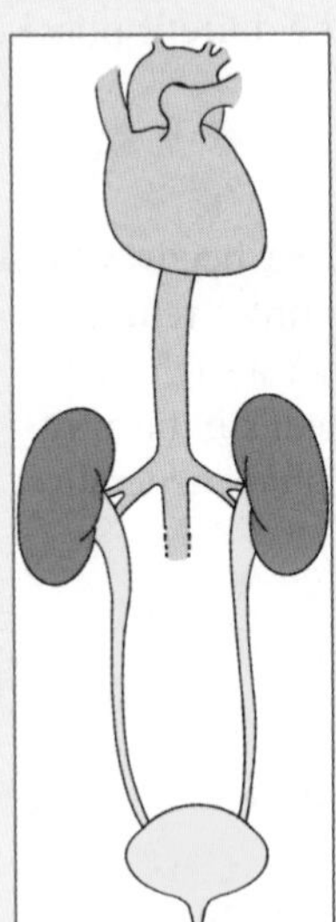

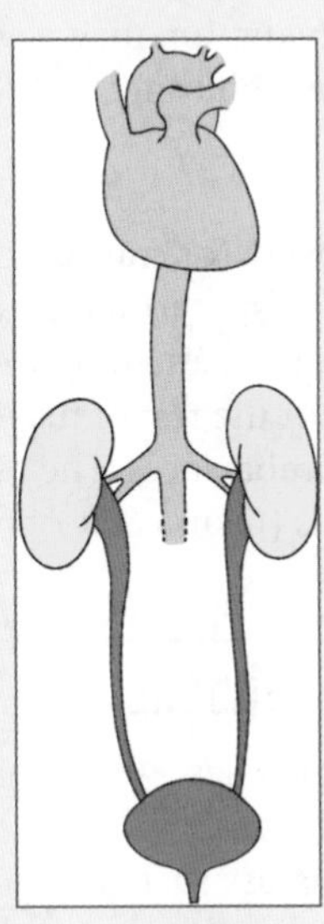

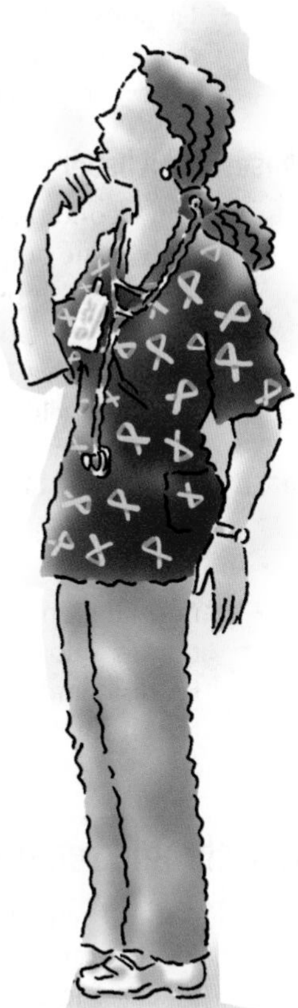

About 5% of hospitalized patients develop acute renal failure at some point during their hospitalizations. Many conditions reduce blood flow or otherwise damage the kidneys' nephrons. Acute renal failure normally passes through three distinct phases: oliguric-anuric, diuretic, and recovery.

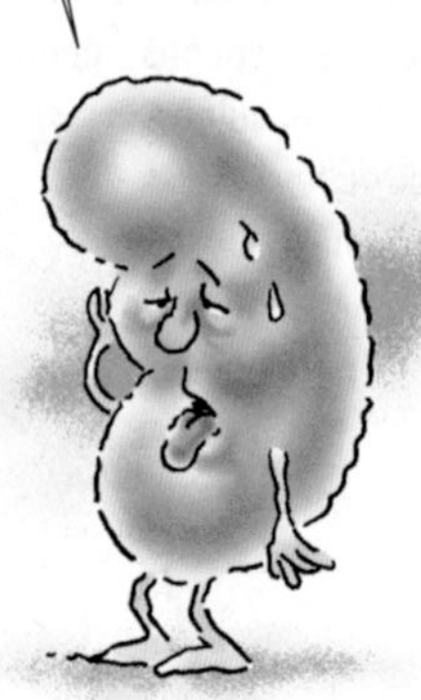
Acute renal failure normally passes through three distinct phases: oliguric-anuric, diuretic, and recovery. The first phase makes me feel terrible!

Phase 1: A dangerous drop-off

A decrease in urine output is the first clinical sign of acute renal failure during the first phase called *the oliguric-anuric phase*. Typically, as the glomerular filtration rate (GFR) decreases, the patient's urine output decreases to less than 400 ml during a 24-hour period.

When the kidneys fail, nitrogenous waste products accumulate in the blood, which causes an elevation in blood urea nitrogen (BUN) and serum creatinine levels. The result is uremia. Electrolyte imbalances, metabolic acidosis, and other symptoms follow as the patient becomes increasingly uremic and renal dysfunction disrupts other body systems. Left untreated, the condition is fatal.

The oliguric-anuric phase generally lasts 1 to 2 weeks but may last for several more. The longer the patient remains in this phase, the poorer the prognosis for a return to normal renal function (Okusa & Rosner, 2013).

Phase 2: A bit better

The second phase, or diuretic phase, starts with a gradual increase in daily urine output from 400 ml/24 hours to 1 to 2 L/24 hours. The BUN level stops rising. Although urine output begins to increase in this phase, a potential for fluid and electrolyte imbalances still exists as GFR increases and dehydration may develop. The diuretic phase lasts about 10 days (Okusa & Rosner, 2013).

Phase 3: On the road to recovery

The third phase, the recovery (or convalescent) phase, begins when fluid and electrolyte values start to stabilize, indicating a return to normal kidney function. The patient may experience a slight reduction in kidney function for the rest of his life, so he'll still be at risk for fluid and electrolyte imbalances. The recovery phase generally lasts from 3 to 12 months (Okusa & Rosner, 2013).

How chronic renal failure happens

Chronic renal failure, which has a more insidious onset than acute renal failure, may result from:

- chronic glomerular disease such as glomerulonephritis
- chronic infections, such as chronic pyelonephritis or tuberculosis

- congenital anomalies such as polycystic kidney disease
- vascular diseases, such as renal nephrosclerosis or hypertension
- obstructions such as those from renal calculi
- collagen diseases such as systemic lupus erythematosus
- long-term therapy with nephrotoxic drugs such as aminoglycosides
- endocrine diseases such as diabetes mellitus.

Setting the stage

Because chronic renal failure has a slow onset, identifying specific time frames for its stages may be difficult. The rate at which kidney function deteriorates depends as well on the specific disease causing the deterioration. It's possible, however, to stage progression of the disease by the degree of kidney function.

Chronic renal failure can be divided into four basic stages:

1. reduced renal reserve (GFR 40 to 70 ml/minute)
2. renal insufficiency (GFR 20 to 40 ml/minute)
3. renal failure (GFR 10 to 20 ml/minute)
4. end-stage renal disease (GFR less than 10 ml/minute).

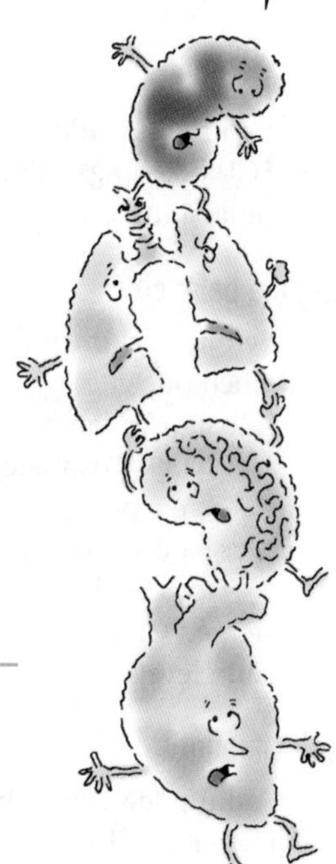
If left unchecked, chronic renal failure can produce potentially fatal physiologic changes in all major organ systems.

Running down the reserve

The kidneys have great functional reserve. Few symptoms develop until more than 75% of GFR is lost. The remaining functional nephrons then deteriorate progressively; signs and symptoms worsen as renal function diminishes. Failing kidneys can't regulate fluid balance or filter solutes or participate effectively in acid-base balance. If chronic renal failure continues unchecked, uremic toxins accumulate and produce potentially fatal physiologic changes in all major organ systems.

Imbalances caused by renal failure

Renal failure—acute or chronic—can cause a number of fluid, electrolyte, and acid-base imbalances, including:

- hypervolemia or hypovolemia
- hyponatremia or hypernatremia
- hypocalcemia
- hyperkalemia
- hypermagnesemia
- hyperphosphatemia
- metabolic acidosis or metabolic alkalosis.

Water, water, everywhere . . . or not

When urine output decreases, especially with the more sudden onset of acute renal failure, the body retains fluid, which can lead to hypervolemia. That condition may also occur if fluid intake exceeds urine output. The resulting fluid retention can lead to hypertension, peripheral edema, heart failure, or pulmonary edema.

Hypovolemic water losses usually occur during the diuretic phase of acute renal failure and can result in hypotension or circulatory collapse.

Pump up the potassium

As the kidneys' ability to excrete potassium is impaired, serum potassium levels increase, resulting in hyperkalemia. In chronic renal failure, a patient tends to tolerate high potassium levels more than a patient with acute renal failure, in which the onset is more sudden.

Metabolic acidosis, which occurs with renal failure, causes potassium to move from inside the cells into the extracellular fluid. The release of potassium from any necrotic or injured cells worsens hyperkalemia. Additional stressors—such as infection, gastrointestinal (GI) bleeding, trauma, and surgery—can also lead to high serum potassium levels.

Tipping the balance

Serum calcium and phosphorus have an inverse relationship, so when one goes out of balance, the other follows suit. Secondary imbalances can occur as a result.

Hyperphosphatemia develops when the kidneys lose the ability to excrete phosphorus. Consequently, high serum phosphorus levels cause a decrease in calcium levels.

Decreased activation of vitamin D by the kidneys results in decreased GI absorption of calcium—another cause for low serum calcium levels.

The salt situation

Sodium levels may be either abnormally high or unusually low during renal failure.

Hyponatremia can occur with acute renal failure because a decreased GFR and damaged tubules increase water and sodium retention. This dilutional hyponatremic state can also be caused by the intracellular–extracellular exchange between sodium and potassium during metabolic acidosis.

Hypernatremia can occur with decreased intravascular volume. A progression in the degree of kidney failure causes less sodium to be excreted, worsening hypernatremia.

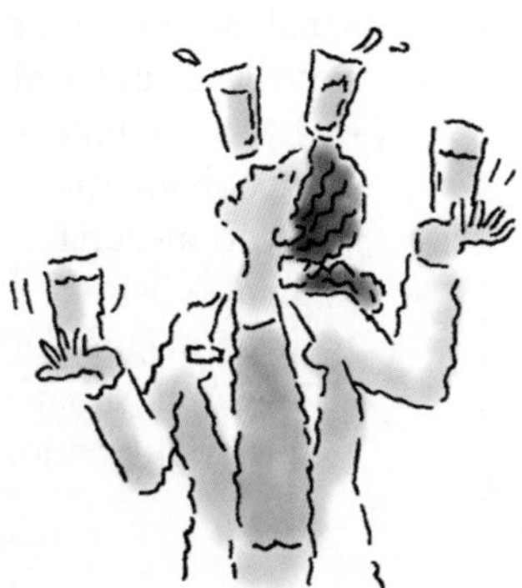
When urine output decreases, the body retains too much fluid. Then, during the diuretic phase, the body can lose so much fluid that it runs the risk of hypotension or circulatory collapse.

Magnesium to the max

The patient with renal failure may retain magnesium as a result of a decreased GFR and destruction of the tubules. However, a high serum magnesium level usually isn't recognized unless the patient receives external sources of magnesium, such as laxatives, antacids, I.V. solutions, or hyperalimentation solutions.

The acid-base seesaw

Metabolic acidosis is the most common acid-base imbalance occurring with renal failure. It develops as the kidneys lose the ability to secrete hydrogen ions—an acid—in the urine. The imbalance is also exacerbated as the kidneys fail to hold onto bicarbonate—a base.

Patients with chronic renal failure have more time to compensate for this acid-base imbalance than patients with acute renal failure. The lungs try to compensate for the excess acid by increasing the depth and rate of respirations in an attempt to blow off carbon dioxide.

Metabolic alkalosis rarely occurs with renal failure. When it does, it usually results from excessive intake of bicarbonate, given in an effort to correct metabolic acidosis.

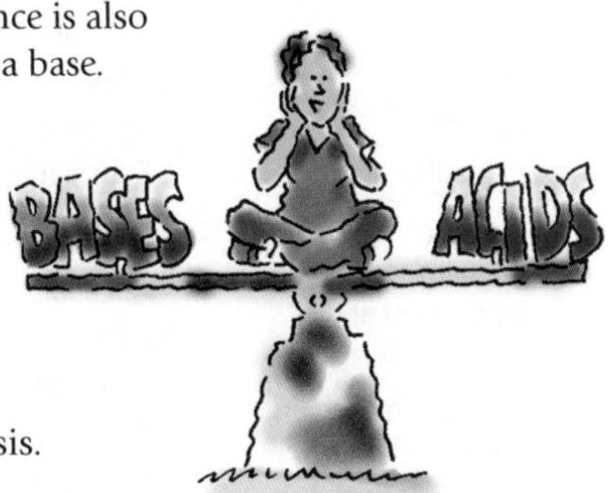

What to look for

The patient's history may reveal a disorder that can cause renal failure; it may also include a recent episode of fever, chills, GI problems (such as anorexia, nausea, vomiting, diarrhea, or constipation), and central nervous system problems such as headache.

Signs and symptoms vary, depending on the length of time in which renal failure develops. (See *Laboratory results associated with acute renal failure*.) Fewer signs may appear in patients with acute renal failure because of the condition's shorter clinical course. In patients with chronic renal failure, however, almost all body systems are affected. Your assessment findings will likely involve several body systems. (See *Recognizing renal failure,* page 306.)

Laboratory results associated with acute renal failure

Keep alert for these early signs of acute renal failure:

- urine output below 400 ml over 24 hours
- increased BUN level
- increased serum creatinine level.

Salt shortage

In cases of renal failure in which the kidneys can't retain salt, hyponatremia may occur. The patient may complain of dry mouth, fatigue, and nausea. You may note hypotension, loss of skin turgor, and listlessness that progresses to somnolence and confusion.

Later, as the number of functioning nephrons decreases, so does the kidney's capacity to excrete sodium and potassium. Urine output decreases. The urine may be dilute, with casts or crystals

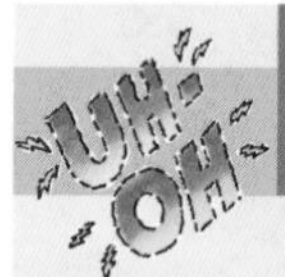

CAUTION!

Recognizing renal failure

Signs and symptoms associated with renal failure are listed here by body system. Keep in mind that your patient may develop some or all of them.

Neurologic
- Burning, itching, and pain in the legs and feet
- Coma
- Confusion
- Fatigue
- Headache
- Hiccups
- Irritability
- Listlessness and somnolence
- Muscle irritability and twitching
- Seizures
- Shortened attention span and memory

Cardiovascular
- Anemia
- Arrhythmias
- Edema
- Heart failure
- Hypertension
- Hypotension
- Irregular pulse
- Pericardial rub
- Tachycardia
- Weight gain with fluid retention

Pulmonary
- Crackles
- Decreased breath sounds if pneumonia is present
- Dyspnea
- Kussmaul's respirations

GI
- Ammonia smell to the breath
- Anorexia
- Bleeding
- Constipation or diarrhea
- Dry mouth
- Inflammation and ulceration of GI mucosa
- Metallic taste in the mouth
- Nausea and vomiting
- Pain on abdominal palpation and percussion

Integumentary
- Dry, brittle hair that may change color or fall out easily
- Dry mucous membranes
- Dry, scaly skin with ecchymoses, petechiae, and purpura
- Loss of skin turgor
- Severe pruritus
- Thin, brittle fingernails with lines
- Uremic frost (in later stages)
- Yellow-bronze skin color

Genitourinary
- Amenorrhea in women
- Anuria or oliguria
- Changes in urinary appearance or patterns
- Decreased libido
- Dilute urine with casts and crystals
- Hematuria
- Impotence in men
- Infertility
- Proteinuria

Musculoskeletal
- Bone and muscle pain
- Gait abnormalities or loss of ambulation
- Inability to ambulate
- Muscle cramps
- Muscle weakness
- Pathologic fractures

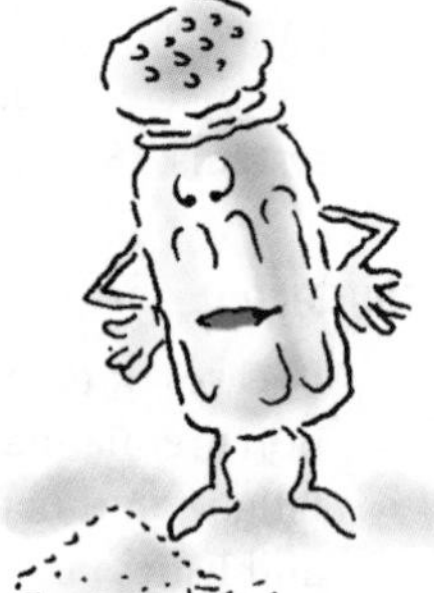

Not enough sodium, too much sodium—it's a delicate balance.

present. Accumulation of potassium causes muscle irritability and then muscle weakness, irregular pulse, and life-threatening cardiac arrhythmias. Sodium retention causes fluid overload, and edema becomes palpable. The patient gains weight from fluid retention. Metabolic acidosis can also occur.

Hard on the heart

When the cardiovascular system is involved with renal failure, you'll find hypertension and an irregular pulse. Tachycardia may occur. You may note signs of a pericardial rub related to pericarditis, especially in patients with chronic renal failure. You may also hear crackles at the bases of the lungs, and you may palpate peripheral edema if heart failure occurs.

The lungs take a plunge

Pulmonary changes include reduced pulmonary macrophage activity with increased susceptibility to infection. If pneumonia is present, breath sounds may decrease over areas of consolidation. Crackles at the lung bases occur with pulmonary edema. Kussmaul's respirations occur with metabolic acidosis.

Down in the mouth

With inflammation and ulceration of GI mucosa, inspection of the mouth may reveal gum ulceration and bleeding. The patient may complain of hiccups, a metallic taste in the mouth, anorexia, nausea, and vomiting (caused by esophageal, stomach, or bowel involvement). You may note an ammonia smell to the breath. Abdominal palpation and percussion may cause pain.

Integumentary indicators

Inspection of the skin typically reveals a yellow-bronze color. The skin is dry and scaly with purpura, ecchymoses, and petechiae that form as a result of thrombocytopenia and platelet dysfunction caused by uremia. In later stages, if untreated, the patient may experience uremic frost (powdery deposits on the skin as a result of urea and uric acid being excreted in sweat) and thin, brittle fingernails with characteristic lines. Mucous membranes are dry. Hair is dry and brittle and may change color and fall out easily. The patient usually complains of severe itching.

Musculoskeletal maladies

The patient may have a history of pathologic fractures and complain of bone and muscle pain, which may be caused by an imbalance in calcium and phosphorus or in the amount of parathyroid hormone (PTH) produced. You may note gait abnormalities or, possibly, that the patient can no longer ambulate.

More problems

With chronic renal failure, the patient may have a history of infertility and decreased libido. Women may have amenorrhea, and men may be impotent.

You may note changes in the patient's level of consciousness that may progress from mild behavior changes, shortened memory and attention span, apathy, drowsiness, and irritability to confusion, coma, and seizures. The patient may complain of muscle cramps and twitching caused by muscle irritability. The patient may also complain of pain, burning, and itching in the legs and feet that may be relieved by voluntarily shaking, moving, or rocking them. Those symptoms may eventually progress to paresthesia and motor nerve dysfunction.

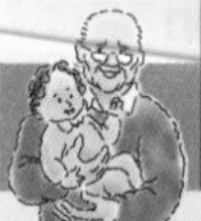
Ages and stages

Age-related kidney changes

As people age, nephrons are lost and the kidneys decrease in size. These changes decrease renal blood flow and may result in doubled BUN levels in older patients.

What tests show

Diagnostic test results typical of patients with renal failure include:

- elevated serum BUN, creatinine, potassium, and phosphorus levels (See *Age-related kidney changes*.)
- arterial blood gas (ABG) results that indicate metabolic acidosis—specifically, a low pH and bicarbonate level
- low hematocrit, low hemoglobin level, and mild thrombocytopenia
- urinalysis showing casts, cellular debris, decreased specific gravity, proteinuria, and hematuria
- electrocardiogram (ECG) showing tall, peaked T waves; a widened QRS complex; and disappearing P waves if hyperkalemia is present.

Other studies, such as kidney biopsy, kidney-ureter-bladder radiography, and kidney ultrasonography, may also be performed to determine the cause of renal failure.

How it's treated

Treatment of renal failure aims to correct specific symptoms and to alter the disease process.

Go low pro

A patient with renal failure needs to make dietary changes. They need to follow a high-calorie diet to meet daily nutritional requirements and to prevent breakdown of body protein. Their diet also needs to restrict phosphorus, sodium, and potassium.

A low-protein diet will reduce end products of protein metabolism that the kidneys are unable to excrete. The protein a patient needs should be consumed only in foods that contain all essential amino acids to prevent breakdown of body protein, such as eggs, milk, poultry, and meat.

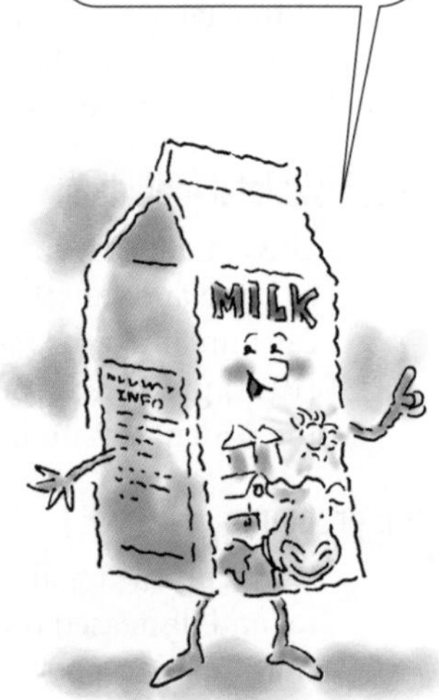
A patient with renal failure should get his protein in foods such as milk that contain all essential amino acids to prevent breakdown of body protein. Drink up!
MILK

Fine-tuning fluids

Maintaining fluid balance requires careful monitoring of vital signs, weight changes, and urine output. Fluid retention can be reduced, if some renal function remains, with the use of a loop diuretic such as furosemide (Lasix) and with restriction of fluid.

Careful monitoring of serum potassium levels is necessary to detect hyperkalemia. If the patient develops this condition, emergency treatment should be initiated. (See *Emergency treatment of hyperkalemia.*) A non–aluminum-containing, phosphate-binding agent may be given to lower serum phosphorus levels.

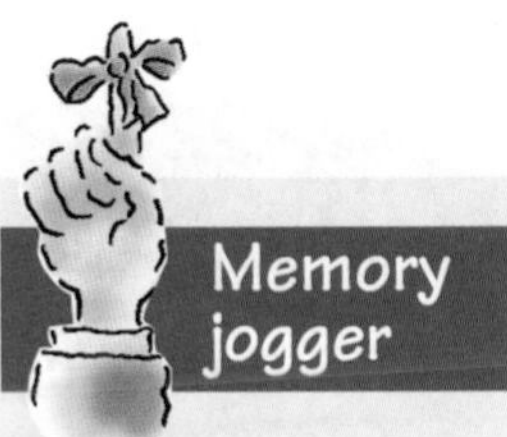

Memory jogger

To remember dietary changes needed to manage renal failure, think **"High, Lo, No."**

High calories

Low protein

No added salt (also watch the potassium)

A kick to the marrow

In patients with chronic renal failure, kidney production of erythropoietin is diminished. This hormone controls the rate of red blood cell (RBC) production in bone marrow and functions as a growth factor and differentiating factor. Treatment includes administration of synthetic erythropoietin to stimulate bone marrow to produce RBCs.

Filling in for the kidneys

Hemodialysis and peritoneal dialysis are used in both acute and chronic renal failure. By assuming the function of the kidneys, these measures help correct fluid and electrolyte disturbances and relieve some of the symptoms of renal failure.

How you intervene

Caring for a patient with renal failure requires careful monitoring, administration of various medicines and therapeutic regimens, and empathic ministering to the patient and family. (See *Teaching about renal failure,* page 310.) Follow these guidelines:

- Assess the patient carefully to determine the type and severity of fluid, electrolyte, and acid-base imbalances.
- Maintain accurate fluid intake and output records.
- Weigh the patient daily, and compare the results with the 24-hour intake and output record.
- Monitor vital signs, including breath sounds and central venous pressure when available, to detect changes in fluid volume. Report hypertension, which may occur as a result of fluid and sodium retention.
- Observe the patient for signs and symptoms of fluid overload, such as edema, bounding pulse, and shortness of breath.
- Monitor serum electrolyte and ABG levels for abnormalities. Report significant changes to the practitioner.

Emergency treatment of hyperkalemia

Emergency treatment of hyperkalemia includes administration of Kayexalate, dialysis, administration of 50% hypertonic glucose I.V., regular insulin, calcium gluconate I.V., and sodium bicarbonate I.V.

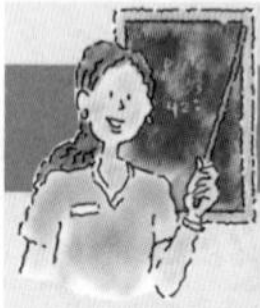

Teaching points

Teaching about renal failure

When teaching a patient with renal failure, be sure to cover the following topics and then evaluate your patient's learning:

- basics of renal failure and its treatment
- prescribed medications
- avoidance of high-sodium and high-potassium foods
- importance of weighing himself daily
- warning signs and symptoms and when to report them
- need for frequent rest for a patient with anemia
- referrals to counseling services, if indicated
- proper methods of caring for shunt, fistula, or vascular access device
- proper method of performing peritoneal dialysis at home, if appropriate.

- Observe the patient for signs and symptoms that may indicate an electrolyte or acid-base imbalance—for example, tetany, paresthesia, muscle weakness, tachypnea, or confusion.
- Monitor ECG readings to detect arrhythmias caused by electrolyte imbalances.
- Monitor hemoglobin levels and hematocrit.
- If the patient requires dialysis, check the vascular access site every 2 hours for patency and signs of clotting. Check the site for bleeding after dialysis.
- Restrict fluids as prescribed.
- Administer prescribed diuretics to patients whose kidneys can still excrete excess fluid.
- Administer other prescribed medications, such as oral or I.V. electrolyte replacement to correct electrolyte imbalances and vitamin supplements to correct nutritional deficiencies.
- Know the route of excretion for medications being given. Drugs excreted through the kidneys or removed during dialysis may require dosage adjustments.
- Expect to administer sodium bicarbonate I.V. to control acute acidosis and orally to control chronic acidosis. Remember that sodium bicarbonate has a high sodium content. Multiple doses of the drug may result in hypernatremia, which could contribute to the onset of heart failure and pulmonary edema.

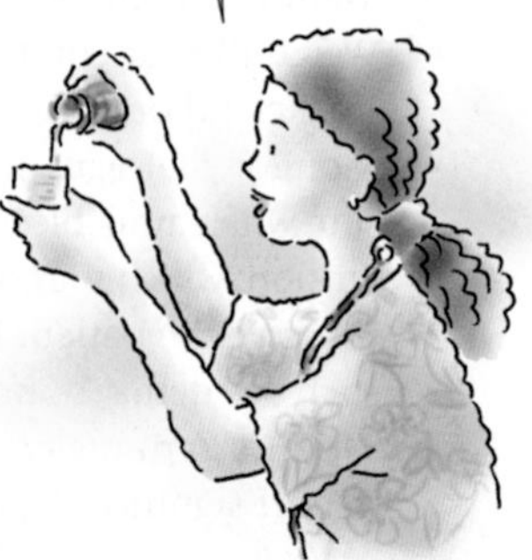
Keep in mind that drugs excreted through the kidneys or removed during dialysis may require dosage adjustments.

- As necessary, restrict electrolyte intake, especially potassium and phosphorus, to prevent imbalances. Monitor and document the patient's response. (See *Documenting renal failure.*)
- Be prepared to initiate dialysis when electrolyte or acid-base imbalances don't respond to drug therapy or when fluid removal isn't possible.
- Maintain nutritional status. Provide a diet high in calories and low in protein, sodium, and potassium. Initiate a nutritional consultation as needed.
- If a graft or fistula for dialysis has been placed in the patient's arm, don't use that extremity for measuring blood pressure, drawing blood, or inserting I.V. catheters.
- Provide emotional support to the patient and his family.
- Teach the patient and his family about renal failure and its treatment (National Institute of Diabetes and Digestive and Kidney Diseases, 2012; National Kidney Foundation, 2013; Workeheh, 2013).

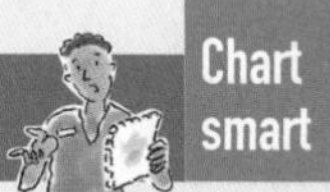

Chart smart

Documenting renal failure

If your patient has renal failure, make sure you document the following information:

- assessment findings, such as those related to fluid, electrolyte, or acid-base imbalances
- vital signs, including breath sounds and central venous pressure readings (if available)
- daily weight
- laboratory test results
- intake and output
- administration of I.V. or oral electrolyte replacement therapy
- dialysis and care of the vascular access site
- notification of the practitioner
- patient and family teaching and patient's response.

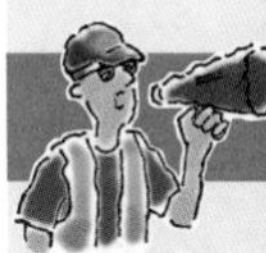

That's a wrap!

Renal failure review

Renal failure basics

- Involves disruption of normal kidney function
- Affects the kidney's functional unit, the nephron, which forms urine
- Results in kidneys losing the ability to excrete water, electrolytes, wastes, and acid-base products through the urine, causing imbalances
- May lead to development of hypertension, anemia, uremia, and renal osteodystrophy
- May be acute or chronic

Acute renal failure

- Occurs suddenly
- Usually reversible
- May stem from prerenal, intrarenal, or obstructive postrenal conditions
- Divided into three phases: oliguric-anuric, diuretic, and recovery

Chronic renal failure

- Occurs slowly
- Irreversible
- May stem from chronic glomerular disease, chronic infections, congenital anomalies, vascular disease, long-term therapy with nephrotoxic drugs, and endocrine diseases
- Divided into four stages: reduced renal reserve, renal insufficiency, renal failure, and end-stage renal disease

Imbalances caused by renal failure

Hypervolemia

- Occurs when urine output decreases and the body retains fluid or when fluid intake exceeds urine output
- May lead to hypertension, peripheral edema, heart failure, or pulmonary edema

(continued)

Renal failure review *(continued)*

Hypovolemia
- Usually occurs during the diuretic phase of acute renal failure
- May result in hypotension or circulatory collapse

Hyperkalemia
- Occurs as the kidneys' ability to excrete potassium is impaired
- May also occur because metabolic acidosis, which occurs with renal failure, causes potassium to move from inside the cells into the extracellular fluid
- May be exacerbated by release of potassium from necrotic or injured cells
- Can also be caused by stressors, such as infection, GI bleeding, trauma, and surgery

Hyperphosphatemia
- Develops when the kidneys lose the ability to excrete phosphorus

Hypocalcemia
- Occurs when phosphorus levels increase (calcium and phosphorus have an inverse relationship)
- May also occur because decreased activation of vitamin D by the kidneys results in decreased GI absorption of calcium

Hyponatremia
- Occurs with acute renal failure because decreased GFR and damaged tubules increase water and sodium retention
- Can also be caused by the intracellular–extracellular exchange between sodium and potassium during metabolic acidosis

Hypernatremia
- Can occur with chronic kidney disease because progressive kidney failure results in the excretion of less sodium

Hypermagnesemia
- May result from decreased GFR and destruction of tubules
- Isn't usually apparent unless the patient is receiving external sources of magnesium, such as laxatives, antacids, I.V. solutions, or hyperalimentation solutions

Metabolic acidosis
- Is the most common acid-base imbalance occurring with renal failure
- Occurs when the kidneys lose their ability to secrete hydrogen ions (acid) in the urine
- Also occurs when the kidneys fail to store bicarbonate (base)

Metabolic alkalosis
- Rarely results from excessive intake of bicarbonate, which may be given to correct metabolic acidosis

Treatment
- Correction of specific symptoms
- Treatment of the underlying disease
- Low-protein, low-sodium, low-potassium, high-calorie diet
- Maintenance of fluid and electrolyte balance
- Erythropoietin to stimulate production of RBCs in the bone marrow
- Possibly hemodialysis or peritoneal dialysis
- Possibly a kidney transplant

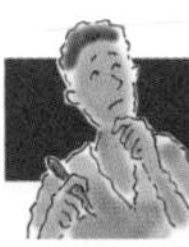

Quick quiz

1. A patient with hyperkalemia may experience several ECG changes, including:
   A. flat T waves, a small QRS complex, and normal P waves.
   B. tall, peaked T waves; a widened QRS complex; and disappearing P waves.
   C. no T waves, a normal QRS complex, and flattened or misshaped P waves.
   D. tall, peaked T waves; a normal QRS complex; and disappearing P waves.

Answer: B. High potassium levels may result in disappearing P waves; a widened QRS complex; and tall, peaked T waves because of the effect on cardiac cells.

2. Which of the following is the optimal diet for a patient with renal failure?
   A. High-calorie, low-protein, low-sodium, low-potassium
   B. High-calorie, high-protein, high-sodium, high-potassium
   C. Low-calorie, high-protein, low-sodium, low-potassium
   D. High-calorie, low-protein, low-sodium, high-potassium

Answer: A. A high-calorie, low-protein, low-sodium, and low-potassium diet is the optimal diet for meeting the metabolic and nutritional requirements of a patient with renal failure.

3. Laboratory results associated with acute renal failure include:
   A. increased BUN level and decreased serum creatinine level.
   B. decreased BUN level and increased urine output.
   C. increased BUN and serum creatinine levels.
   D. increased BUN level and increased urine output.

Answer: C. The patient with acute renal failure has increased BUN and serum creatinine levels and decreased urine output.

Scoring

☆☆☆ If you answered all three questions correctly, great job! You're dominant in the renal arena!

☆☆ If you answered two questions correctly, way to go! Your intelligence is still acute and your diagnosis is one of chronic success!

☆ If you answered fewer than two questions correctly, don't look so glum. Shake it off and good luck with the next chapter.

References

National Institute of Diabetes and Digestive and Kidney Diseases. (2012). *Kidney disease statistics for the United States.* Retrieved from http://kidney.niddk.nih.gov/KUDiseases/pubs/kustats/index.aspx#9

National Kidney Foundation. (2013). *Nephrology essentials.* Retrieved from http://www.kidney.org/professionals/CAP/nephEssentials.cfm

Okusa, M., & Rosner, M. (2013). *Overview of the management of acute kidney injury (acute renal failure).* Retrieved from http://www.uptodate.com/contents/overview-of-the-management-of-acute-kidney-injury-acute-renal-failure

Workeheh, B. (2013). *Acute kidney injury: Practice essentials.* Retrieved from http://emedicine.medscape.com/article/243492-overview

Chapter 18

Burns

Just the facts

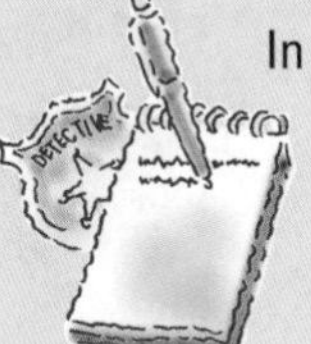

In this chapter, you'll learn:

- the physiologic changes that occur with severe burn injuries
- fluid, electrolyte, and acid-base imbalances that occur as a result of severe burn injuries
- signs and symptoms of burn injuries
- treatments for managing burn injuries
- appropriate nursing care for burn patients.

A look at burns

A major burn is a horrifying injury, requiring painful treatment and a long period of rehabilitation. Destruction of the epidermis, dermis, or subcutaneous layers of the skin can affect the entire body and, in many cases, is life-threatening. If not fatal, a burn can be permanently disfiguring and incapacitating, both emotionally and physically.

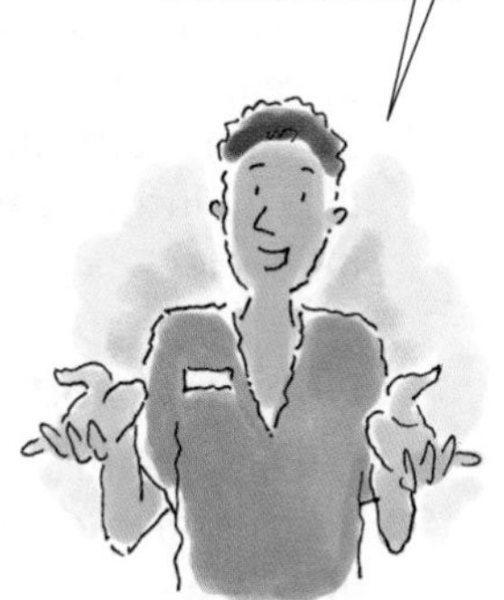

Burns are serious injuries that require painful treatment and long periods of rehabilitation.

Disrupting duties

Like any injury to the skin, a burn interferes with the skin's ability to help keep out infectious organisms, maintain fluid balance, and regulate body temperature. Burn injuries cause major changes in the body's fluid and electrolyte balance. Many of those imbalances change over time as the initial injury progresses.

The extreme heat from a burn can be severe enough to completely destroy cells. Even with a lesser injury, normal cell activity is disrupted. With minimal injury, the cell may recover its function. The burn patient's prognosis depends on the size and severity of the burn.

Several factors determine the severity of a burn, including the cause, degree, and extent of the burn as well as the part of the body involved. The outcome for a burn patient is also affected by the presence of preexisting medical conditions and the patient's age.

Types of burns

Burns can result from thermal or electrical injuries as well as from exposure to chemicals and radiation.

Thermal burns

The most common type of burn injury, thermal burns result from exposure to either dry (flames) or moist (steam, hot liquids) heat. They commonly occur with residential fires, motor vehicle accidents, childhood accidents, exposure to improperly stored gasoline, exposure to space heaters, electrical malfunctions, and arson. Other causes may include the improper handling of firecrackers, contact with scalding liquids, hot tar, and kitchen accidents.

Because its effects are similar to those of a thermal burn, frostbite is included in this category.

Electrical burns

Electrical burns commonly occur after contact with faulty electrical wiring, high-voltage power lines, or immersion in water that has been electrified. Those injuries may also be caused by lightning strikes. An electrical burn that ignites the patient's clothing may cause thermal burns as well.

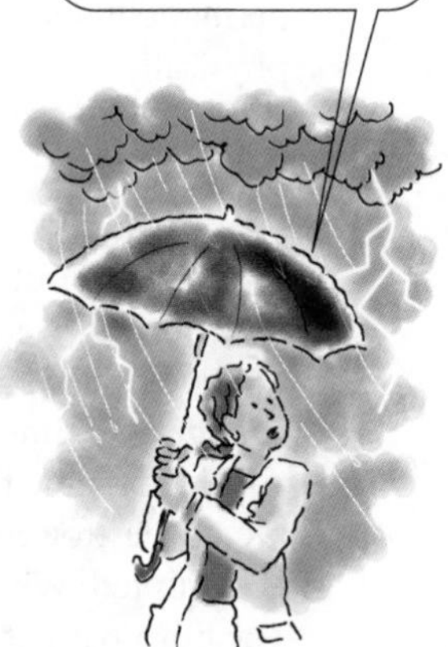
Faulty electrical wiring, high-voltage power lines, immersion in electrified water, and lightning strikes can all cause electrical burns.

Hidden hurt

When caring for a patient with an electrical burn, keep in mind that there may be more damage internally than meets the eye. Check the patient for entrance and exit wounds and be aware that there may be cardiac dysrhythmias. Tissue damage from an electrical burn is difficult to assess because internal destruction along the conduction pathway is usually greater than the surface burn indicates.

Chemical and radiation burns

Chemical burns result from the direct contact, ingestion, inhalation, or injection of acids, alkalies, or vesicants. These chemicals destroy protein in tissues, leading to necrosis. The type and extent of damage caused depends on the properties of the particular chemical.

Radiation burns are typically associated with sunburn or radiation treatment for cancer. These burns tend to be superficial, involving only the outer layer of skin.

Classification of burns

Burn thickness affects cell function. Therefore, classifying the degree of a burn helps to determine the type of intervention needed.

First-degree

Superficial (first-degree) burns affect the epidermis. These burns are usually pink or red, dry, and painful. No blistering occurs with this burn; however, some edema may be present. These burns aren't classified as severe because the epidermis remains intact and continues to prevent water loss from the skin, so they don't affect fluid and electrolyte balance. Regrowth of the epidermis occurs, and healing is generally rapid without scarring.

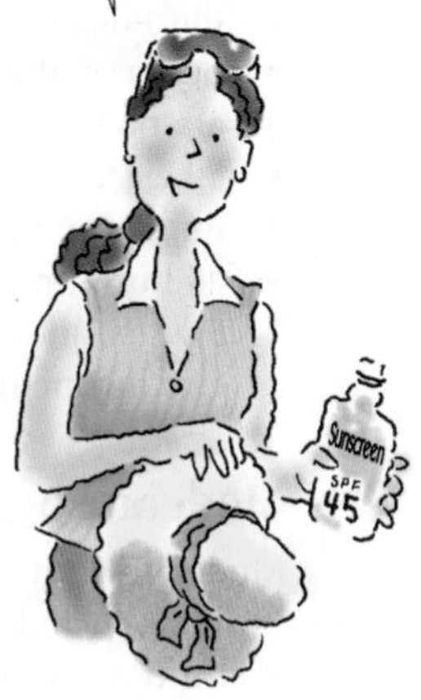
First-degree burns—for example, most sunburns—affect the superficial layer of the epidermis.
Sunscreen
SPF 45

Second-degree

Superficial partial-thickness and deep partial-thickness burns are the two types of second-degree burns and affect both the epidermis and dermis. These burns are caused by brief exposure to flames, hot liquids or solids, dilute chemicals, or intense radiation. Deep partial-thickness burns can progress to third-degree burns over the course of several days after injury.

To identify a superficial partial-thickness burn, look for pink, moist, and tender skin accompanied by thin-walled, fluid-filled blisters. Deep partial-thickness burns can be painful, swollen, and red, with thick-walled blister formation. When pressure is applied to the burn, it blanches and refills. Regeneration of the epithelial layer may occur. The amount of scarring varies with this type of burn. Second-degree burns that cover significant areas of the body may lead to fluid and electrolyte imbalances.

Third-degree

Full-thickness (third-degree) burns destroy the epidermis and the dermis and may affect subcutaneous tissue. These burns look dry and leathery, are painless (because nerve endings are destroyed), and don't blanch when pressure is applied. The color of the burned area varies from white to black or charred.

Full-thickness burns require skin grafting and carry the greatest risk of fluid and electrolyte imbalance.

Fourth-degree

Deep full-thickness (fourth-degree) burns extend beyond the dermis and subcutaneous tissue to the muscle layer and can include tendon or bone.

Fourth-degree burns are charred and hard. The burned areas do not blanch. Surgery is required, but even so, they have a poor prognosis.

Burn severity

The severity of a burn can be estimated by correlating its depth and size. Burns are categorized as major, moderate, and minor. Assessment tools, such as the Rule of Nines or the Lund-Browder classification, are used to estimate the percentage of body surface area involved in a burn. (See *Estimating the extent of a burn.*)

Major burns

Major burns, which require treatment in a specialized burn care facility, include:

- second-degree burns covering more than 25% of an adult's body surface area or more than 20% of a child's body surface area
- third-degree burns covering more than 10% of the body surface area
- burns on the hands, face, eyes, ears, feet, or genitalia
- all inhalation burns
- all electrical burns
- burns complicated by fractures or other major trauma
- all burns in poor-risk patients, such as children younger than age 5 years, adults older than age 60 years, and patients who have pre-existing medical conditions such as heart disease.

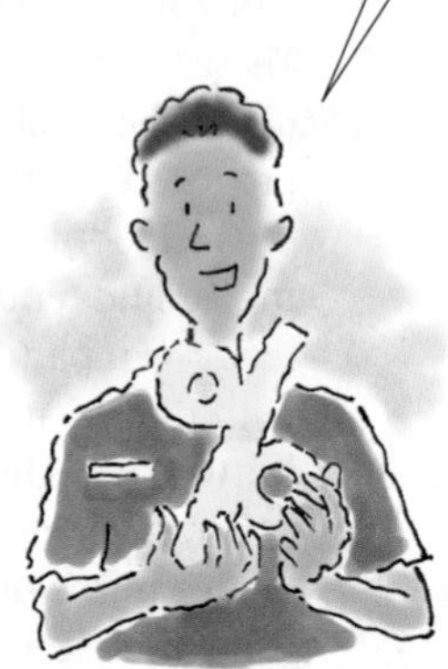

One of the major factors in determining whether a burn is major, moderate, or minor is estimating what percentage of the body is burned.

Moderate burns

Moderate burns, which require treatment in a burn care facility or hospital, include:

- third-degree burns on 2% to 10% of the body surface area, regardless of body size
- second-degree burns on 15% to 25% of an adult's body surface area and 10% to 20% of a child's.

Minor burns

Minor burns, which may be hospitalized but not necessarily at a burn center or can be treated on an outpatient basis, include:

- third-degree burns that appear on less than 2% of the body surface area, regardless of body size
- second-degree burns on less than 15% of an adult's body surface area and 10% of a child's body surface area (most children are transferred to a burn center).

Phases of burns

Burn phases describe the physiologic changes that occur after a burn and include the fluid accumulation, fluid remobilization, and convalescent phases in burns, which are greater than 20% total body

Estimating the extent of a burn

Because body surface area varies with age, two different methods are used to estimate burn size in adult and pediatric patients.

Rule of Nines

You can quickly estimate the extent of an adult patient's burn by using the Rule of Nines. This method quantifies body surface area in multiples of 9, thus the name. To use this method, mentally transfer the burns on your patient to the body charts below. Add the corresponding percentages for each body section burned. Use the total—a rough estimate of burn extent—to calculate initial fluid replacement needs. If the burn doesn't completely cover a body area, the burn can be estimated about the size of the patient's palm which equals 1% of the body.

Lund-Browder Classification

The Rule of Nines isn't accurate for infants or children because their body shapes, and therefore BSA, differ from those of adults. For example, an infant's head accounts for about 17% of his total body surface area, compared with 7% for an adult. Instead, use the Lund-Browder classification to determine burn size for infants and children.

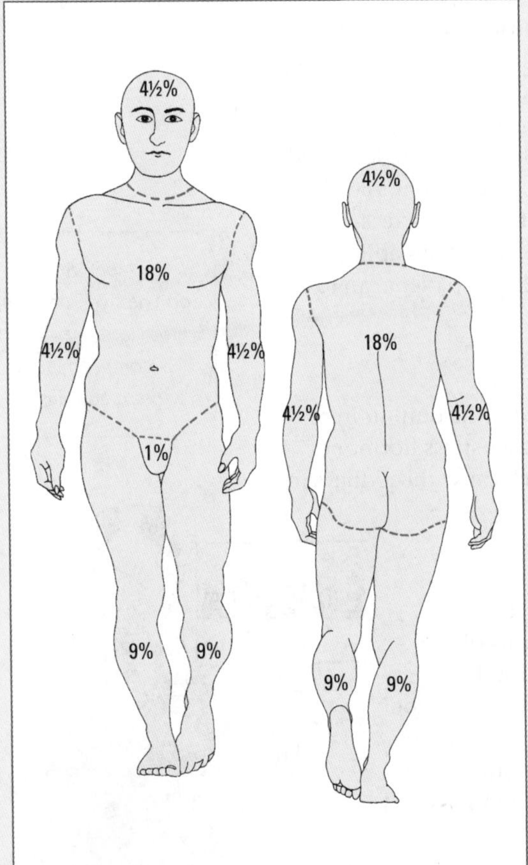

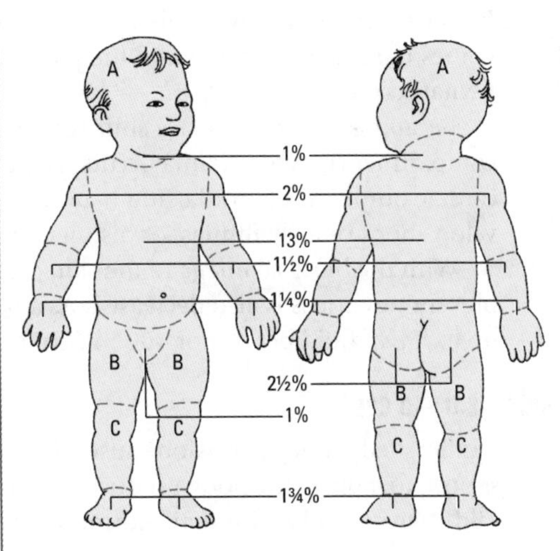

Percentage of burned body surface by age

At birth	1 year	5 years	10 years	15 years	Adult
A: Half of head					
9½%	8½%	6½%	5½%	4½%	3½%
B: Half of one thigh					
2¾%	3¼%	4%	4¼%	4½%	4¾%
C: Half of one leg					
2½%	2½%	2 ¾%	3%	3¼%	3½%

surface area. Burns affect many body systems and can lead to several serious fluid and electrolyte imbalances, which vary depending on the phase of the burn.

Fluid accumulation phase

The fluid accumulation phase, also known as the *burn shock phase* or *emergent phase,* occurs within the first 24 to 36 hours after a burn injury, with its peak occurring between 6 and 8 hours. During this phase, fluid shifts from the vascular compartment to the interstitial space, a process known as *third-space shift*. This shift of fluids causes edema. Severe edema may compromise circulation and diminish pulses in the extremities.

Permeability and plasma

Because of the burn injury, capillary damage alters the permeability of the vessels. Plasma—the liquid and protein part of blood—escapes from the vascular compartment into the interstitium. Because less fluid is available to dilute the blood, the blood becomes hemoconcentrated and the patient's hemoglobin level and hematocrit rise.

Because of the third-space shift (fluids moving out of the vascular compartment), hypovolemia occurs. Hypovolemia causes decreased cardiac output, tachycardia, and hypotension. The patient may develop shock or arrhythmias, or his mental status may decrease.

With the burn's damage to the skin surface, the skin's ability to prevent water loss is also decreased. As a result, the patient can lose up to 8 L of fluid per day or 400 ml/hour.

Depending on the type of burn, a patient may have a compromised, edematous airway.

EDEMA

The kidneys try to cope

Diminished kidney perfusion causes decreased urine output. In response to a burn, the body produces and releases stress hormones (aldosterone and antidiuretic hormone), which cause the kidneys to retain sodium and water.

Uneasy breathing

Depending on the type of burn, a patient may have a compromised, edematous airway. Look for burns of the head or neck, singed nasal hairs, soot in the mouth or nose, coughing, voice changes, mucosal burns, and stridor. You may hear crackles or wheezes over the lung fields. The patient may breathe rapidly or pant. Circumferential burns and edema of the neck or chest can restrict respirations and cause shortness of breath.

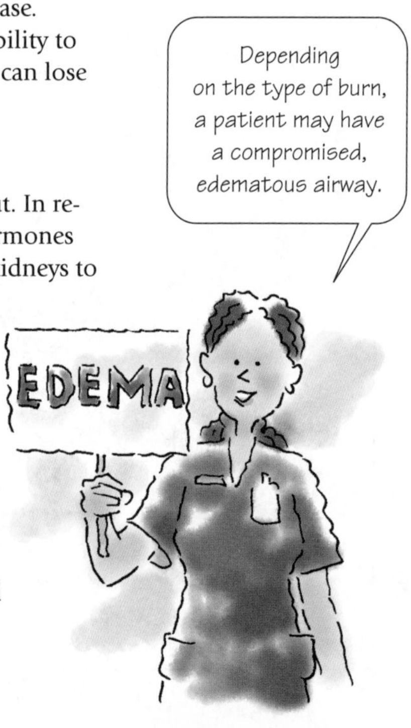

Tissue turmoil

Injured tissue releases acids that can cause a drop in the pH level of blood and subsequently lead to metabolic acidosis. Damage to muscle tissue in full-thickness burns and electrical burns results in release of myoglobin, which can cause renal damage and acute tubular necrosis. Myoglobin gives urine a darkened appearance.

The GI takes a hit

Hypovolemia can lead to decreased circulation to the GI system, resulting in paralytic ileus. This is manifested by decreased or absent peristalsis and bowel sounds.

Stress ulcers, or Curling's ulcers, can develop in the antrum of the stomach or in the duodenum as a result of the intense physiologic stress associated with burn trauma. These ulcers can be observed by endoscopy approximately 72 hours after injury.

Curling's ulcers are most likely caused during the fluid accumulation phase as a result of decreased blood flow to the stomach along with reflux of duodenal contents. Large amounts of pepsin are also released. The combined ischemia, pepsin, and acid leads to ulceration.

Signs of Curling's ulcer include bloody or coffee-ground emesis and occult blood in the stool. Histamine blockers and antacids are used to reduce gastric acidity and ulceration. These lesions usually heal once the patient recovers from the acute injury.

The body's metabolic needs also increase because of the burn injury, usually in proportion to the size of the burn wound. A negative nitrogen balance can occur as well as a result of tissue destruction, protein loss, and the body's stress response.

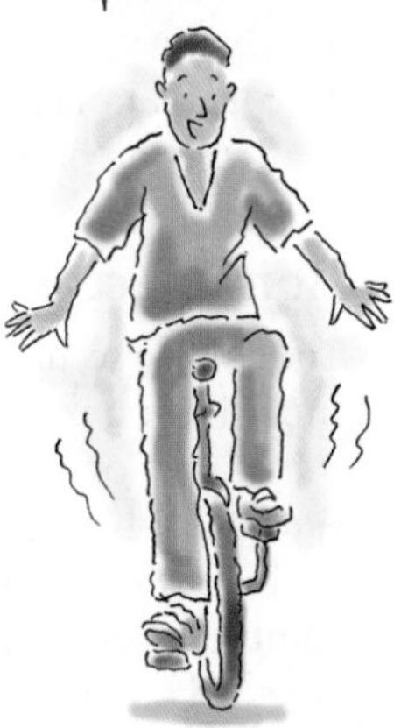
All of these burn phases can lead to several fluid and electrolyte imbalances. Whoa!

Unbalanced!

Many electrolyte imbalances can occur during the fluid accumulation phase because of the hypermetabolic needs and the priority that fluid replacement takes over nutritional needs during the emergent phase:

- Hyperkalemia can result from massive cellular trauma, metabolic acidosis, or renal failure. The condition develops as potassium is released into the extracellular fluid in the initial days following the injury.
- Hypovolemia can occur as a result of fluid losses and fluids moving from the vascular space to the interstitial space. Lost fluid resembles intravascular fluid in composition and contains proteins and electrolytes.
- Hyponatremia can result from increased loss of sodium and water from the cells. Large amounts of sodium become trapped in edematous fluid during the fluid accumulation phase. Aqueous silver nitrate dressings may also contribute to this electrolyte imbalance.

- Hypernatremia can occur as a result of the aggressive use of hypertonic sodium solutions during fluid replacement therapy.
- Hypocalcemia can occur because calcium travels to the damaged tissue and becomes immobilized at the burn site. That movement can occur 12 to 24 hours after the burn injury. It can also occur because of an inadequate dietary intake of calcium or inadequate supplementation during treatment.
- Metabolic acidosis can develop as a result of the accumulation of acids released from the burned tissue. It can also occur as a result of decreased tissue perfusion from hypovolemia.
- Respiratory acidosis can result from inadequate ventilation, as happens in inhalation burns.

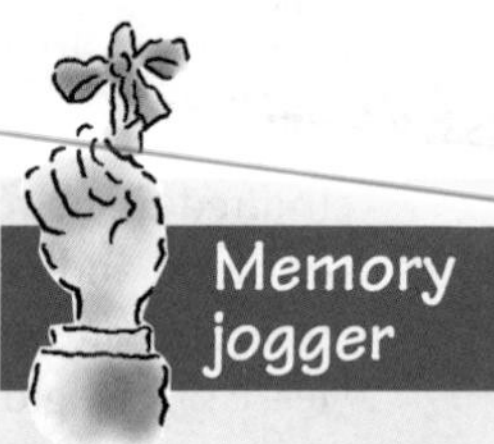

To remember how fluids shift following a burn injury (the burn phases), think of an **ARC**:

Accumulation phase—fluids shift from the vascular compartment into the interstitial spaces.

Remobilization phase—fluid moves back to the vascular compartment.

Convalescent phase—major fluid shifts have been resolved and healing can begin.

Fluid remobilization phase

The fluid remobilization phase, also known as the *diuresis stage* or *acute stage*, starts about 48 hours after the initial burn. During this phase, fluid shifts back to the vascular compartment. Edema at the burn site decreases, and blood flow to the kidneys increases, which promotes urine output. Sodium is lost through the increase in diuresis, and potassium either moves back into the cells or is lost through urine.

Shifty business

Fluid and electrolyte imbalances present during the initial phase after a burn can change during the fluid remobilization phase. Here's a rundown of these imbalances:

- Hypokalemia can develop as potassium shifts from the extracellular fluid back into the cells. The condition usually occurs 4 to 5 days after a major burn.
- Hypervolemia can occur as fluid shifts back to the vascular compartment. Excessive administration of I.V. fluids may exacerbate the condition.
- Hyponatremia may occur when sodium is lost during diuresis.
- Metabolic acidosis can occur when loss of sodium results in the depletion of bicarbonate.

Convalescent phase

The convalescent phase begins after the fluid accumulation and remobilization phases have resolved. During this phase, the focus is on the healing or reconstruction of the burn wound. Although the major fluid shifts have been resolved, further fluid and electrolyte imbalances may continue as a result of inadequate dietary intake. Anemia commonly develops at this time because severe burns typically destroy red blood cells.

What tests show

Diagnostic test results you may see when caring for a burn patient include:

- increased hemoglobin levels and hematocrit
- increased serum potassium levels
- decreased serum sodium levels
- decreased serum calcium levels
- increased blood urea nitrogen and creatinine levels, indicating renal failure
- low pH and bicarbonate levels, indicating metabolic acidosis
- increased carboxyhemoglobin levels, indicating smoke inhalation
- electrocardiogram (ECG) changes reflecting electrolyte imbalances or myocardial damage
- myoglobin in the urine.

Edema alert!

Watch for signs and symptoms of pulmonary edema, which can result from fluid replacement therapy and the shift of fluid back to the vascular compartment. Check for decreased hemoglobin levels and hematocrit due to hemodilution from that fluid shift.

Inspect for infection

Skin impairment leads not only to body temperature alterations and chills but also to infection. Blisters, charring, and scarring may appear, depending on the type and age of the burn. With infected wounds, you may note a foul odor and purulent drainage.

When caring for a burn patient, always remember your ABCs—airway, breathing, and circulation.

How they're treated

Priorities in treating a burn patient reflect the ABCs—airway, breathing, and circulation. For a patient with severe facial burns or suspected inhalation injury, treatment to prevent hypoxia includes endotracheal (ET) intubation, administration of high concentrations of oxygen, and positive-pressure ventilation. Be aware that acute respiratory distress syndrome may develop from both the body's immune response to injury and fluid leakage across the alveolocapillary membrane.

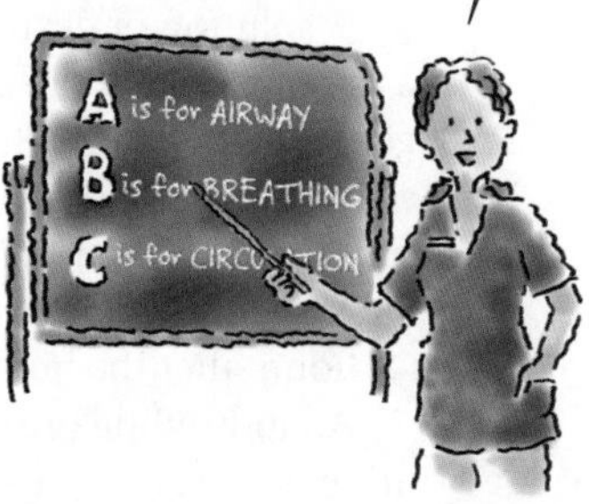

Let it flow, let it flow, let it flow

Fluid resuscitation is a vital part of burn treatment. Several formulas have been created to guide initial treatment for burn patients. The Parkland formula is one of the more commonly used formulas. (See *Fluid replacement formula*, page 324.)

Fluid replacement formula

Here's a commonly used formula, the modified Parkland formula, for calculating fluid replacement in burn patients. Always base fluid replacement on the patient's response, especially urine output. Urine output of 30 to 50 ml/hour is a sign of adequate renal perfusion in an adult and 1 ml/kg/hour in small children.

Formula

Use 4 ml of lactated Ringer's solution per kilogram of body weight per percentage of body surface area over 24 hours.

Example: for a 68-kg (150-lb) person with 27% body surface area burns, 4 ml × 68 kg × 27 = 7,344 ml over 24 hours. Give one-half of the total over the first 8 hours after the burn and the remainder over the next 16 hours.

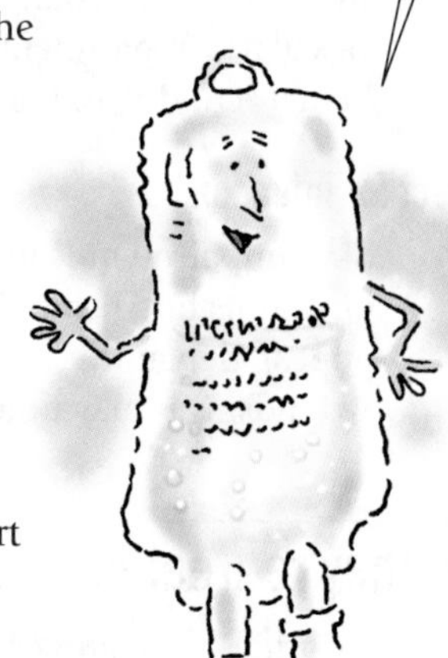
Fluid resuscitation is a vital part of burn treatment.

Initial treatment includes administration of lactated Ringer's solution through a large-bore I.V. line to expand vascular volume. This balanced isotonic solution supplies water, sodium, and other electrolytes; it can help correct metabolic acidosis because the lactate in the solution is quickly metabolized into bicarbonate.

Colloid controversy

Hypertonic solutions called *colloids* may be used to increase blood volume. Colloids draw water from the interstitial space into the vasculature. However, the use of colloids in the immediate postburn period is controversial because they increase colloid osmotic pressure in the interstitial space, which may worsen edema at the burn site. Patients who may benefit from colloid solutions are those requiring lower volume resuscitation such as preexisting heart disease, geriatric patients, and inhalation injuries. Examples of colloid solutions are plasma, albumin, and dextran.

A solution of dextrose 5% in lactated Ringer's is typically reserved as a maintenance dose for children to prevent life-threatening hypoglycemia. Dextrose 5% in water may be used to replace normal insensible water loss as well as water loss associated with damage to the skin barrier after the first 24 hours. Central and peripheral I.V. lines are inserted as necessary. Potassium may be added to I.V. fluids 48 to 72 hours after the burn injury.

An indwelling urinary catheter permits accurate monitoring of urine output. Administration of 2 to 4 mg of morphine I.V. alleviates pain and anxiety. The patient may need a nasogastric (NG) tube to prevent gastric distention from paralytic ileus, along with histamine blockers and antacids to prevent Curling's ulcers.

All burn patients need a booster of 0.5 ml of tetanus toxoid given I.M. Burn care facilities don't recommend administering a prophylactic antibiotic because overuse of antibiotics fosters the development of resistant bacteria.

Treatment tips

Treatment of the burn wound includes:

- initial debridement by washing the surface of the wound area with mild soap
- sharp debridement of loose tissue and blisters because blister fluid contains vasospastic agents that can worsen tissue ischemia
- coverage of the wound with an antibacterial agent, such as silver sulfadiazine (Silvadene), and an occlusive cotton gauze dressing
- removal of eschar (escharotomy) if the patient is at risk for vascular, circulatory, or respiratory compromise—for example, if the patient has a circumferential burn that circles around an extremity, the chest cavity, or the abdomen, skin grafts may also be required. If the patient is going to be transferred to a burn center, defer to their treatment criteria prior to transfer. Most burn centers request that no antibacterial agent is applied to the burn but require dry dressings applied to the wound.

How you intervene

For a burn patient, proper intervention and good nursing care can make the difference between life and death. During the emergent phase, immediate, aggressive burn treatment to increase the patient's chance for survival takes first priority. Later, the priority shifts to providing supportive measures and using strict aseptic technique to minimize the risk of infection. (For tips on how to handle burns outside the health care system, see *Emergency burn care*, page 326.)

Here are some general burn care guidelines:

- Maintain head and spinal alignment until head and spinal cord injuries have been ruled out.

Shocking situation

- Give emergency treatment for electric shock if needed. If an electric shock caused ventricular fibrillation and subsequent cardiac and respiratory arrest, begin cardiopulmonary resuscitation at once. Try to obtain an estimate of the voltage that caused the injury.
- Make sure the patient has adequate airway and effective breathing and circulation. If needed, assist with ET intubation. The patient may have a tracheostomy tube inserted if ET intubation isn't possible. Administer 100% oxygen as ordered, and adjust the flow to maintain adequate gas exchange. Draw blood for arterial blood gas (ABG) analyses as ordered.

Emergency burn care

Here's what you should do if you encounter a person who has just been burned:

- Extinguish any remaining flames on the patient's clothing.
- Don't directly touch the patient if he's still connected to live electricity. Unplug or disconnect the electrical source if possible.
- Assess the ABCs (airway, breathing, circulation), and initiate cardiopulmonary resuscitation if necessary.
- Assess the scope of the burns and other injuries.
- Remove the patient's clothing; cut around clothing that sticks to the skin.
- Irrigate areas of chemical burns with copious amounts of water.
- Remove from the patient any jewelry or other metal objects that can retain heat and constrict patient movement.
- Cover the patient with a blanket.
- Send for emergency medical assistance.

- Assess vital signs every 15 minutes. Assess breath sounds, and watch for signs of hypoxia and pulmonary edema.
- Take steps to control bleeding, and remove clothing that's still smoldering. Cut around clothing stuck to the patient's skin. Remove rings and other constricting items.
- Assess the skin for the location, depth, and extent of the burn.
- Assist with the insertion of a central venous line and additional arterial and I.V. lines.
- Start I.V. therapy at once to prevent hypovolemic shock and maintain cardiac output. Follow the Parkland formula or another fluid resuscitation formula, as ordered by the doctor.
- Insert an indwelling urinary catheter as ordered, and monitor intake and output every 15 to 30 minutes.
- Maintain adequate pulmonary hygiene by turning the patient and performing postural drainage regularly.
- Watch for signs of decreased tissue perfusion, increased confusion, and agitation. Assess peripheral pulses for adequacy.
- Assess the patient's heart and hemodynamic status for changes that might indicate fluid imbalances, such as hypervolemia or hypovolemia.
- Observe the pattern of third-space shifting (generalized edema, ascites, and pulmonary or intracranial edema), and document your findings.
- Monitor potassium levels, and watch for signs and symptoms of hyperkalemia, such as cardiac rhythm strip changes; weakness; diarrhea; and a slowed, irregular heart rate.

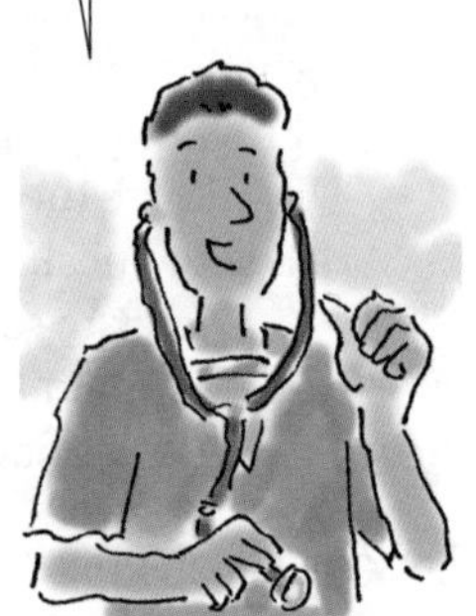
Assess the patient's heart and hemodynamic status for changes that might indicate fluid imbalance.

- Monitor sodium levels, and watch for signs and symptoms of hyponatremia, such as increasing confusion, twitching, seizures, abdominal pain, nausea, and vomiting.
- Watch for signs and symptoms of metabolic acidosis, such as headache; disorientation; drowsiness; nausea; vomiting; and rapid, shallow breathing.
- Monitor oxygen saturation and ABG results.
- Monitor other laboratory results.
- Monitor ECG results for arrhythmias.
- Anticipate the need to administer maintenance I.V. replacement fluids based on daily assessment of fluid, electrolyte, acid-base, and nutritional status.
- Maintain core body temperature by covering the patient with a sterile blanket and exposing only small areas of his body at a time.
- Insert an NG tube, if ordered, to decompress the stomach. Avoid aspiration of stomach contents during the procedure.
- Obtain a preburn weight from the patient or from a family member or friend.
- If bowel sounds are present, provide a diet high in potassium, protein, vitamins, fats, nitrogen, and calories to maintain the patient's preburn weight. If necessary, feed the patient enterally until he can tolerate oral feedings. If he can't tolerate oral or enteral feedings, administer hyperalimentation as ordered.
- Weigh the patient every day at the same time with the same amount of linen, clothes, and dressings.
- Explain all procedures to the patient before performing them. Speak calmly and clearly to help alleviate anxiety. Encourage the patient to participate in self-care as much as possible. (See *Teaching about burns.*)
- Use strict aseptic technique for all patient care, including routinely washing your hands and using protective isolation clothing.
- Observe the patient for signs of infection, such as fever, tachycardia, and purulent wound drainage. Burn patients have an increased risk of infection from destruction of the skin barrier and the loss of nutrients.
- Administer an analgesic 30 minutes before wound care.
- Culture wounds before applying a topical antibiotic for the first time.
- Cover burns with a dry, sterile dressing. Never cover large burns with saline-soaked dressings because they can drastically lower body temperature. A topical ointment and an antibiotic may be applied as appropriate. Silver nitrate and mafenide acetate (Sulfamylon) can cause electrolyte imbalances and metabolic alterations.
- Maintain joint function with physical therapy and use of support garments and splints.

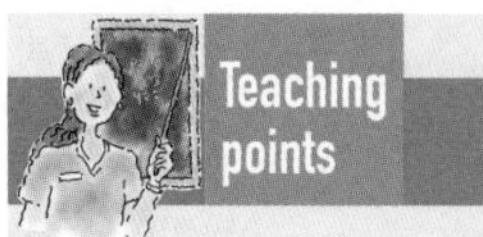
Teaching points

Teaching about burns

When teaching a patient about burns, be sure to cover the following topics and then evaluate your patient's learning:

- burn basics and prevention
- the patient's particular plan of treatment and wound management
- signs and symptoms to report to the practitioner
- long-term care issues, such as home care follow-up and rehabilitation.

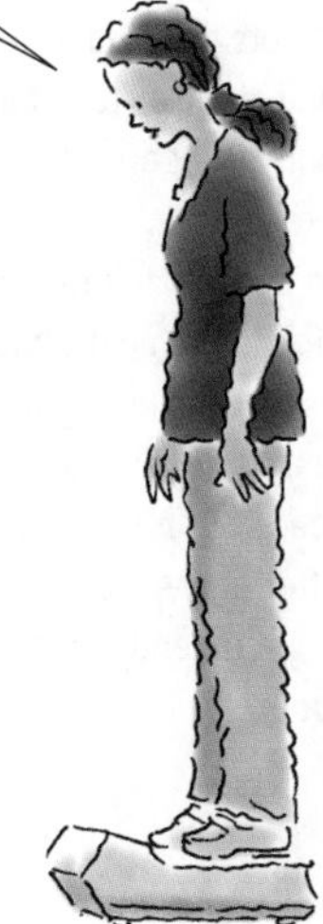
Obtain a preburn weight from the patient.

- Notify the practitioner of significant changes in the patient's condition and pertinent laboratory test results.
- Provide opportunities for the patient to voice concerns, especially about altered body image. If appropriate, arrange a meeting with another burn patient with similar injuries or refer the patient to a burn support group. When possible, show the patient how bodily functions are improving. If necessary, refer him for mental health counseling.
- Prepare the patient and family to go home.
- Document all care given, all teaching done, and the patient's reaction to each. (See *Documenting burn care.*)

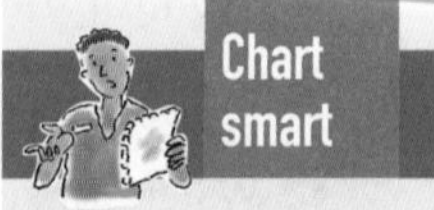

Chart smart

Documenting burn care

If your patient has burns, make sure you document the following information:

- assessment findings
- depth, extent, and severity of burn injury
- extent of edema
- pertinent laboratory results
- I.V. therapy
- urinary output
- other interventions such as wound care
- support made available to the patient and family
- patient and family teaching along with the patient's response.

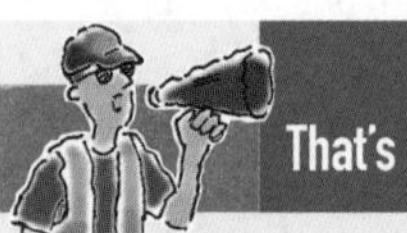

That's a wrap!

Burns review

Burn basics

- Usually cause major changes in the body's fluid and electrolyte balance, which may change over time as the initial injury progresses
- Types: thermal, electrical, chemical, and radiation

Classification of burns

- First-degree: superficial burn that affects the epidermis; fluid and electrolyte balance isn't affected
- Second-degree: partial-thickness burn that affects the epidermis and dermis; fluid and electrolyte imbalances occur with burns that cover significant areas of the body
- Third-degree: full-thickness burn that affects the epidermis, dermis, and tissues below the dermis; carries the greatest risk of fluid and electrolyte imbalances
- Fourth-degree: deep full-thickness burns that extend to the muscle; prognosis is poor

Burn severity

- Requires the use of assessment tools, such as the Rule of Nines or the Lund-Browder classification, to estimate the percentage of body surface area involved
- May be categorized as major, moderate, or minor

Phases of burns

Fluid accumulation phase

- Occurs within first 24 to 36 hours after a burn; also known as *burn shock phase*
- Causes fluid to shift from the vascular compartment to interstitial space (third-space shift), resulting in edema
- Produces stress hormones that cause the kidneys to retain sodium and water, leading to diminished kidney perfusion and decreased urine output
- Causes such fluid and electrolyte imbalances as:
  - Hyperkalemia—results from massive cellular trauma, metabolic acidosis, or renal failure; develops as potassium is released into extracellular fluid during initial days following injury

(continued)

Burns review *(continued)*

- Hypovolemia—results from fluid losses and third-space shift
- Hyponatremia—results from increased cellular loss of sodium and water; causes large amounts of sodium to become trapped in edematous fluid
- Hypernatremia—can result from aggressive use of hypertonic sodium solutions during fluid replacement therapy
- Hypocalcemia—can result when calcium travels to the damaged tissue and becomes immobilized at burn site; may also result from inadequate dietary intake of calcium or inadequate supplementation during treatment
- Metabolic acidosis—may result from accumulation of acids released by burned tissue; may also result from decreased perfusion due to hypovolemia

Fluid remobilization phase

- Begins about 48 hours after the initial burn
- Causes fluid to shift back into the vascular compartment
- Causes such fluid and electrolyte imbalances as:
  - Hypokalemia—can develop as potassium shifts from extracellular fluid back into the cells; usually occurs 4 to 5 days after a major burn
  - Hypervolemia—can occur as fluid shifts back to the vascular compartment; may result from giving too much I.V. fluid
  - Hyponatremia—may occur when sodium is lost during diuresis
  - Metabolic acidosis—occurs when loss of sodium results in the depletion of bicarbonate

Convalescent phase

- Begins after first two phases have been resolved
- May cause further fluid and electrolyte imbalances as a result of inadequate dietary intake

Treatment

- Depends on the severity of the burn
- For severe burns, airway, breathing, and circulation are priorities
- Involves rehydration with fluid resuscitation
- Requires monitoring of urine output with catheter
- May require pain relief measures
- Involves wound care

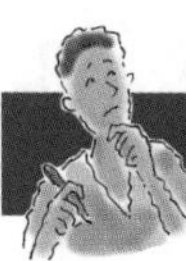

Quick quiz

1. During the fluid accumulation phase of a major burn injury, fluids shift from the:
   A. intravascular space to the interstitial space.
   B. interstitial space to the intravascular space.
   C. intracellular space to the interstitial space.
   D. intravascular space to the intracellular space.

Answer: A. During the fluid accumulation phase, fluids shift from the intravascular space to the interstitial space.

2. Hypovolemia usually occurs during which major burn phase?
   A. Fluid remobilization
   B. Fluid accumulation
   C. Convalescent
   D. Acute

Answer: B. Hypovolemia usually occurs during the fluid accumulation phase as fluid moves from the intravascular space to the interstitial space, a process known as third-space shift.

3. You insert an I.V. line and begin fluid resuscitation. The doctor wants you to use the Parkland formula. The patient is a 155-lb (70-kg) male and is estimated at having 50% of his total body surface area burned. What amount of lactated Ringer's solution should you administer over the first 8 hours?
   A. 700 ml
   B. 7,000 ml
   C. 1,400 ml
   D. 6,000 ml

Answer: B. The Parkland formula is 4 ml × the percentage of total body surface area burned × weight in kilograms. So, 4 ml × 50% × 70 kg = 14,000 ml or 14 L of lactated Ringer's solution in the first 24 hours. Therefore, you would give 7,000 ml (or half) in the first 8 hours.

4. During the fluid remobilization phase of a patient with burn injuries, the nurse would expect to see signs of which electrolyte imbalance?
   A. Hypokalemia
   B. Hyperkalemia
   C. Hypernatremia
   D. Hypovolemia

Answer: A. Hypokalemia occurs in the fluid remobilization (diuresis) phase as potassium shifts from the extracellular fluid back into the cells.

Scoring

☆☆☆ If you answered all four questions correctly, outstanding! You've learned how to beat the heat!

☆☆ If you answered three questions correctly, way to go! You don't have much left to learn when it comes to burns!

☆ If you answered fewer than three questions correctly, don't feel the heat just yet. There are still a couple more chapters to go!

References

Bacomo, F. K., & Chung, K. K., (2011). A primer on burn resuscitation. *Journal of Emergencies, Trauma, and Shock, 4*(1), 109–113.

Edlich, R. F. (2013). *Thermal burns*. Retrieved from http://emedicine.medscape.com/article/1278244-overview

Haberal, M., Abali, A. E., & Karakayali, H. (2010). Fluid management in major burn injuries. *Indian Journal of Plastic Surgery*, 43(Suppl), S29–S36. Retrieved from http://www.ncbi.nlm.nih.gov/pmc/articles/PMC3038406/

Jenkins, J. A. (2013). *Emergent management of thermal burns*. Retrieved from http://emedicine.medscape.com/article/769193-overview

Jeschke, M. G., Pinto, R., Herndon, D. N., Finnerty, C. C., & Kraft, R. (2014). Hypoglycemia is associated with increased postburn morbidity and mortality in pediatric patients. *Critical Care Medicine, 42*(5), 1221–1331. doi:10.1097/CCM.0000000000000138

Jeschke, M. G., Shahrokhi, S., Finnerty, C. C., Branski, L. K., & Dibildox, M. (2013). Wound coverage technologies in burn care: Established techniques. *Journal of Burn Care & Research*. Advance online publication. doi:10.1097/BCR.0b013e3182920d29

Kraft, R., Herndon, D. N., Finnerty, C. C., Shahrokhi, S., & Jeschke, M. G. (2013). Occurrence of multiorgan dysfunction in pediatric burn patients: Incidence and clinical outcome. *Annals of Surgery, 259*(2), 381–387. doi:10.1097/SLA.0b013e31828c4d04

Mitchell, K. B., Khalil, E., Brennan, A., Shao, H., Rabbitts, A., Leahy, N. E., . . . Gallagher, J. J. (2013). New management strategy for fluid resuscitation: Quantifying volume in the first 48 hours after burn injury. *Journal of Burn Care & Research, 34*(1), 196–202. doi;10.1097/BCR.0b013e3182700965

Namdar, T., Stollwerck, P. L., Stang, F. H., Siemers, F., Mailänder, P., & Lange, T. (2010). Transdermal fluid loss in severely burned patients. *German Medical Science, 8*, Doc28. Retrieved from http://www.ncbi.nlm.nih.gov/pmc/articles/PMC2975262/

Oliver, R.I. (2013). *Burn resuscitation and early management*. Retrieved from http://emedicine.medscape.com/article/1277360-overview

Sheridan, R. L. (2012). *Burn rehabilitation*. Retrieved from http://emedicine.medscape.com/article/318436-overview#aw2aab6b5

Sheridan, R. L. (2013). *Initial evaluation and management of the burn patient*. Retrieved from http://emedicine.medscape.com/article/435402-overview#a1

Part IV

Treating imbalances

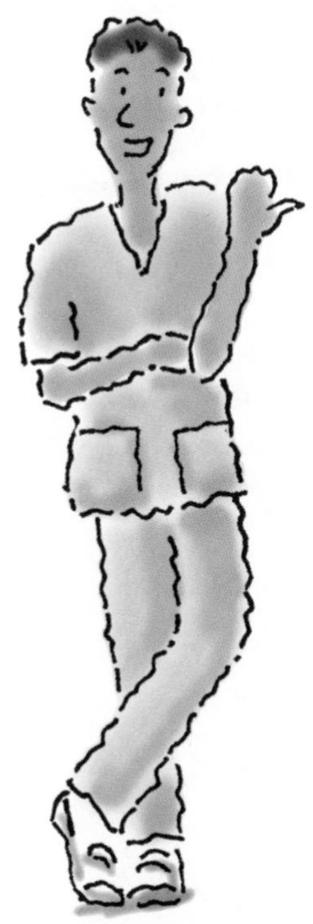

Chapter 19

I.V. fluid replacement

Just the facts

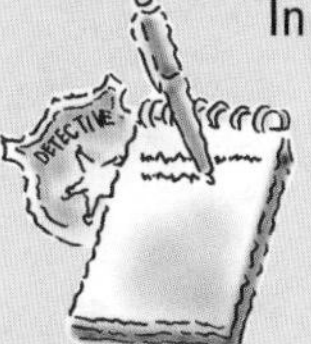

In this chapter, you'll learn:

- types of I.V. fluids and their uses
- methods used to administer I.V. fluids
- complications associated with I.V. therapy
- proper care for patients receiving I.V. therapy.

A look at I.V. therapy

To maintain health, the balance of fluids and electrolytes in the intracellular and extracellular spaces needs to remain relatively constant. Whenever a person experiences an illness or a condition that prevents normal fluid intake or causes excessive fluid loss, I.V. fluid replacement may be necessary.

A lot to offer

I.V. therapy that provides the patient with life-sustaining fluids, electrolytes, and medications offers the advantages of immediate and predictable therapeutic effects. The I.V. route is, therefore, the preferred route, especially for administering fluids, blood products, electrolytes, and drugs in an emergency.

This route also allows for fluid intake when a patient has GI malabsorption. I.V. therapy permits accurate dosage titration for analgesics and other medications. Potential disadvantages associated with I.V. therapy include drug and solution incompatibility, adverse reactions to various medications, localized infection, sepsis, and other complications.

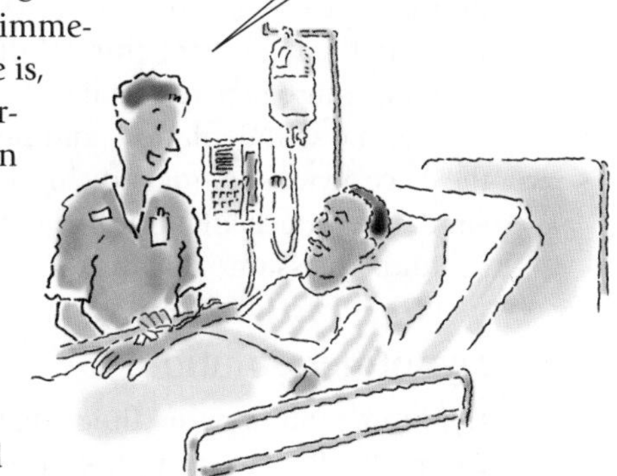

I.V. therapy has its advantages and disadvantages. Keep reading to find out more.

Types of I.V. solutions

Solutions used for I.V. fluid replacement fall into the broad categories of crystalloids (which may be isotonic, hypotonic, or hypertonic) and colloids (which are always hypertonic).

Crystalloids

Crystalloids are solutions with small molecules that flow easily from the bloodstream into cells and tissues. Isotonic crystalloids contain about the same concentration of osmotically active particles as extracellular fluid, so fluid doesn't shift between the extracellular and intracellular areas.

Concentrating on concentration

Hypotonic crystalloids are less concentrated than extracellular fluid, so they move from the bloodstream into cells, causing cells to swell. In contrast, hypertonic crystalloids are more highly concentrated than extracellular fluid, so fluid is pulled into the bloodstream from the cells, causing cells to shrink. (See *Comparing fluid tonicity*.)

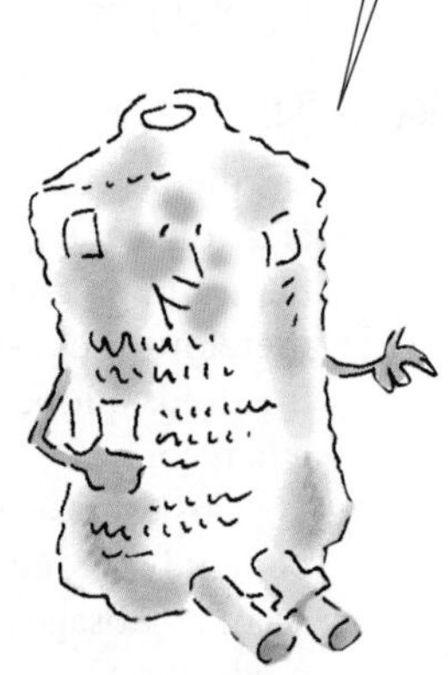

I.V. fluid replacement falls into two broad categories: crystalloids and colloids.

Isotonic solutions

Isotonic solutions have an osmolality (concentration) between 240 and 340 mOsm/kg. Dextrose 5% in water (D_5W), a commonly administered isotonic fluid, has an osmolality of 252 mOsm/kg. The dextrose metabolizes quickly, however, acting like a hypotonic solution and leaving water behind. Infusing large amounts of the solution may cause hyperglycemia.

Normal saline solution, another isotonic solution, contains only the electrolytes sodium and chloride. Other isotonic fluids are more similar to extracellular fluid. For instance, Ringer's solution contains sodium, potassium, calcium, and chloride.

Hypotonic solutions

Hypotonic solutions are fluids that have an osmolality less than 240 mOsm/kg. An example of a commonly used hypotonic solution is half-normal saline solution.

It makes a cell swell

Hypotonic solutions should be given cautiously because fluid then moves from the extracellular space into cells, causing them to swell. That fluid shift can cause cardiovascular collapse from vascular fluid

Comparing fluid tonicity

The illustrations below show the effects of different types of I.V. fluids on fluid movement and cell size.

Isotonic

Isotonic fluids, such as normal saline solution, have a concentration of dissolved particles, or tonicity, equal to that of the intracellular fluid. Osmotic pressure is therefore the same inside and outside the cells, so they neither shrink nor swell with fluid movement.

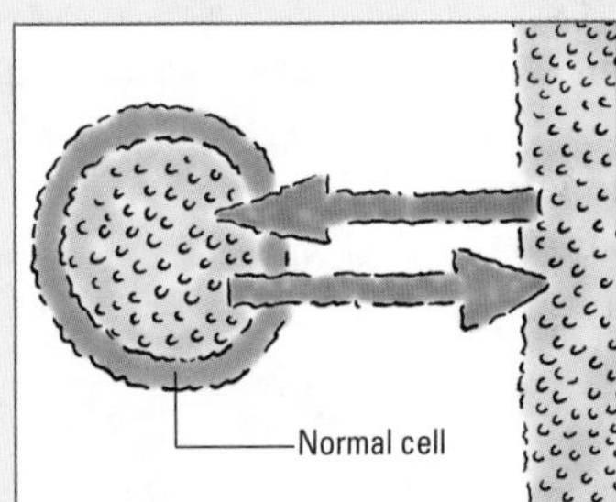

Hypertonic

Hypertonic fluid has a tonicity greater than that of intracellular fluid, so osmotic pressure is unequal inside and outside the cells. Dehydration or rapid infusion of hypertonic fluids, such as 3% saline or 50% dextrose, draws water out of the cells into the more highly concentrated extracellular fluid.

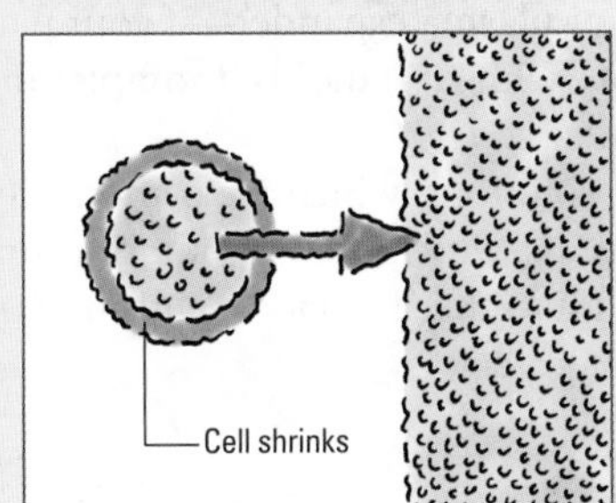

Hypotonic

Hypotonic fluids, such as half-normal saline solution, have a tonicity less than that of intracellular fluid, so osmotic pressure draws water into the cells from the extracellular fluid. Severe electrolyte losses or inappropriate use of I.V. fluids can make body fluids hypotonic.

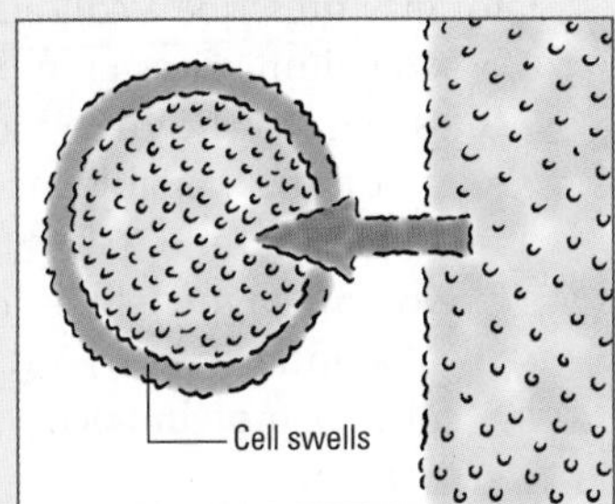

depletion. It can also cause increased intracranial pressure (ICP) from fluid shifting into brain cells.

Hypotonic solutions shouldn't be given to patients at risk for increased ICP—for example, those who have had a stroke, head trauma, or neurosurgery (Abunnaja, Cuviello, & Sanchez, 2013). Signs of increased ICP include a change in the patient's level of consciousness; motor or sensory deficits; and changes in the size, shape, or response to light in the pupils. Hypotonic solutions also shouldn't be used for patients who suffer from abnormal fluid shifts into the interstitial space or the body cavities—for example, as a result of liver disease, a burn, or trauma.

Hypertonic solutions

Hypertonic solutions are those that have an osmolality greater than 340 mOsm/kg. Examples include:

- dextrose 5% in half-normal saline solution
- 3% sodium chloride solution
- dextrose 10% in normal saline solution.

The incredible shrinking cell

A hypertonic solution draws fluids from the intracellular space, causing cells to shrink and the extracellular space to expand. Patients with cardiac or renal disease may be unable to tolerate extra fluid. Watch for fluid overload and pulmonary edema.

Because hypertonic solutions draw fluids from cells, patients at risk for cellular dehydration (patients with diabetic ketoacidosis [DKA], for example) shouldn't receive them. (See *A look at I.V. solutions*.)

Colloids

The use of colloids over crystalloids is controversial. Still, the doctor may prescribe a colloid—or plasma expander—if your patient's blood volume doesn't improve with crystalloids. Examples of colloids that may be given include:

- albumin (available in 5% solutions, which are osmotically equal to plasma, and 25% solutions, which draw about four times their volume in interstitial fluid into the circulation within 15 minutes of administration)
- plasma protein fraction
- dextran
- hetastarch.

Flowing into the stream

Colloids pull fluid into the bloodstream. The effects of colloids last several days if the lining of the capillaries is normal. The patient needs to be closely monitored during a colloid infusion for increased blood pressure, dyspnea, and bounding pulse, which are all signs of hypervolemia.

If neither crystalloids nor colloids are effective in treating the imbalance, the patient may require a blood transfusion or other treatment.

Delivery methods

The choice of I.V. delivery is based on the purpose of the therapy and its duration; the patient's diagnosis, age, and health history; and the condition of the patient's veins. I.V. solutions can be delivered through a peripheral or central vein. Catheters and tubing are chosen based on the therapy and site to be used. Here's a look at how to choose a site—peripheral or central—and which equipment you'll need for each.

A look at I.V. solutions

This chart shows examples of some commonly used I.V. fluids and includes some of their clinical uses and special considerations.

Solution	Uses	Special considerations
Isotonic		
Dextrose 5% in water	• Fluid loss and dehydration • Hypernatremia	• Solution is isotonic initially; becomes hypotonic when dextrose is metabolized. • Don't use for resuscitation; can cause hyperglycemia. • Use cautiously in renal or cardiac disease; can cause fluid overload. • Doesn't provide enough daily calories for prolonged use; may cause eventual breakdown of protein.
0.9% sodium chloride (normal saline solution)	• Shock • Hyponatremia • Blood transfusions • Resuscitation • Fluid challenges • Metabolic alkalosis • Hypercalcemia • Fluid replacement in patients with diabetic ketoacidosis (DKA)	• Because this replaces extracellular fluid, don't use in patients with heart failure, edema, or hypernatremia; can lead to overload.
Hypotonic		
0.45% sodium chloride (half-normal saline solution)	• Water replacement • DKA after initial normal saline solution and before dextrose infusion • Hypertonic dehydration • Sodium and chloride depletion • Gastric fluid loss from nasogastric suctioning or vomiting	• Use cautiously; may cause cardiovascular collapse or increased intracranial pressure. • Don't use in patients with liver disease, trauma, or burns.
Hypertonic		
Dextrose 5% in half-normal saline solution	• DKA after initial treatment with normal saline solution and half-normal saline solution—prevents hypoglycemia and cerebral edema (occurs when serum osmolality is reduced too rapidly)	• In patients with DKA, use only when glucose falls $<$ 250 mg/dl.

(continued)

A look at I.V. solutions *(continued)*

Solution	Uses	Special considerations
Dextrose 5% in normal saline solution	• Hypotonic dehydration • Temporary treatment of circulatory insufficiency and shock if plasma expanders aren't available • Syndrome of inappropriate antidiuretic hormone (or use 3% sodium chloride) • Addisonian crisis	• Don't use in patients with cardiac or renal disease because of danger of heart failure and pulmonary edema.
3% sodium chloride solution	• Severe dilutional hyponatremia • Severe sodium depletion	• Administer cautiously to prevent pulmonary edema. • Observe infusion site closely for signs of infiltration and tissues damage.
Dextrose 10% in normal saline solution	• Conditions in which some nutrition with glucose is required	• Monitor serum glucose levels. • Observe infusion site closely for signs of infiltration and damage to tissues (Kuwahara, Kaneda, Shimono, & Inoue, 2013).

Peripheral lines

Peripheral I.V. therapy is administered for short-term or intermittent therapy through a vein in the arm or hand. Potential I.V. sites include the metacarpal, cephalic, and basilic veins. In an adult, using veins in the leg or foot is unusual because of the risk of thrombophlebitis and should be avoided if at all possible. For neonatal and pediatric patients, other sites include veins of the head, neck, and lower extremities.

Give the green light to the right site

Choose a site that meets the patient's need for fluids while keeping the patient as comfortable as possible. Place I.V. catheters in the hand or lower arm so sites can be moved upward as needed. Use the patient's nondominant hand if possible. For a patient who has suffered trauma or cardiac arrest, use a large vein in the antecubital area to gain rapid access. Avoid the antecubital site in a mobile patient because the catheter may kink with movement or cause other discomfort. Avoid using veins over joints. Catheters in those veins are uncomfortable and awkward and can be displaced easily.

Avoid using veins in the feet of a child who is able to walk. Also avoid using veins in the arm of a patient who has an injury, loss of sensation, or arteriovenous fistula in the arm. Remember, don't insert an I.V. in the arm on the same side as a mastectomy with axillary node removal or on the affected side of a person who suffered a stroke. If the patient is unable to speak coherently, perform a basic head-to-toe assessment prior to starting an I.V. because the patient may have a central access such as an implanted port or peripherally inserted central catheter that can be used instead.

Pick a cath, not just any cath

Three main types of catheters are used for insertion into a peripheral vein:

- Steel-winged infusion needles are inserted easily, but infiltration is common. These catheters are small, nonflexible, and used only when access with another device proves unsuccessful. The catheters are also used for short-term therapy in adults, especially for giving medications by I.V. push (through a syringe over a short period of time).
- Indwelling catheters inserted over a steel needle are easy to use and less likely to infiltrate. Once in place, these catheters are more comfortable for the patient.
- Plastic catheters inserted through a hollow needle are longer and are more commonly used for central vein infusions. The catheter must be threaded through the vein for a greater distance, which makes these catheters more difficult to use.

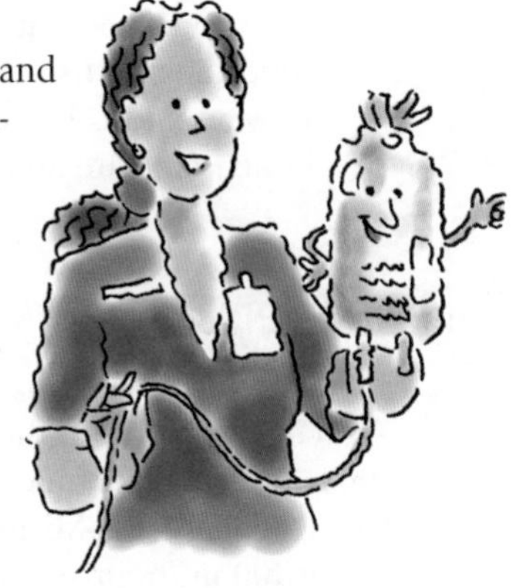
Choose an I.V. site that meets the patient's needs for fluids while keeping him as comfortable as possible.

Needle size matters

Choosing the right diameter (or gauge) needle or catheter is important for ensuring adequate flow and patient comfort. The higher the gauge, the smaller the diameter of the needle.

If you want to give a lot of fluid over a short period of time, or if you will be giving more viscous fluids (such as blood), use a catheter with a lower gauge (such as 14G, 16G, or 18G) and a shorter length, which offers less resistance to fluid flow. For routine I.V. fluid administration, use higher gauge catheters, such as a 20G or a 22G. French catheters are the exception to the needle gauge rule: The higher the number, the *greater* the diameter.

Central lines

Central venous therapy involves administering solutions through a catheter placed in a central vein, typically the subclavian or internal jugular vein, less commonly the femoral vein. Central venous therapy is used for patients who have inadequate peripheral veins, need access for blood sampling, require a large volume of fluid, need a hypertonic solution to be diluted by rapid blood flow in a larger vein, or need a high-calorie nutritional supplement (Kuwahara et al. 2013).

Pick a cath, part 2

Three main types of catheters are used for short- and long-term central venous therapy:

- The traditional central venous catheter is a multilumen catheter usually used for short-term therapy. Although the lumen size may vary, a multilumen catheter provides multiple I.V. access using one insertion site.
- A peripherally inserted central catheter is now commonly used in health care facilities and in home care. A certified nurse can insert this catheter through a vein in the antecubital area, cephalic or basilic veins, at bedside. Fewer, less severe adverse effects occur with these catheters than with traditional central venous catheters. Also, the catheters can be left in place for several months, making them ideal for long-term therapy (Seres, Valcarcel, & Guillaume, 2013).
- For extended long-term therapy, the patient may receive a vascular access port implanted in a pocket surgically constructed in the subcutaneous tissue or a tunneled catheter, such as a Hickman, Broviac, and Groshong. Some of these catheters have multiple lumens and are used in the health care facility and at home.

Tubing systems

The mechanics of infusing a solution require a tubing system that can deliver a drug at the correct infusion rate. I.V. tubing is available principally in microdrip sets, which are designed so that 60 gtt equal 1 ml. Microdrip sets are useful for infusion rates lower than 100 ml/hour—for instance, when using a solution to keep a vein open.

A macrodrip set, on the other hand, is designed so that 10 to15 gtt equal 1 ml, depending on the manufacturer. Macrodrip sets are preferred for infusion rates greater than 100 ml/hour—for instance, when treating a patient with shock.

When infusing a solution, make sure you choose the right tubing system. This is my favorite "tubing" system!

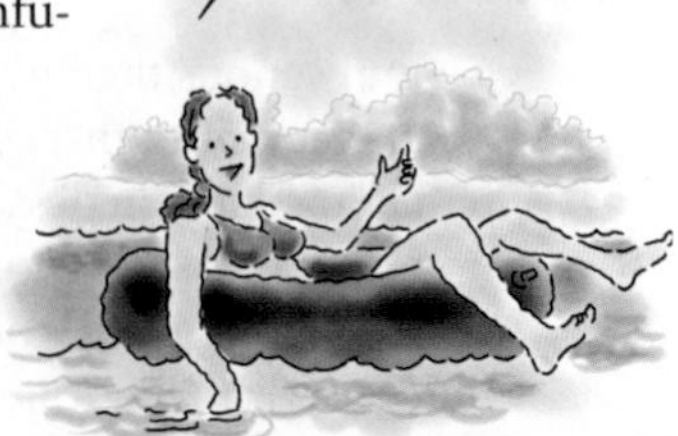

Getting pumped

Electronic infusion pumps deliver fluids at precisely controlled infusion rates. Because each machine requires its own type of tubing, check the manufacturer's directions before use.

Most tubings contain anti–free-flow protection to prevent fluid overload and back-check valves to prevent drugs from mixing inside piggyback systems (one I.V. line plugged into another at a piggyback port). Filters on some tubing eliminate particulate matter, bacteria, and air bubbles. Other types of tubing are available specifically for administering individual drugs or for piggybacking multiple drugs.

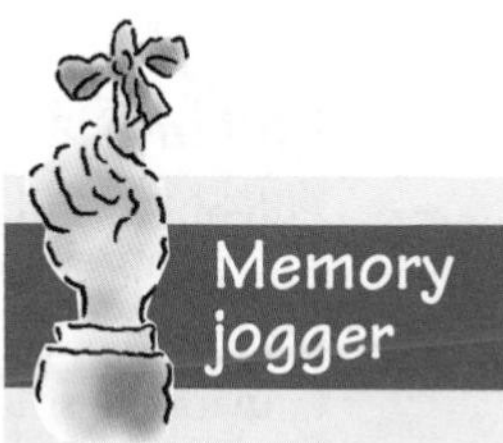

When you're trying to think of the four most common complications of I.V. therapy, remember that getting any complication is a **PITI**:

Phlebitis

Infiltration

Thrombophlebitis

Infection.

Complications of I.V. therapy

Caring for a patient with an I.V. line requires careful monitoring as well as a clear understanding of what the possible complications are, what to do if they arise, and how to deal with flow issues.

Infiltration, infection, phlebitis, and thrombophlebitis are the most common complications of I.V. therapy. Other complications include extravasation, a severed catheter, an allergic reaction, an air embolism, speed shock, and fluid overload.

Infiltration

During infiltration, fluid may leak from the vein into surrounding tissue. This occurs when the access device dislodges from the vein. Look for coolness at the site, pain, swelling, leaking, and lack of blood return. Also, look for a sluggish flow that continues even if a tourniquet is applied above the site. If you see infiltration, stop the infusion, remove the I.V. catheter, elevate the extremity, and apply warm soaks.

Go small

To prevent infiltration, use the smallest catheter that will accomplish the infusion, avoid placement in joint areas, and anchor the catheter in place.

Infection

I.V. therapy involves puncturing the skin, the body's barrier to infection. As a result, the patient may develop an infection. Look for purulent drainage at the site, tenderness, erythema, warmth, or hardness on palpation. Signs and symptoms that the infection has become systemic include fever, chills, and an elevated white blood cell count.

Infection interventions

Nursing actions for an infected I.V. site include monitoring vital signs and notifying the doctor. Swab the site for culture, and remove the catheter as ordered. To prevent infection, provide adequate dressing changes and continuous assessment of the site, and always maintain aseptic technique.

Phlebitis and thrombophlebitis

Phlebitis is inflammation of the vein; thrombophlebitis is an irritation of the vein with the formation of a clot and is usually more painful than phlebitis. Poor insertion technique or the pH or osmolality of the solution or medication can cause these complications. Look for pain, redness, swelling, or induration at the site; a red line streaking along the vein; fever; or a sluggish flow of the solution.

Fighting off phlebitis

When phlebitis or thrombophlebitis occurs, remove the I.V., monitor the patient's vital signs, notify the doctor, and apply warm soaks to the site. To prevent these complications, choose large bore veins and change the catheter every 72 hours when infusing a medication or solution with high osmolality.

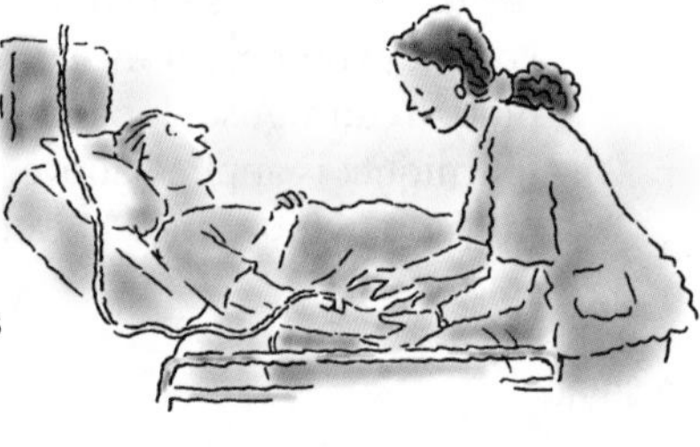
Phlebitis and thrombophlebitis can cause pain, redness, swelling, or induration at the I.V. site.

Extravasation

Similar to infiltration, extravasation is the leakage of fluid into surrounding tissues. It results when medications seep through veins and produce blistering and, eventually, necrosis. Initially, the patient may experience discomfort, burning, or pain at the site. Also look for skin tightness, blanching, and lack of blood return. Delayed reactions include inflammation and pain within 3 to 5 days and ulcers or necrosis within 2 weeks.

Eliminating extravasation

When administering medications that may extravasate, know your facility's policy. When giving caustic agents, such as chemotherapy, check for blood return frequently and stop the infusion if blood return is lost (Akbulut, 2011). Nursing actions include notifying the practitioner, infiltrating the site with an antidote as ordered, applying ice early and warm soaks later, and elevating the extremity. Assess the circulation and nerve function of the limb.

Severed catheter

A severed catheter can occur when a piece of catheter becomes dislodged and is set free in the vein. Look for pain at the fragment site; decreased blood pressure; cyanosis; loss of consciousness; and a weak, rapid pulse. If this extremely rare but serious complication occurs, apply a tourniquet above the site of pain, notify the doctor immediately, monitor the patient, and provide support as needed. To avoid the problem altogether, don't reinsert a needle through its plastic catheter once the needle has been withdrawn.

Allergic reaction

A patient may suffer an allergic reaction to the fluid, medication, I.V. catheter, or even the latex port in the I.V. tubing. However, the source of the reaction may not be known. Look for a red streak extending up the arm, rash, itching, watery eyes and nose, shortness of breath, and wheezing.

On the lookout for anaphylaxis

Left untreated, the condition may progress rapidly to anaphylaxis. Nursing measures for allergic reaction include stopping the I.V. immediately, notifying the doctor, monitoring the patient, and giving oxygen and medications as ordered.

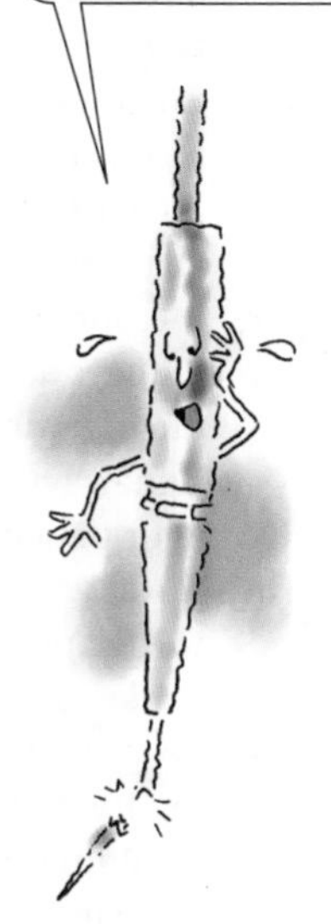
A severed catheter is an extremely rare but serious complication. It's best to avoid the problem altogether.

Air embolism

An air embolism occurs when air enters the vein and can cause a decrease in blood pressure, an increase in the pulse rate, respiratory distress, an increase in ICP, and a loss of consciousness.

When air is apparent

If the patient develops an air embolism, notify the doctor and clamp off the I.V. Place the patient on his left side, and lower his head to allow the air to enter the right atrium, where it can disperse more safely by way of the pulmonary artery. Monitor him, and administer oxygen. To avoid this serious complication, prime all tubing completely, tighten all connections securely, and use an air detection device on an I.V. pump.

Speed shock

Speed shock occurs when I.V. solutions or medications are given too rapidly. Almost immediately, the patient will have facial flushing, an irregular pulse, a severe headache, and decreased blood pressure. Loss of consciousness and cardiac arrest may also occur.

If speed shock occurs, clamp off the I.V., and notify the practitioner immediately. Provide oxygen, obtain vital signs frequently, and administer medications as ordered. Also, keep in mind that the use of infusion control devices can prevent this complication.

Fluid overload

Fluid overload can happen gradually or suddenly, depending on how well the patient's circulatory system can accommodate the fluid. Look for neck vein distention, puffy eyelids, edema, weight gain, increased blood pressure, increased respirations, shortness of breath, cough, and crackles in the lungs on auscultation.

Slow the flow

If the patient develops fluid overload, slow the I.V. rate, notify the practitioner, and monitor vital signs. Keep the patient warm, keep the head of the bed elevated, and give oxygen and other medications (such as a diuretic) as ordered.

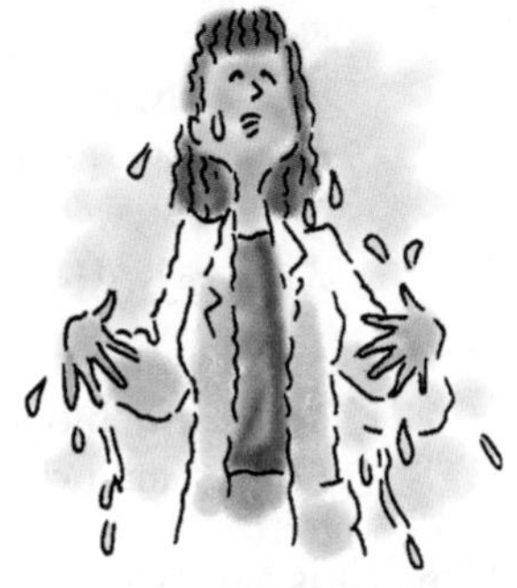
Fluid overload can happen gradually or suddenly. This one happened rather suddenly . . .

How you intervene

Nursing care for the patient with an I.V. includes the following actions:

- Check the I.V. order for completeness and accuracy. Most I.V. orders expire after 24 hours. A complete order should specify the amount and type of solution, all additives and their concentrations, and the rate and duration of the infusion. If the order is incomplete or confusing, clarify the order before proceeding.
- Monitor daily weights to document fluid retention or loss. A 2% increase or decrease in body weight is significant. A 2.2-lb (1-kg) change corresponds to 1 qt (1 L) of fluid gained or lost.
- Measure intake and output carefully at scheduled intervals. The kidneys attempt to restore fluid balance during dehydration by reducing urine production. A urine output of less than 30 ml/hour signals retention of metabolic wastes. Notify the practitioner if your patient's urine output falls below 30 ml/hour.
- Always carefully monitor the infusion of solutions that contain medication because rapid infusion and circulation of the drug can be dangerous.
- Keep in mind the size, age, and history of your patient when giving I.V. fluids to prevent fluid overload. For pediatric patients, use a volume control I.V. delivery device to limit the amount of fluid the patient receives hourly and to prevent the accidental administration of excessive amounts of fluid.
- Note the pH of the I.V. solution. The pH can alter the effect and stability of drugs mixed in the I.V. bag. Consult medication literature or the practitioner if you have questions.
- Change the site, dressing, and tubing as often as facility policy requires. Solutions should be changed at least every 24 hours. (See *Documenting an I.V. infusion*.)

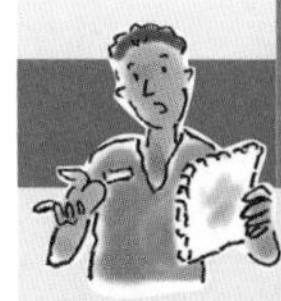

Chart smart

Documenting an I.V. infusion

If your patient has an I.V. infusion, make sure you document the following information:
- the date, time, and type of catheter inserted
- the site of insertion and its appearance
- the type and amount of fluid infused
- the patient's tolerance of, and response to, therapy
- patient and the patient's response (Altun, 2010)

- When changing I.V. tubing, don't move or dislodge the I.V. device. If you have trouble disconnecting the tubing, use a hemostat to hold the I.V. hub while twisting the tubing. Don't clamp the hemostat shut because doing so may crack the hub.
- Always report needlestick injuries. Exposure to a patient's blood increases the risk of infection with bloodborne viruses such as HIV, hepatitis B virus, hepatitis C virus, and cytomegalovirus. About 1 out of 300 people with occupational needlestick injuries become HIV-seropositive.

Catching clues

- Always listen to your patient carefully. Subtle statements such as "I just don't feel right" may be your clue to the beginning of an allergic reaction.
- Keep in mind that a candidate for home I.V. therapy must have a family member or friend who can safely and competently administer the I.V. fluids as well as a backup person; a suitable home environment; a telephone; available transportation; adequate reading skills; and the ability to prepare, handle, store, and dispose of equipment properly. Procedures for caring for the I.V. are the same at home as in a health care facility, except at home, the patient uses clean technique instead of sterile technique. (See *Teaching about I.V. therapy*.)

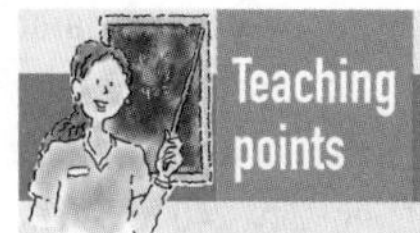

Teaching points

Teaching about I.V. therapy

When teaching a patient who is receiving I.V. therapy, be sure to cover the following topics and then evaluate your patient's learning:
- expectations before, during, and after the I.V. procedure
- signs and symptoms of complications and when to report them
- activity or diet restrictions
- care for an I.V. line at home.

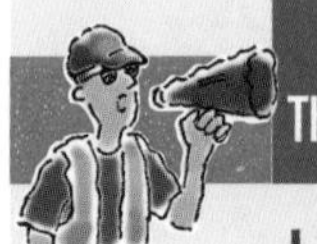

That's a wrap!

I.V. fluid replacement review

Types of I.V. solutions

- Broadly classified as crystalloids or colloids

Crystalloids

- Solutions with small molecules that flow easily from the bloodstream into cells and tissues
- May be isotonic, hypotonic, or hypertonic

Isotonic solutions

- Contain about the same concentration of osmotically active particles as extracellular fluid, so fluid doesn't shift between extracellular and intracellular spaces
- Osmolality: 240 to 340 mOsm/kg
- Example: D_5W, normal saline solution, and dextrose 5% in normal saline solution

Hypotonic solutions

- Are less concentrated than extracellular fluid, which allows movement from the bloodstream into the cells, causing cells to expand
- Osmolality: less than 240 mOsm/kg
- Example: half-normal saline solution
- Can cause cardiovascular collapse from vascular fluid depletion or increased ICP from fluid shifting into brain cells
- Avoid using in patients at risk for increased ICP, such as those who have had a stroke, head trauma, or neurosurgery (Abunnaja et al., 2013).
- Also, avoid using in patients who suffer from abnormal fluid shifts into the interstitial space or body cavities, such as in liver disease, burns, or trauma

Hypertonic solutions

- Are more concentrated than extracellular fluid, which allows movement of fluid from cells into the bloodstream, causing cells to shrink
- Osmolality greater than 340 mOsm/kg
- Examples include dextrose 5% in half-normal saline solution, 3% sodium chloride solution, and dextrose 10% in normal saline solution
- May not be tolerated by those with cardiac or renal disease
- May cause fluid overload and pulmonary edema
- Should not be used in patients at risk for cellular dehydration, such as those with DKA

Colloids

- Act as plasma expanders
- Are always hypertonic, pulling fluid from cells into the bloodstream
- Examples: albumin, plasma protein fraction, dextran, and hetastarch
- Require close monitoring for signs and symptoms of hypervolemia, such as increased blood pressure, dyspnea, and bounding pulse

Delivery methods

- Methods include peripheral and central I.V. therapy
- Choice based on purpose and duration of therapy; patient's diagnosis, age, and health history; condition of the veins
- Catheters and tubings are selected according to type of therapy and site used

(continued)

I.V. fluid replacement review *(continued)*

Complications of I.V. therapy

- Infiltration: leakage of fluid from vein into surrounding tissue when access device dislodges from the vein
- Infection: may occur at the insertion site; requires monitoring for purulent drainage, tenderness, erythema, warmth, or hardness at the site
- Phlebitis: inflammation of the vein
- Thrombophlebitis: irritation of the vein with clot formation
- Extravasation: leakage of fluid into surrounding tissues; results when medications seep through veins, producing blistering and eventually necrosis
- Severed catheter: dislodgment of a piece of catheter into the vein (rare)
- Allergic reaction: may result from I.V. fluid, medication, catheter, or latex port in the I.V. tubing
- Air embolism: entry of air into a vein; results in decreased blood pressure, increased pulse, respiratory distress, increased ICP, and loss of consciousness
- Speed shock: too rapid infusion of I.V. solutions or medications; results in facial flushing, irregular pulse, decreased blood pressure, and possibly loss of consciousness and cardiac arrest
- Fluid overload: gradual or sudden occurrence; produces neck vein distention, increased blood pressure, puffy eyelids, edema, weight gain, and respiratory symptoms

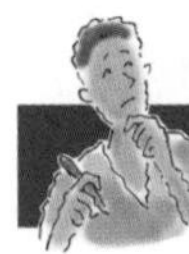

Quick quiz

1. Hypertonic solutions cause fluids to move from the:
   A. interstitial space to the intracellular space.
   B. intracellular space to the extracellular space.
   C. extracellular space to the intracellular space.
   D. intracellular space to the interstitial space.

Answer: B. Hypertonic solutions, because of their increased osmolality, draw fluids out of the cells and into the extracellular space.

2. Hypotonic fluids shouldn't be used for a patient with:
   A. increased ICP.
   B. DKA whose blood glucose level is 200 mg/dl or more.
   C. blood loss as a result of trauma.
   D. water replacement.

Answer: A. Hypotonic fluids cause swelling of the cells and can further increase ICP.

3. Which of the following is a sign of an allergy to I.V. tubing?
   A. Shortness of breath
   B. Dry throat
   C. Slow, bounding pulse
   D. Hypertension

Answer: A. Signs and symptoms of an allergic reaction include shortness of breath, rash, and itching.

4. Your patient is a 90-year-old male with a history of heart failure. When you make rounds, you notice that an I.V. of normal saline solution was mistakenly given an hour before and has infused 600 ml since then. You should observe this patient for signs of:
   A. septic shock.
   B. decreased ICP.
   C. circulatory overload.
   D. increased ICP.

Answer: C. Because of his advanced age and cardiac condition, the type of fluid infused, and the infusion rate, the patient is at risk for circulatory overload.

5. When a hypotonic crystalloid solution is infused into the bloodstream, it causes the cells to:
   A. shrink.
   B. swell.
   C. release chloride.
   D. release potassium.

Answer: B. Hypotonic crystalloids are less concentrated than extracellular fluids, so they move from the bloodstream into the cell and cause the cell to expand with fluid.

6. Hypertonic solutions should be used cautiously in patients with:
   A. cancer or burns.
   B. cardiac or renal disease.
   C. respiratory or GI disease.
   D. hepatic or renal disease.

Answer: B. A hypertonic solution draws fluids from the intracellular space into the bloodstream. Patients with cardiac or renal disease may be unable to tolerate that extra fluid volume.

Scoring

☆☆☆ If you answered all six questions correctly, bravo! You've absorbed the information well.

☆☆ If you answered four or five questions correctly, excellent! You infusion hot shot, you!

☆ If you answered fewer than four questions correctly, no biggie. With a little more I.V. training, you'll be inserting 18 gaugers in no time!

References

Abunnaja, S., Cuviello, A., & Sanchez, J. (2013). Enteral and nutrition in the perioperative period: State of the art. *Nutrients, 5*(2), 608–623. doi:10.3390/nu5020608

Akbulut, G. (2011). New perspective for nutritional support of cancer patients: Enteral/parenteral nutrition. *Experimental and Therapeutic Medicine, 2*(4), 675–684. doi:10.3892/etm.2011.426

Altun, I. (2010). The efficacy of workshop on body fluids in health and disease and its impact on nurses training. *Pakistan Journal of Medical Sciences, 26*(2), 426–429.

Crawford, A., & Harris, H. (2013). IV fluids: What nurses need to know. *Nursing 2013, 41*(5), 30–38.

Earhart, A., & McMahon, P. (2011). Vascular access and contrast media. *Journal of Infusion Nursing, 34*(2), 97–105.

Gonzales, E. (2008). Fluid resuscitation in the trauma patient. *Journal of Trauma Nursing, 15*(3), 149–157.

Infusion Nurses Society. (2011). Infusion nursing standards of practice. *Journal of Infusion Nursing, 34*(1S), S1–S110.

Kuwahara, T., Kaneda, S., Shimono, K., & Inoue, Y. (2013). Effects of lipid emulsion and multivitamins on the growth of microorganisms in peripheral parenteral nutrition solutions. *International Journal of Medical Sciences, 10*(9), 1079–1084. doi:10.7150/ijms.6407

Lancaster, S., Owens, A. Bryant, A., Ramey, L., Nicholson, J., Gossett, K., . . . Padgett, T. (2010). Emergency: Upper extremity deep vein thrombosis. *American Journal of Nursing, 110*(5), 48–52.

Perlow, M. (2013). Perfusion, hypoperfusion, and ischemia processes: The effect on bodily function. *Journal of Infusion Nursing, 36*(5), 336–340.

Rosenthal, K. (2013). Intravenous fluids: The whys and wherefores. *Nursing, 36*(7), 26–27.

Seres, D., Valcarcel, M., & Guillaume, A. (2013). Advantages of enteral nutrition over parenteral nutrition. *Therapeutic Advances in Gastroenterology, 6*(2), 157–167. doi:10.1177/1756283X12467564

Simmons, S. (2013). Taking the sting out of anaphylaxis. *Nursing Critical Care, 5*(3), 10–16.

Singh, A., Carlin, B., Shade, D., & Kaplan, P. (2009). The use of hypertonic saline for fluid resuscitation in sepsis: A review. *Critical Care Nursing Quarterly, 32*(1), 10–13.

Chapter 20

Total parenteral nutrition

Just the facts

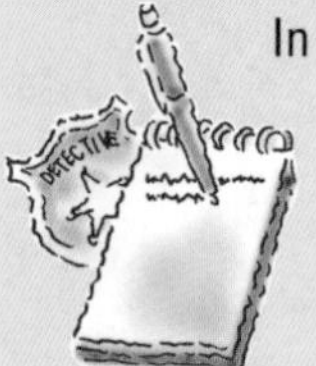

In this chapter, you'll learn:

- ways to identify patients who could benefit from total parenteral nutrition (TPN)
- the types of TPN components and their delivery methods
- complications associated with TPN
- appropriate care for patients receiving TPN.

A look at TPN

TPN is a highly concentrated, hypertonic nutrient solution administered by way of an infusion pump through a large central vein. For patients with high caloric and nutritional needs due to illness or injury, TPN provides crucial calories; restores nitrogen balance; and replaces essential fluids, vitamins, electrolytes, minerals, and trace elements (Mofidi & Kronn, 2009). (See *Understanding common TPN additives*.)

TPN also promotes tissue and wound healing and normal metabolic function; gives the bowel a chance to heal; reduces activity in the gallbladder, pancreas, and small intestine; and is used to improve a patient's response to surgery.

Who needs TPN?

Patients who can't meet their nutritional needs by oral or enteral feedings may require I.V. nutritional supplementation or TPN. Generally, this treatment is prescribed for any patient who can't absorb nutrients from the gastrointestinal (GI) tract for more than 10 days. More specific indications include:

- debilitating illnesses lasting longer than 2 weeks
- loss of 10% or more of preillness weight

Understanding common TPN additives

Common components of TPN solutions—such as glucose, amino acids, and other additives—are used for specific purposes. For instance, glucose provides calories for metabolism. Here's a list of other common additives and the purposes each serves.

Electrolytes

- *Calcium* promotes development and maintenance of bones and teeth and aids in blood clotting.
- *Chloride* regulates acid-base balance and maintains osmotic pressure.
- *Magnesium* helps the body absorb carbohydrates and protein.
- *Phosphorus* is essential for cell energy and calcium balance.
- *Potassium* is needed for cellular activity and cardiac function.
- *Sodium* helps control water distribution and maintains normal fluid balance.

Vitamins

- *Folic acid* is needed for DNA formation and promotes growth and development.
- *Vitamin B complex* helps the final absorption of carbohydrates and protein.
- *Vitamin C* helps in wound healing.
- *Vitamin D* is essential for bone metabolism and maintenance of serum calcium levels.
- *Vitamin K* helps prevent bleeding disorders.

Other additives

- *Micronutrients* (such as zinc, copper, chromium, selenium, and manganese) help in wound healing and red blood cell synthesis.
- *Amino acids* provide the proteins necessary for tissue repair and immune functions.
- *Lipids* support hormone and prostaglandin synthesis and prevent essential fatty acid deficiency.

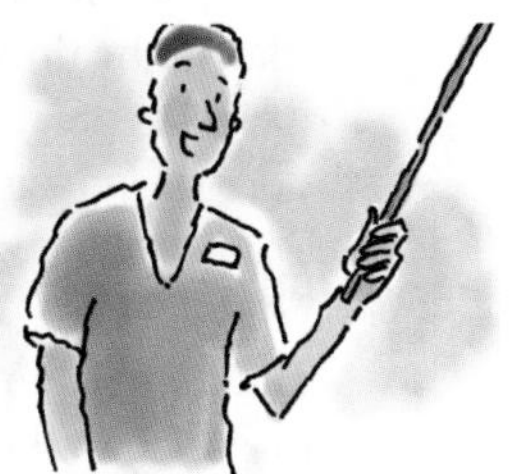

Study this list of common additives and learn the purpose each serves.

- serum albumin level below 3.5 g/dl
- excessive nitrogen loss from a wound infection, a fistula, or an abscess
- renal or hepatic failure
- nonfunction of the GI tract lasting for 5 to 7 days (American Society of Parenteral and Enteral Nutrition, 2014). (See *Key facts about PPN*, see page 354.)

TPN triggers

Common illnesses or treatments that can trigger the need for TPN include inflammatory bowel disease, ulcerative colitis, bowel obstruction or resection, radiation enteritis, severe diarrhea or vomiting, AIDS, chemotherapy, and severe pancreatitis, all of which hinder a patient's ability to absorb nutrients. Also, patients may benefit from TPN if they've undergone major surgery or if they have a high metabolic rate resulting from sepsis, trauma, or burns of more than 40% of total body surface area. Infants with congenital or acquired disorders may need TPN to promote proper growth and development.

TPN has limited value for well-nourished patients with GI tracts that are healthy or are likely to resume normal function within 10 days. The treatment also may be inappropriate for a patient with a poor prognosis or when the risks of TPN outweigh its benefits.

Key facts about PPN

Peripheral parenteral nutrition (PPN) is prescribed for patients who have a malfunctioning GI tract and need short-term nutrition lasting less than 2 weeks. It may be used to provide partial or total nutritional support. PPN is infused peripherally in various combinations of lipid (fat) emulsions and amino acid–dextrose solutions. To ensure adequate nutrition, PPN solutions in final concentrations of less than or equal to 10% dextrose and less than or equal to 5% protein shouldn't be administered for longer than 10 days unless they're supplemented with oral or enteral feedings.

Today's TPN trends

The trend of today's nutritional supplementation is to tailor TPN formulas to the patient's specific needs. As a result, standard TPN mixtures are becoming less popular. Nutritional support teams consisting of nurses, doctors, pharmacists, and dietitians assess, prescribe for, and monitor patients receiving TPN. The solutions may consist of:

- protein (essential and nonessential amino acids), with varying types available for patients with renal or liver failure
- dextrose (10% to 35% concentration)
- fat emulsions (20% to 30% solution)
- electrolytes
- vitamins
- trace element mixtures.

Lipid emulsions

Lipid emulsions are thick emulsions that supply patients with both essential fatty acids and calories. These emulsions assist in wound healing, red blood cell (RBC) production, and prostaglandin synthesis. They may be piggybacked with TPN, given alone through a separate peripheral or central venous line, or mixed with amino acids and dextrose in one container (total nutrient admixtures) and infused over 24 hours.

The limits on lipids

Lipid emulsions should be given cautiously to patients with hepatic or pulmonary disease, acute pancreatitis, anemia, or a coagulation disorder and to patients at risk for developing a fat embolism. These emulsions shouldn't be given to patients who have conditions that disrupt normal fat metabolism, such as pathologic hyperlipidemia, or lipid nephrosis.

Also, make sure you report any adverse reactions to the practitioner so the TPN regimen can be changed as needed. (See *Adverse reactions to lipid emulsions*.)

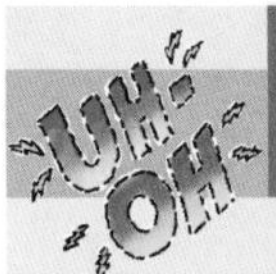

CAUTION!

Adverse reactions to lipid emulsions

Lipid emulsions can cause immediate adverse reactions as well as delayed complications.

Immediate or early adverse reactions to lipid emulsions

- Back and chest pain
- Cyanosis
- Diaphoresis or flushing
- Dyspnea
- Headache
- Hypercoagulability
- Irritation at the site
- Lethargy or syncope
- Nausea or vomiting
- Slight pressure over the eyes
- Thrombocytopenia

Delayed complications associated with prolonged administration

- Blood dyscrasias
- Fatty liver syndrome
- Hepatomegaly
- Jaundice
- Splenomegaly

How to infuse TPN

TPN must be infused through a central vein. As a hypertonic solution, it may be up to six times the concentration of blood and, therefore, too irritating for a peripheral vein.

TPN may be infused around the clock or for part of the day—for instance, as the patient sleeps at night. A sterile catheter made of polyurethane or silicone is inserted into the subclavian or jugular vein. A polyurethane catheter is rigid during insertion but softens at body temperature. It's biocompatible, so tissues don't react to the material and it's less thrombogenic than earlier types of manufactured catheters. A Silastic catheter may be a better alternative for therapy lasting months or years because it's more flexible and durable and it's compatible with many medications and solutions.

Looking to the peripheral

A peripherally inserted central catheter, a variation of central venous therapy, can be used for therapy lasting 3 months or more. The catheter is inserted through the basilic or cephalic vein and threaded so that the tip lies in the superior vena cava.

The patient generally experiences less discomfort with a peripheral catheter, especially if he can move around easily. Movement stimulates blood flow and decreases the risk of phlebitis. Peripherally inserted central catheters are often used for intermediate-term therapy, both at home and in the health care facility.

What to look for

Signs and symptoms of electrolyte imbalances caused by TPN administration include abdominal cramps, lethargy, confusion, malaise, muscle weakness, tetany, convulsions, and cardiac arrhythmias. Acid-base imbalances can also occur as a result of the patient's condition or the TPN content. Look for these other complications:

- heart failure or pulmonary edema from fluid and electrolyte administration, conditions that can lead to tachycardia, lethargy, confusion, weakness, and labored breathing
- hyperglycemia from dextrose infusing too quickly, a condition that may require an adjustment in the patient's insulin dosage
- adverse reactions to medications added to TPN—for example, added insulin can cause hypoglycemia, which can result in confusion, restlessness, lethargy, pallor, and tachycardia
- catheter-related infections and catheter occlusion.

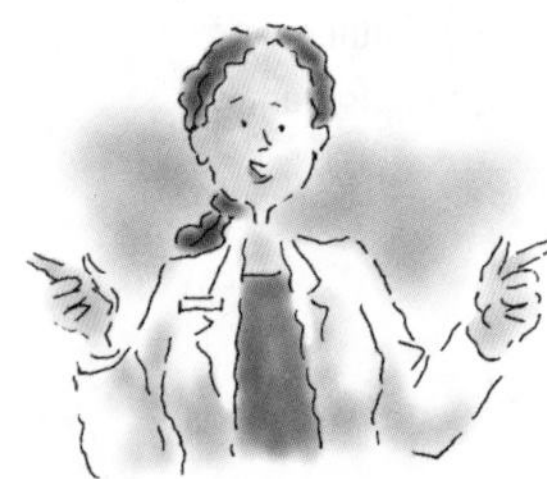
Constant assessment and rapid intervention are critical for patients receiving TPN.

How you intervene

Constant assessment and rapid intervention are critical for patients receiving TPN. When caring for a patient receiving TPN, you'll want to take these actions:

- Carefully monitor patients receiving TPN to detect early signs of complications, such as infection, metabolic problems, heart failure, pulmonary edema, or allergic reactions. Adjust the TPN regimen as needed. (See *Teaching about TPN*.)
- Assess the patient's nutritional status, and weigh the patient at the same time each morning in similar clothing, after he voids, and on the same scale. Weight indicates nutritional progress and also determines fluid overload. Patients ideally should gain 1 to 2 lb (0.5 to 1 kg)/week. Weight gain greater than 1 lb (0.5 kg)/day indicates fluid retention.
- Assess the patient for peripheral and pulmonary edema. Edema is a sign of fluid overload.

The sugar situation

- Monitor serum glucose levels every 6 hours initially, then once a day. Watch for thirst and polyuria, which are indications that the patient may have hyperglycemia. Periodically, confirm glucometer readings with laboratory test results. Serum glucose levels should be less than 200 mg/dl. This indicates the patient's tolerance of the glucose solution.
- Monitor for signs and symptoms of glucose metabolism disturbance, fluid and electrolyte imbalances, and nutritional problems. Some patients may require insulin added directly to the TPN for the duration of treatment.
- Monitor electrolyte levels daily at first and then twice a week. Keep in mind that when a patient is severely malnourished, starting TPN may spark refeeding syndrome, which includes a rapid drop in potassium, magnesium, and phosphorus levels. To avoid compromising cardiac function, initiate feeding slowly and monitor the patient's electrolyte levels closely until they stabilize.
- Monitor protein levels twice a week. Albumin levels may drop initially as treatment restores hydration.
- Check renal function by monitoring blood urea nitrogen (BUN) and creatinine levels; increases may indicate excess amino acid intake.
- Assess nitrogen balance with 24-hour urine collection.
- Assess liver function with liver function tests, bilirubin, triglyceride, and cholesterol levels. Abnormal values may indicate intolerance.
- Review the patient's serum chemistry and nutritional studies, and alert the practitioner of abnormal results, which may indicate that the TPN fluid concentration or ingredients may need to be adjusted to meet the patient's specific needs.

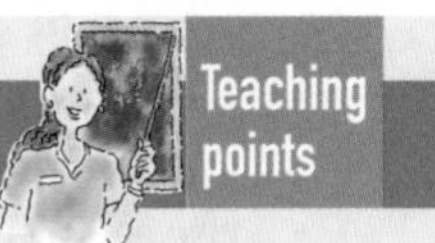

Teaching about TPN

When teaching a patient about TPN, be sure to cover the following topics and then evaluate your patient's learning:

- basics of TPN and its specific use
- adverse reactions or catheter complications and when to report them
- basic care of a TPN line
- maintenance of equipment
- weight, calorie count, intake and output, and glucose level monitoring.

- Avoid an adverse reaction by starting TPN slowly—usually 60 to 80 ml/hour for the first 24 hours—and increasing gradually. Continually monitor the patient's cardiac and respiratory status.
- Use an infusion pump for rate control.

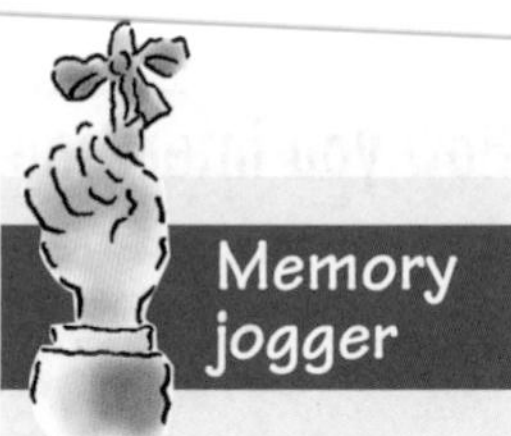

To remember how to avoid the complication of refeeding syndrome when giving TPN to a severely malnourished patient, think "Start low and go slow."

TPN technique

- Use a 1.2-micron filter when administering TPN containing an I.V. fat emulsion (IVFE). Use a 0.2-micron filter when administering a TPN solution that doesn't contain an IVFE.
- Remove the TPN solution from the refrigerator 1 hour before administering it so that it can warm to room temperature.
- Examine the TPN solution before administration. It should be clear or pale yellow if multivitamins are added to the solution. If you see particulate matter, cloudiness, or an oily layer in the bag when preparing to hang a TPN solution, return the bag to the pharmacy.
- Flush central lines according to protocol.
- If using a single-lumen central venous line, *don't* use the line for blood or blood products or to give a bolus injection, administer simultaneous I.V. solutions, measure the central venous pressure, or draw blood for laboratory tests.
- Never add medications to a TPN solution container once it's actively infusing.
- Don't use add-on devices such as a three-way stopcock unless absolutely necessary; they increase the risk of infection.
- Infuse or discard any TPN solution within 24 hours once the administration set is attached. If the next TPN infusion is not available when the infusion is completed, provide 10% dextrose solution until the next TPN infusion is available.
- Perform site care and dressing changes at least three times a week (once a week for transparent semipermeable dressings), or whenever the dressing becomes wet, soiled, or nonocclusive. Use strict aseptic technique.
- Monitor the patient for signs of inflammation and infection, and document anything you find. TPN provides the perfect medium for microbial growth (both local and systemic).
- Change the I.V. administration set according to facility policy, and always use aseptic technique. Changes of I.V. administration sets are usually done every 24 to 72 hours, depending on the type of solution.

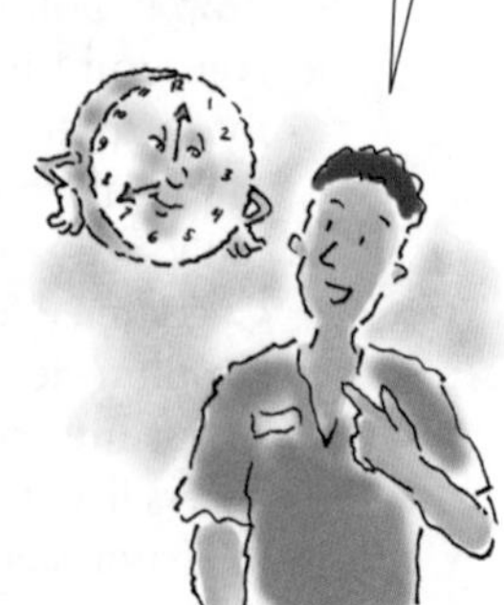

Don't allow TPN solutions to hang for more than 24 hours.

Timing out the TPN

- Record vital signs at least every 4 hours. Temperature elevation is one of the earliest signs of catheter-related sepsis.
- Provide emotional support, especially if eating is restricted because of the patient's condition.
- Provide frequent mouth care.
- While weaning the patient from TPN, document his dietary intake and total calorie and protein intake. Use percentages when

recording food intake. For instance, chart that, "The patient ate 50% of a baked potato," rather than "The patient had a good appetite."

- When discontinuing TPN, decrease the infusion slowly, depending on current glucose intake. Slowly decreasing the infusion minimizes the risk of hyperinsulinemia and resulting hypoglycemia. Weaning usually takes place over 24 to 48 hours but can be completed in 4 to 6 hours if the patient receives sufficient oral or I.V. carbohydrates.
- Promptly report any adverse reactions to the practitioner.
- Prepare your patient for home care.
- Accurately document all aspects of care, according to facility policy. (See *Documenting TPN*.)

Chart smart

Documenting TPN

If your patient is receiving TPN, make sure you document the following information:

- adverse reactions or catheter complications
- signs of inflammation or infection at the I.V. site
- nursing interventions (including infusion rate) and the patient's response
- time and date of administration set changes
- specific dietary intake
- patient teaching

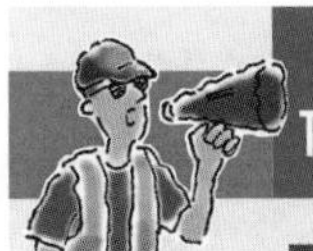

That's a wrap!

Total parenteral nutrition review

Total parenteral nutrition

- Highly concentrated, hypertonic nutrient solution used for patients with high caloric and nutritional needs due to illness or injury
- Provides crucial calories; restores nitrogen balance; and replaces essential fluids, vitamins, electrolytes, minerals, and trace elements
- Promotes tissue and wound healing and normal metabolic function; gives the bowel a chance to heal; reduces activity in the gallbladder, pancreas, and small intestine; and improves a patient's response to surgery
- Used in patients who can't meet their nutritional needs by oral or enteral feedings, including those with inflammatory bowel disease, ulcerative colitis, bowel obstruction or resection, radiation enteritis, severe diarrhea or vomiting, AIDS, chemotherapy, and severe pancreatitis
- Typically has limited value in well-nourished patients with GI tracts that are healthy or are likely to resume normal function within 10 days
- Must be infused through a central vein

Common TPN additives

Electrolytes

- Calcium: promotes development and maintenance of bones and teeth and aids in blood clotting
- Chloride: regulates acid-base balance and maintains osmotic pressure
- Magnesium: helps the body absorb carbohydrates and protein
- Phosphorus: essential for cell energy and calcium balance
- Sodium: helps control water distribution and maintains normal fluid balance (National Institutes of Health, 2014)

Vitamins

- Folic acid: helps with DNA formation and promotes growth and development
- Vitamin B complex: helps the final absorption of carbohydrates and protein

(continued)

Total parenteral nutrition review *(continued)*

- Vitamin C: helps in wound healing
- Vitamin D: essential for bone metabolism and maintenance of serum calcium levels
- Vitamin K: helps prevent bleeding disorders (National Institutes of Health, 2014)

Other additives

- Micronutrients (zinc, copper, chromium, selenium, manganese): help in wound healing and RBC synthesis
- Amino acids: provide the proteins necessary for tissue repair and immune functions
- Lipids: support hormone and prostaglandin synthesis; prevent essential fatty acid deficiency (National Institutes of Health, 2014)

Lipid emulsions

- Thick preparations that supply patients with essential fatty acids and calories
- Assist in wound healing, RBC production, and prostaglandin synthesis
- May be piggybacked with TPN
- Should be used cautiously in patients with hepatic or pulmonary disease, acute pancreatitis, anemia, or a coagulation disorder and in patients at risk for developing a fat embolism
- Should be avoided in patients with pathologic hyperlipidemia or lipid nephrosis (National Institutes of Health, 2014)

TPN complications

- Electrolyte imbalances
- Acid-base imbalances
- Heart failure or pulmonary edema
- Hyperglycemia
- Rebound hypoglycemia
- Refeeding syndrome (in severely malnourished patients), which includes a rapid drop in potassium, magnesium, and phosphorus levels

Monitoring

- Assess nutritional status and daily weight.
- Assess for edema, a sign of fluid overload.
- Monitor serum glucose level every 6 hours initially, then once daily.
- Monitor electrolyte levels daily at first, then twice weekly.
- Monitor protein levels twice weekly.
- Monitor BUN and creatinine levels, liver function tests, and nitrogen balance.

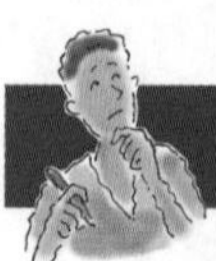

Quick quiz

1. When a severely malnourished patient starts receiving TPN, his laboratory tests show a rapid drop in potassium, magnesium, and phosphorus levels. The findings indicate which of the following conditions?

   A. Fluid shock
   B. Hypervolemia
   C. Hypovolemia
   D. Refeeding syndrome

Answer: D. These findings are signs of refeeding syndrome.

2. When preparing to hang a TPN solution, you see an oily layer in the bag. You should:

A. gently agitate the solution to disperse the contents.
B. hang the solution; the oily layer will disperse in time.
C. return the solution to the pharmacy.
D. squeeze the bag to mix the solution.

Answer: C. The solution should be clear or pale yellow. An oily layer indicates that the fluid may have been contaminated or improperly prepared and it should be returned to the pharmacy.

3. Site care and dressing changes for a patient with TPN should be performed at least:

A. once a week.
B. every other week.
C. every day.
D. three times a week.

Answer: D. It's recommended that site care and dressing changes be performed three times a week; however, the patient's condition or facility policy may dictate the need for more frequent care.

4. Infusions of lipid emulsions are useful for promoting:

A. wound healing.
B. coagulation in bleeding disorders.
C. a reduction in inflammation from pancreatitis.
D. decreased hemoglobin level and hematocrit in anemia.

Answer: A. Lipid emulsions assist in wound healing, in the production of RBCs, and in prostaglandin synthesis. They should be avoided in patients with acute pancreatitis or a coagulation disorder and used cautiously in patients with acute pancreatitis.

Scoring

☆☆☆ If you answered all four questions correctly, totally cool! Your daily nutritional intake must include plenty of brain food!

☆☆ If you answered three questions correctly, you should still be pumped up! Your TPN knowledge is top 10!

☆ If you answered fewer than three questions correctly, let me give you some "parenteral" advice: Get your energy up and review the chapter!

References

American Society of Parenteral and Enteral Nutrition. (2014). *What is parenteral nutrition?* Retrieved from http://www.nutritioncare.org/wcontent.aspx?id=270

Mofidi, S., & Kronn, D. (2009). Emergency management of inherited metabolic disorders. *Topics in Clinical Nutrition, 24*(4), 374–384.

National Institutes of Health. (2014). *Total parenteral nutrition.* Retrieved from http://www.nlm.nih.gov/medlineplus/druginfo/meds/a601166.html

Appendices and index

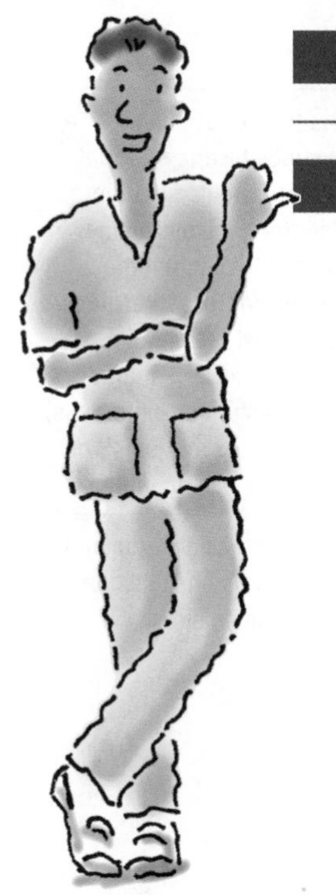

Common fluid and electrolyte imbalances in pediatric patients

Imbalance	Causes	Signs and symptoms	Treatment
Hypovolemia (fluid volume deficit)	Dehydration, vomiting, diarrhea, decreased oral intake, and excessive fluid loss	Thirst, oliguria or anuria, dry mucous membranes, weight loss, sunken eyes, decreased tears, depressed fontanels (in infants), tachycardia, and altered level of consciousness	Oral rehydration (in mild to moderate dehydration), I.V. fluid administration (in severe dehydration), or electrolyte replacement
Hypernatremia (serum sodium > 145 mEq/L [> 145 mmol/L])	Water loss in excess of sodium loss, diabetes insipidus (insufficient antidiuretic hormone [ADH] production or reduced response to ADH), insufficient water intake, diarrhea, vomiting, fever, renal disease, and hyperglycemia	Decreased skin turgor; tachycardia; flushed skin; intense thirst; dry, sticky mucous membranes; hoarseness; nausea; vomiting; decreased blood pressure; confusion; and seizures	Gradual replacement of water (in excess of sodium) or ADH replacement or vasopressin administration (for patients with diabetes insipidus)
Hyponatremia (serum sodium < 136 mEq/L [< 136 mmol/L])	Syndrome of inappropriate antidiuretic hormone (SIADH), edema (from cardiac failure), hypotonic fluid replacement (for diarrhea), cystic fibrosis, malnutrition, fever, and excess sweating	Dehydration, dizziness, nausea, abdominal cramps, and apprehension	Sodium replacement, water restriction, diuretic administration, or fluid replacement (with ongoing fluid loss, such as with diarrhea)
Hyperkalemia (serum potassium > 4.7 mEq/L [> 4.7 mmol/L])	Acute acidosis, hemolysis or rhabdomyolysis, renal failure, administration of large volume of packed red blood cells or older units of blood, excessive administration of I.V. potassium supplement, and Addison's disease	Arrhythmias; weakness; paresthesia; electrocardiogram (ECG) changes (tall, tented T waves; ST segment depression; prolonged PR interval and QRS complex; and absent P waves); nausea; vomiting; hoarseness; flushed skin; intense thirst; and dry, sticky mucous membranes	Dialysis (for renal failure), sodium polystyrene sulfonate (Kayexalate) (to remove potassium via the gastrointestinal [GI] tract), I.V. calcium gluconate (antagonizes cardiac abnormalities), I.V. insulin with hypertonic dextrose solution (shifts potassium into the cells), bicarbonate (for acidosis), or restricted potassium intake
Hypokalemia (serum potassium < 3.4 mEq/L [< 3.4 mmol/L])	Vomiting, diarrhea, nasogastric suctioning, diuretic use, acute alkalosis, kidney disease, starvation, and malabsorption	Fatigue, muscle weakness, muscle cramping, paralysis, hyporeflexia, hypotension, tachycardia or bradycardia, apathy, drowsiness, irritability, decreased bowel motility, and ECG changes (flattened or inverted T waves, presence of U waves, and ST segment depression)	Oral or I.V. potassium administration (I.V. infusions must be diluted and given slowly)

Common fluid and electrolyte imbalances in elderly patients

Imbalance	Causes	Signs and symptoms	Treatment
Hypervolemia (fluid volume excess)	Renal failure, heart failure, cirrhosis, increased oral or I.V. sodium intake, mental confusion, seizures, and coma	Edema, weight gain, jugular vein distention, crackles, shortness of breath, bounding pulse, elevated blood pressure, and increased central venous pressure	Diuretics, fluid restriction (< 1 qt [1 L]/day), sodium restriction, or hemodialysis (for patients with renal failure)
Hypovolemia (fluid volume deficit)	Dehydration; vomiting; diarrhea; fever; polyuria; chronic kidney disease; diabetes mellitus; diuretic use; hot weather; and decreased oral intake secondary to anorexia, nausea, diminished thirst mechanism, or inadequate water intake (common in nursing home patients)	Dry mucous membranes; oliguria or concentrated urine; anuria; orthostatic hypotension; dizziness; weakness; confusion or altered mental status; and possible severe hypotension, increased hemoglobin, hematocrit, blood urea nitrogen, and serum creatinine levels	Fluid administration (may be oral or I.V., depending on degree of deficit and patient's response; a urine output of 30 to 50 ml/hour usually signals adequate renal perfusion)
Hypernatremia (serum sodium > 145 mEq/L [> 145 mmol/L])	Water deprivation, hypertonic tube feedings without adequate water replacement, diarrhea, and low body weight	Dry mucous membranes, restlessness, irritability, weakness, lethargy, hyperreflexia, seizures, hallucinations, and coma	Gradual infusion of hypotonic electrolyte solution or isotonic saline solution
Hyponatremia (serum sodium < 135 mEq/L [< 135 mmol/L])	Diuretics, loss of GI fluids, kidney disease, excessive water intake, and excessive I.V. fluids or parenteral feedings	Nausea and vomiting, lethargy, confusion, muscle cramps, diarrhea, delirium, weakness, seizures, and coma	Gradual sodium replacement, water restriction (1 to 1.5 L/day), or discontinuation of diuretic therapy (if ordered)
Hyperkalemia (serum potassium > 5 mEq/L [> 5 mmol/L])	Renal failure, impaired tubular function, potassium-conserving diuretic use (in patients with renal insufficiency), rapid I.V. potassium administration, metabolic acidosis, and diabetic ketoacidosis	Arrhythmias, weakness, paresthesia, electrocardiogram (ECG) changes (tall, tented T waves; ST segment depression; prolonged PR interval and QRS complex; shortened QT interval; absent P waves)	Dialysis (for renal failure), sodium polystyrene sulfonate (Kayexalate) (to remove potassium), I.V. calcium gluconate (antagonizes cardiac abnormalities), I.V. insulin or hypertonic dextrose solution (shifts potassium into the cells), bicarbonate (for patients with acidosis), or potassium intake restriction
Hypokalemia (serum potassium < 3.5 mEq/L [< 3.5 mmol/L])	Vomiting, diarrhea, nasogastric suction, diuretic use, digoxin toxicity, and decreased potassium intake	Fatigue, weakness, confusion, muscle cramps, ECG changes (flattened T waves, presence of U waves, ST segment depression, prolonged PR interval), and ventricular tachycardia or fibrillation	Oral or I.V. potassium administration (I.V. infusions must be diluted and given slowly)

Transfusing blood and selected components

Blood component	Indications	Compatibility	Nursing considerations
Packed red blood cells (RBCs)			
Same RBC mass as whole blood but with 80% of the plasma removed	• To restore or maintain oxygen-carrying capacity • To correct anemia and surgical blood loss • To increase RBC mass • Red cell exchange	• Group A receives A or O • Group B receives B or O • Group AB receives AB, A, B, or O • Group O receives O • Rh type must match	• Use blood administration tubing to infuse over less than 4 hours. • Use only with normal saline solution. • Avoid administering packed RBCs for anemic conditions correctable by nutritional or drug therapy.
Leukocyte-poor RBCs			
Same as packed RBCs with about 70% of the leukocytes removed	• Same as packed RBCs • To prevent febrile reactions from leukocyte antibodies • To treat immunocompromised patients • To restore RBCs to patients who have had two or more nonhemolytic febrile reactions	• Same as packed RBCs • Rh type must match	• Use blood administration tubing. • May require a 40-micron filter suitable for hard-spun, leukocyte-poor RBCs. • Other considerations are same as those for packed RBCs. • Cells expire 24 hours after washing.
Platelets			
Platelet sediment from RBCs or plasma platelets	• To treat bleeding caused by decreased circulating platelets or functionally abnormal platelets • To improve platelet count preoperatively in a patient whose count is 50,000/μl or less	• ABO compatibility identical; Rh-negative recipients should receive Rh-negative platelets	• Use a blood filter or leukocyte reduction filter. • As prescribed, premedicate with antipyretics and antihistamines if patient's history includes a platelet transfusion reaction or to reduce chills, fever, and allergic reactions. • Use single donor platelets if patient has a need for repeated transfusions. • Platelets aren't used to treat autoimmune thrombocytopenia or thrombocytopenic purpura unless patient has a life-threatening hemorrhage.

Fresh frozen plasma (FFP)			
Uncoagulated plasma separated from RBCs and rich in coagulation factors V, VIII, and IX	• To treat postoperative hemorrhage • To correct an undetermined coagulation factor deficiency • To replace a specific factor when that factor isn't available • Warfarin reversal	• ABO compatibility required • Rh match not required	• Use a blood administration set and administer infusion rapidly. • Keep in mind that large-volume transfusions of FFP may require correction for hypocalcemia because citric acid in FFP binds calcium. • Must be infused within 24 hours of being thawed.
Albumin 5% (buffered saline); albumin 25% (salt-poor)			
A small plasma protein prepared by fractionating pooled plasma	• To replace volume lost because of shock from burns, trauma, surgery, or infections • To treat hypoproteinemia (with or without edema)	• Not required	• Use administration set supplied by manufacturer and set rate based on patient's condition and response. • Keep in mind that albumin is contraindicated in severe anemia. • Administer cautiously in cardiac and pulmonary disease because heart failure may result from circulatory overload.
Factor VIII concentrate (antihemophilic factor)			
Cold insoluble portion of plasma recovered from FFP	• To treat a patient with hemophilia A • To treat a patient with von Willebrand's disease	• ABO compatibility not required	• Administer by I.V. injection using a filter needle, or use administration set supplied by manufacturer.
Cryoprecipitate			
Insoluble plasma portion of FFP containing fibrinogen, factor VIIIc, factor VIIvWF, factor XIII, and fibronectin	• To treat factor VIII deficiency and fibrinogen disorders • To treat significant factor XIII deficiency • To treat a patient with hemophilia A • To treat a patient with von Willebrand's disease	• ABO compatibility required • Rh match not required	• Administer by I. V. injection using a filter needle, or use administration set supplied by the manufacturer. • Administer with a blood administration set. • Add normal saline solution to each bag of cryoprecipitate, as necessary, to facilitate infusion. • Keep in mind that thawed cryoprecipitate must be kept at room temperature and administered as soon as possible after thawing. • Before administration, check laboratory studies to confirm a deficiency of one of specific clotting factors present in cryoprecipitate. • Be aware that patients with hemophilia A or von Willebrand's disease should only be treated with cryoprecipitate when appropriate factor VIII concentrates aren't available.

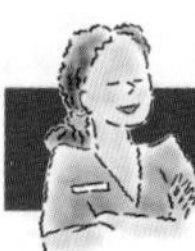

Practice makes perfect

1. A construction worker labors outside in 90° F (32.2° C) temperatures. What hormone will his body release in larger quantities to help him retain water?
   - A. Insulin
   - B. Antidiuretic hormone
   - C. Renin
   - D. Cortisol

2. A postoperative patient is ordered an I.V. solution of dextrose 5% in normal saline solution. What type of fluid is this solution?
   - A. Hypertonic
   - B. Hypotonic
   - C. Isotonic
   - D. Colloid

3. You're teaching a group of athletes how to prevent excessive fluid loss. You should tell them to consume fluids when they:
   - A. experience dry mouth.
   - B. feel light-headed or dizzy.
   - C. are thirsty.
   - D. sweat.

4. A patient with hyponatremia caused by diabetes insipidus requires I.V. fluid replacement. Which I.V. fluid would provide the greatest concentration of sodium replacement if the patient were to develop a subnormal serum sodium level?
   - A. Dextrose 5% in water
   - B. Half-normal saline solution
   - C. Ringer's solution
   - D. Dextrose 5% in lactated Ringer's solution

5. A 29-year-old patient comes to the emergency department after being involved in a motor vehicle accident. Chest radiography reveals a right pneumothorax. You expect his arterial blood gas results to reflect which of the following?
   - A. His pH is low, $Paco_2$ is high, and bicarbonate is normal.
   - B. His pH is low, $Paco_2$ is low, and bicarbonate is low.
   - C. His pH is low, $Paco_2$ is high, and bicarbonate is low.
   - D. His pH is high, $Paco_2$ is low, and bicarbonate is low.

6. A patient is transferred to the intensive care unit in septic shock. Arterial blood gas results show that the patient is acidotic. You expect the anion gap to be:
   A. 0 to 4 mEq/L.
   B. 4 to 8 mEq/L.
   C. 8 to 14 mEq/L.
   D. greater than 14 mEq/L.

7. A patient who sustained multiple abdominal injuries in a motor vehicle accident 2 days ago becomes hypotensive. His urine output for the past 4 hours totals 45 ml. The doctor decides to insert a pulmonary artery (PA) catheter. During measurement of PA pressures, what specific information is being obtained when the balloon is wedged in a branch of the PA?
   A. Left-sided heart function
   B. Central venous pressure
   C. Cardiac output
   D. Right-sided heart function

8. A patient with Alzheimer's disease is admitted with suspected dehydration after her daughter reports that the patient has refused to drink anything for the past 3 days. The doctor orders several laboratory tests. Which laboratory test result is most expected with dehydration?
   A. Urine specific gravity of 1.005
   B. Serum sodium level of 150 mEq/L
   C. Hematocrit of 38%
   D. Serum creatinine level of 0.8 to 1.5 mg/dl

9. A 53-year-old homeless person is admitted with dehydration. Which type of I.V. fluid should be avoided when treating this patient?
   A. Isotonic fluid
   B. Colloid fluid
   C. Hypotonic fluid
   D. Hypertonic fluid

10. A 78-year-old patient is admitted with pulmonary edema. The patient is given I.V. morphine. Why?
   A. To lower his blood pressure
   B. To promote diuresis
   C. To slow his breathing
   D. To remove fluid from his lungs

11. A patient diagnosed with lung cancer develops syndrome of inappropriate antidiuretic hormone, which puts him at risk for hyponatremia. Which serum sodium level indicates hyponatremia?
   A. 128 mEq/L
   B. 135 mEq/L
   C. 142 mEq/L
   D. 150 mEq/L

12. While being treated for hyponatremia, a patient develops iatrogenic hypernatremia. Which treatment is appropriate for resolving this problem?
    A. Fluid restriction
    B. Hypotonic fluid administration
    C. Hypertonic fluid administration
    D. Diuretic therapy

13. A 35-year-old man with a history of food poisoning and subsequent vomiting complains of weakness, palpitations, abdominal pain, and cramping. His body temperature is 99.6° F (37.6° C). Electrocardiogram results show irregularities. Which imbalance is he most likely to have?
    A. Hypervolemia
    B. Hypokalemia
    C. Acidosis
    D. Hyperchloremia

14. A 65-year-old patient receives daily doses of furosemide (Lasix) and digoxin (Lanoxin) for treatment of heart failure. His serum potassium level is 3.1 mEq/L. Which associated electrocardiogram (ECG) changes would you expect?
    A. Peaked T wave
    B. Depressed ST segment
    C. Narrow QRS complexes
    D. Absent P waves

15. As part of a patient's treatment for hypokalemia, the doctor prescribes I.V. potassium supplementation. At which rate should it be administered?
    A. 5 mEq/hour
    B. 10 mEq/hour
    C. 15 mEq/hour
    D. 20 mEq/hour

16. A patient with a history of systemic lupus erythematosus develops hyperkalemia. The doctor prescribes sodium polystyrene sulfonate (Kayexalate) to reduce the patient's serum potassium level. This drug works by:
    A. forcing potassium into the cells.
    B. promoting renal excretion of potassium.
    C. pulling potassium out of the bowel for excretion.
    D. pulling potassium into the bowel for excretion.

17. A 28-year-old patient is seen in the obstetrics clinic with a blood pressure of 220/130 mm Hg and abnormal reflexes. The nurse-midwife caring for her suspects preeclampsia. A urinalysis for protein is ordered immediately, and proteinuria is detected. The patient is transported to the obstetric unit in the medical center. On admission, the nurse assesses the patient's deep tendon reflexes as 4+. This value means the reflexes are:

A. normal and active.
B. present but diminished.
C. slow to respond.
D. hyperactive.

18. Which intervention is most appropriate for the patient receiving a continuous magnesium sulfate infusion?

A. Insert an indwelling urinary catheter.
B. Attach the patient to a continuous cardiac monitor.
C. Administer calcium gluconate every 4 hours.
D. Perform neurologic checks every 2 hours.

19. Which finding suggests that a patient has received too much magnesium sulfate?

A. Muscle weakness
B. Tetany
C. Tachycardia
D. Hyperreflexia

20. A patient develops hypermagnesemia. Which intervention is most effective in reducing serum magnesium levels?

A. Administer a cation-exchange resin.
B. Infuse a bolus of calcium gluconate.
C. Increase the volume of I.V. and oral fluids.
D. Administer antidiuretic hormone.

21. A 36-year-old woman with a history of hyperthyroidism has undergone a total thyroidectomy. After surgery, she experiences hypotension, irritability, and circumoral paresthesia. Her surgical wound has well-approximated borders, no bleeding, and minimal swelling. Her speech and breathing are unimpaired. Based on the patient's signs and symptoms, her serum calcium level is likely to be:

A. greater than 10.1 mg/dl.
B. 10 mg/dl.
C. 9 mg/dl.
D. 8 mg/dl.

22. A 35-year-old patient with a history of alcohol abuse is admitted with acute pancreatitis. His calcium level on admission is 7.6 mg/dl. Which finding also suggests hypocalcemia?

A. Prolonged ST segment on an electrocardiogram (ECG)
B. Constipation
C. Flaccid reflexes
D. Increased cardiac output

23. A patient with acute hypocalcemia develops torsades de pointes. Which drug is most commonly given to treat acute hypocalcemia?

A. Calcium carbonate
B. Calcium gluconate
C. Calcium chloride
D. Calcitonin

24. You need to prepare a calcium infusion for a patient with hypocalcemia. You should mix the drug in which solution?

A. Normal saline solution
B. Dextrose 5% in water
C. Half-normal saline solution
D. Dextrose 5% in half-normal saline solution

25. A public health nurse in a homeless shelter assesses a 57-year-old man with chronic alcoholism. He has a productive cough and a low-grade fever. He's 5′10″ (1.8 m) and weighs 135 lb (61.2 kg). The nurse's nutritional assessment reveals he's malnourished. The patient is admitted to a respiratory isolation room in a community hospital because tuberculosis is suspected. Based on his history of alcohol abuse, you expect his serum phosphorous level to be:

A. below normal.
B. above normal.
C. in the normal range.
D. unaffected.

26. A patient's phosphorus level is elevated. Which of the following electrolytes should you expect to be decreased?

A. Calcium
B. Potassium
C. Sodium
D. Magnesium

27. You're teaching a patient with hypophosphatemia about the importance of consuming phosphorus-rich foods. You should recommend:

A. pumpkin.
B. cranberries.
C. trout.
D. green beans.

28. A 10-year-old girl who recently returned from traveling abroad complains that she's experienced frequent episodes of diarrhea and weakness for the last 3 days. She's diagnosed with gastroenteritis. Her temperature is 102.4° F (39.1° C), her pulses are weak, and her blood pressure is 76/40 mm Hg. She has poor skin turgor, low urine output, and dry mucous membranes. Serum laboratory studies reveal the child's chloride level to be 88 mEq/L. The direct cause of the child's hypochloremia is most likely:

A. fever.
B. low urine output.
C. diarrhea.
D. dry mucous membranes.

29. A 39-year-old patient is admitted with severe vomiting and abdominal pain. His admission laboratory findings reveal hypochloremia. Which other electrolyte would you expect to be deficient?

A. Calcium
B. Sodium
C. Magnesium
D. Phosphorus

30. A 62-year-old patient who underwent a partial gastrectomy 2 days ago develops hypochloremia. This places the patient at risk for:

A. respiratory acidosis.
B. respiratory alkalosis.
C. metabolic acidosis.
D. metabolic alkalosis.

31. A 16-year-old male with a recent history of weight loss, increased appetite, and urinary frequency is seen in the clinic. He complains of weakness and syncope. On initial observation, the nurse notes that his skin and mucous membranes are dry and that his eyeballs appear sunken. The teen's mother reports that he gets up a lot at night to go to the bathroom. His capillary blood glucose measurement is 480 mg/dl. Which acid-base imbalance should you suspect?

A. Metabolic acidosis
B. Metabolic alkalosis
C. Respiratory acidosis
D. Respiratory alkalosis

32. A 23-year-old patient is admitted with diabetic ketoacidosis. Which value from the arterial blood gas analysis supports the diagnosis?

A. pH: 7.48
B. $Paco_2$: 48 mm Hg
C. Bicarbonate: 28 mEq/L
D. Anion gap: 17 mEq/L

33. You're caring for a 33-year-old patient who developed Guillain-Barré syndrome 1 week after contracting an upper respiratory infection. This places the patient at risk for which acid-base imbalance?

A. Metabolic acidosis
B. Metabolic alkalosis
C. Respiratory acidosis
D. Respiratory alkalosis

34. A patient with a history of heart failure calls you to her room because she's short of breath. You assess her and find that her heart failure is worsening. Which type of fluid volume excess is the patient experiencing because of her heart failure?

A. Intravascular
B. Extracellular
C. Intracellular
D. Interstitial

35. A 27-year-old woman in her 38th week of pregnancy is admitted to the obstetric unit after her bag of water broke at home. You perform a vaginal examination and note that her cervix is 6 cm dilated. You attach the fetal monitor and find that the fetal heart rate is normal. As her labor progresses, she hyperventilates. Which acid-base imbalance is she most likely to experience if she continues to hyperventilate?

A. Metabolic acidosis
B. Metabolic alkalosis
C. Respiratory acidosis
D. Respiratory alkalosis

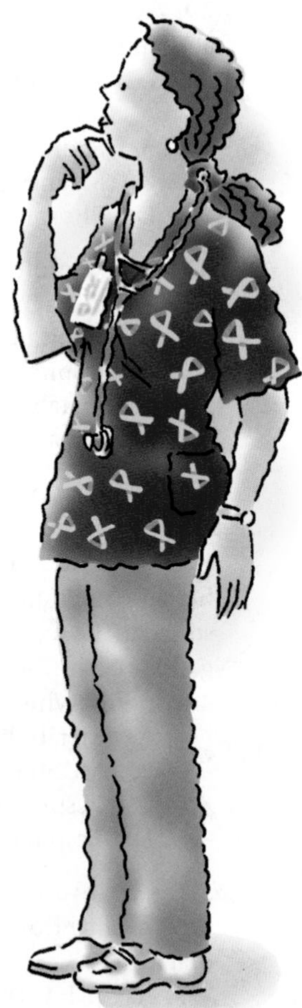

36. A 58-year-old man calls for emergency medical services from his home after he experiences excruciating substernal chest pain. He's rushed to the emergency department where he's given nitroglycerin and morphine for the pain. Electrocardiogram results show changes consistent with an acute anterior wall myocardial infarction (MI). A main complication of an anterior wall MI is heart failure. Which chamber of the heart is most likely to fail in this patient?

A. Right atrium
B. Right ventricle
C. Left atrium
D. Left ventricle

37. A 74-year-old man with a 3-day history of worsening chronic obstructive pulmonary disease is hospitalized. His breathing is labored, breath sounds are congested with rhonchi throughout, and his Sao_2 (as measured by pulse oximetry) is 89%. He's placed on a 35% aerosol mask, and blood is drawn for arterial blood gas analysis. The results are pH, 7.33; Pao_2, 68 mm Hg; $Paco_2$, 53 mm Hg; and bicarbonate, 18 mEq/L. Which acid-base imbalance does the patient most likely have?

A. Metabolic acidosis
B. Metabolic alkalosis
C. Respiratory acidosis
D. Respiratory alkalosis

38. You're caring for a 54-year-old patient who has smoked two packs of cigarettes per day for the past 35 years. He's been admitted with worsening chronic obstructive pulmonary disease (COPD). Why is it important for supplemental oxygen to be carefully monitored in this patient?

A. Increasing the Pao_2 beyond what's needed will lead to oxygen toxicity.
B. High oxygen levels will promote microbial growth in the patient's lungs.
C. Increased Pao_2 levels can depress the drive to breathe in patients with COPD.
D. Increased Pao_2 levels can elevate the drive to breathe in patients with COPD.

39. A patient returned from the postanesthesia care unit with a nasogastric (NG) tube in place. The doctor's order states *irrigate NG tube q4h.* Which solution is the best irrigant?

A. Saline solution
B. Distilled water
C. Tap water
D. Sterile water

40. A 66-year-old woman who survived a cardiac arrest was admitted to the intensive care unit. She experienced a prolonged episode of hypotension and is now in acute renal failure. Frequent electrolyte levels are ordered. Hemodialysis is scheduled to begin within 24 hours. Which type of renal failure did the patient experience?

A. Intrarenal
B. Prerenal
C. Postrenal
D. Renal

41. A patient with a history of hypertension develops chronic renal failure. What should you expect the glomerular filtration rate (GFR) to be?

A. 10 to 20 ml/minute
B. 20 to 40 ml/minute
C. 40 to 60 ml/minute
D. Greater than 60 ml/minute

42. A patient who sustained massive internal injuries in a motor vehicle accident becomes hypotensive and develops acute renal failure. Which acid-base imbalance is this patient most likely to experience?

A. Respiratory acidosis
B. Respiratory alkalosis
C. Metabolic acidosis
D. Metabolic alkalosis

43. A patient received burn injuries 48 hours ago. He's entering the second phase of burn injury. What physiologic changes can be expected?

A. Edema development
B. Increased blood volume
C. Decreased hemoglobin level
D. Profuse urination

44. A fireman sustains burns while fighting an apartment fire. He receives fluid resuscitation using the Parkland formula. Which type of fluid is used?

A. Normal saline solution
B. Half-normal saline solution
C. Lactated Ringer's solution
D. Dextrose 5% in lactated Ringer's solution

45. A 42-year-old man with end-stage AIDS has frequent episodes of watery stool. He's nauseated and refuses to drink fluids. His body temperature is 102° F (38.9° C), his blood pressure is 88/52 mm Hg, and his pulse is 112 beats/minute. Normal saline solution is infusing at 150 ml/hour through a large-bore I.V. catheter. Which type of fluid is normal saline solution?

A. Isotonic
B. Hypotonic
C. Hypertonic
D. Colloid

46. A patient's blood volume doesn't improve after the administration of crystalloids. The doctor prescribes a colloid for this patient. Which of the following solutions is a colloid?

A. Dextrose 5% in half-normal saline solution
B. Hetastarch
C. Dextrose 10% in water
D. Dextrose 5% in lactated Ringer's solution

47. An 18-year-old patient with Crohn's disease is unable to tolerate an elemental diet. Total parenteral nutrition (TPN) is indicated when the patient's serum albumin is less than:
   A. 5 g/dl.
   B. 4.5 g/dl.
   C. 4 g/dl.
   D. 3.5 g/dl.

48. A patient receiving total parenteral nutrition (TPN) requires a transfusion of packed red blood cells. Before you begin the transfusion, you should:
   A. infuse the blood directly into the TPN line.
   B. start a separate I.V. line for the blood transfusion.
   C. stop the TPN, infuse the blood at the TPN site, and then restart the TPN.
   D. use a Y connector and infuse the blood simultaneously with the TPN.

49. A patient's postoperative hemoglobin level is 7.9 g/dl. The doctor orders 2 units of packed red blood cells (RBCs) for the patient. By what percentage should this increase the patient's hematocrit?
   A. 3%
   B. 6%
   C. 9%
   D. 12%

50. A patient experiences a transfusion reaction 15 minutes after you begin a blood transfusion. You collect the appropriate laboratory specimens. Laboratory results reveal hemoglobinuria. Which type of reaction has the patient most likely experienced?
   A. Hemolytic
   B. Febrile
   C. Allergic
   D. Vasogenic

51. You're caring for a patient with a decreased calcium level of 7.4 mg/dl. Which treatment would you expect to provide? (Select all that apply.)
   A. I.V. calcium gluconate or I.V. calcium chloride
   B. Loop diuretics
   C. Magnesium supplements
   D. Vitamin D
   E. Normal saline solution
   F. Hemodialysis or peritoneal dialysis

52. You're caring for a patient with a suspected overdose of magnesium-containing antacids and laxatives. On admission, her laboratory values for magnesium were greater than 3 mg/dl. Which signs and symptoms would you expect to see? (Select all that apply.)

   A. Flushing
   B. Hypertension
   C. Hypotension
   D. Seizures
   E. Nausea and vomiting
   F. Bradycardia

53. A newly admitted patient is being treated for acute pancreatitis. Which electrolyte disorder may be noted?

   A. Hypokalemia
   B. Hypercalcemia
   C. Hypermagnesemia
   D. Hypophosphatemia

54. The major extracellular anion is:

   A. potassium.
   B. sodium.
   C. chloride.
   D. magnesium.

55. Water composes what percentage of total body weight, depending on the amount of fat present?

   A. 20% to 30%
   B. 20% to 40%
   C. 30% to 50%
   D. 45% to 75%

56. A patient arrives at the emergency department with gastroenteritis caused by dehydration. The admitting nurse records that the patient has been experiencing vomiting and diarrhea for the past 3 days. The doctor orders a continuous I.V. infusion. Which I.V. solution is best to administer?

   A. Dextrose 5% in 0.45% saline solution
   B. Dextrose 5% in lactated Ringer's solution
   C. 0.45% saline solution
   D. Lactated Ringer's solution

57. A 65-year-old woman is admitted to the emergency department after vomiting excessively at home. After checking the patient's arterial blood gas (ABG) levels, the doctor diagnoses severe dehydration. Using the ABG results as guide, which acid-base imbalance would you expect the patient to have?

A. Respiratory acidosis
B. Metabolic alkalosis
C. Respiratory alkalosis
D. Metabolic acidosis

58. A malnourished 55-year-old patient with a history of alcohol abuse arrives in the emergency department complaining of muscle weakness and cramps. Electrocardiogram tracings show evidence of arrhythmias, and laboratory tests reveal hypomagnesemia. Which electrolytes are typically depleted with magnesium deficiency?

A. Calcium and phosphorus
B. Potassium and phosphorus
C. Potassium and chloride
D. Chloride and calcium

59. The doctor orders tap water enemas until clear for a patient scheduled for a colonoscopy in the morning. The nurse is aware that after three such enemas, electrolyte imbalances are likely to occur. Signs of which imbalance should cause the most concern?

A. Hypocalcemia
B. Hypercalcemia
C. Hypernatremia
D. Hypokalemia

60. Electrolytes are made up of:

A. glucose, bases, and salts.
B. lipids, acids, and bases.
C. bases, acids, and salts.
D. salts, glucose, and lipids.

Answers

1. B. One way the body conserves water is to release more antidiuretic hormone, which reduces diuresis.

2. A. A solution of dextrose 5% in normal saline is considered hypertonic because its osmolality is 560 mOsm/L.

3. C. The simplest mechanism for maintaining fluid balance is the thirst mechanism. When an individual senses thirst, he should drink to replace lost fluid.

4. C. Ringer's solution contains 147 mEq of sodium per liter. Half-normal saline solution contains 77 mEq/L. Dextrose 5% in water contains no sodium. Dextrose 5% in lactated Ringer's solution contains 130 mEq/L.

5. A. In patients with respiratory acidosis, pH is low, $Paco_2$ is high, and bicarbonate is normal.

6. D. Patients who are in an acidotic state typically have higher than normal amounts of organic acids, which leads to an elevated anion gap ($>$ 14 mEq/L).

7. A. When the tip of the PA catheter is wedged in a branch of the pulmonary artery, it measures pressures that reflect left-sided heart function.

8. B. Because some of the water present in the serum is lost, causing dehydration, the serum sodium level becomes elevated.

9. D. Dehydration is a hypertonic state; therefore, hypertonic fluid should be avoided because it would worsen the patient's condition. Free water or isotonic or hypotonic fluid would be a safer choice.

10. C. Morphine is given to the patient with pulmonary edema because it relieves air hunger and dilates blood vessels, which in turn reduces pulmonary congestion and the amount of blood that returns to the heart.

11. A. Normal serum sodium level is 135 to 145 mEq/L. A serum sodium level less than 135 mEq/L indicates hyponatremia.

12. D. Diuretics increase sodium loss in the urine, thereby lowering the serum sodium level.

13. B. Conditions such as vomiting that lead to loss of gastric acids can cause hypokalemia and alkalosis.

14. B. Hypokalemia causes various ECG changes, including a flattened or inverted T wave, a depressed ST segment, and a characteristic U wave.

15. B. When supplemental potassium is given by I.V. infusion, it should be administered at a rate of 10 mEq/hour.

16. D. Sodium polystyrene sulfonate is a cation-exchange resin that causes potassium to move out of the blood into the intestines. It's then excreted in the stool.

17. D. Deep tendon reflexes are graded on a 0 to 4+ scale. 0 is absent, 1+ is present but diminished, 2+ is normal, 3+ is increased but not necessarily abnormal, and 4+ is hyperactive.

18. B. Magnesium affects cardiac function and can cause arrhythmias. Therefore, any patient receiving a magnesium sulfate infusion should be on continuous cardiac monitoring.

19. A. Hypermagnesemia causes muscle weakness. Therefore, if a patient develops muscle weakness while receiving magnesium, most likely the dose is too great.

20. C. The best method of reducing serum magnesium levels is to increase urinary excretion of magnesium by increasing the patient's fluid intake.

21. D. Hypotension, irritability, and circumoral paresthesia are signs and symptoms of hypocalcemia. Because 8.9 to 10.1 mg/dl is the normal range for total serum calcium levels, 8 mg/dl is the only value here that indicates hypocalcemia.

22. A. The patient with hypocalcemia may experience diarrhea, hyperactive deep tendon reflexes, a diminished response to digoxin (Lanoxin), decreased cardiac output, prolonged ST segment on an ECG, and a lengthened QT interval, which places the patient at risk for torsades de pointes (polymorphic ventricular tachycardia).

23. B. With acute cases of hypocalcemia, I.V. calcium gluconate is usually given. Calcium chloride is a less common alternative.

24. B. When preparing a calcium infusion, add calcium to a solution containing dextrose 5% in water. Solutions containing normal saline cause renal calcium loss.

25. A. Patients who abuse alcohol typically have serum phosphorous levels that fall below normal.

26. A. Phosphorus and calcium have an inverse relationship: When the levels of one are increased, the levels of the other are decreased. No such relationship exists between phosphorus and potassium, sodium, or magnesium.

27. C. Fish is a food source that's rich in phosphorus, so trout would be helpful to a patient with hypophosphatemia.

28. C. The child's low serum chloride level is probably caused by her diarrhea.

29. B. Chloride is a negatively charged ion that has an electrical attraction to sodium. Therefore, if chloride levels become low, so do serum sodium levels.

30. D. To compensate for a chloride loss (hypochloremia), the kidneys retain bicarbonate. The accumulation of excess bicarbonate in extracellular fluid can raise the arterial pH above 7.45, causing metabolic alkalosis.

31. A. The patient has signs and symptoms of type 1 diabetes mellitus. Because of the accumulation of metabolic wastes (e.g., ketones), type 1 diabetes mellitus is most commonly associated with metabolic acidosis.

32. D. Metabolic acidosis causes the anion gap to be greater than 14 mEq/L. With metabolic acidosis, pH will be less than 7.35, bicarbonate will be less than 22 mEq/L, and $Paco_2$ will typically be unaffected.

33. C. In certain neuromuscular diseases, such as Guillain-Barré syndrome, the respiratory muscles fail to respond properly to the respiratory drive, leading to respiratory acidosis.

34. B. Because the heart doesn't pump effectively in a patient with heart failure, fluid imbalances develop. The most common fluid imbalance associated with heart failure is extracellular volume excess. This results from the heart's failure to propel blood forward, consequent vascular pooling, and the sodium and water reabsorption triggered by the renin-angiotensin-aldosterone system.

35. D. When a patient hyperventilates, excess carbon dioxide is blown off. This raises the arterial pH above 7.45 causing respiratory alkalosis.

36. D. With an anterior wall MI, the left ventricle usually fails, causing heart failure.

37. C. When a patient's $Paco_2$ is elevated, carbonic acid is retained, leading to acidosis. Because the acidosis is respiratory in origin, the patient most likely has respiratory acidosis.

38. C. Increased Pao_2 can depress the patient's drive to breathe, which is largely driven by hypoxemia.

39. A. The best solution for gastric irrigation is an isotonic solution such as saline solution.

40. B. The patient's renal failure was due to hypotension, which is a prerenal cause. Prerenal causes are those conditions outside of the kidneys that diminish blood flow to the kidneys.

41. A. Renal failure occurs when the GFR is 10 to 20 ml/minute. A rate of 40 to 70 ml/minute indicates renal reserve; 20 to 40 ml/minute, renal insufficiency; and less than 10 ml/minute, end-stage renal disease.

42. C. As the kidneys lose their ability to excrete hydrogen ions, there's a buildup of hydrogen, which leads to metabolic acidosis.

43. D. The second phase of the burn injury, known as the *remobilization phase*, starts about 48 hours after the initial injury. During this phase, fluid shifts back to the vascular compartment. Edema at the burn site decreases and blood flow to kidneys increases, which increases diuresis.

44. C. The Parkland formula, which is widely used for burn resuscitation, uses lactated Ringer's solution.

45. A. Normal saline solution is an isotonic crystalloid fluid.

46. B. Examples of colloids include albumin, hetastarch, dextran, and plasma protein fraction.

47. D. TPN is typically indicated when the serum albumin level is less than 3.5 g/dl.

48. B. Blood transfusions shouldn't be infused with TPN; therefore, a separate I.V. line should be secured for the blood transfusion.

49. B. One unit of packed RBCs will increase hematocrit by 3%; 2 units, by 6%.

50. A. Hemoglobinuria is a sign of a hemolytic reaction to a blood transfusion and isn't representative of other reaction types.

51. A, C, D. Treatment of hypocalcemia focuses on correcting the imbalance as quickly as possible. I.V. calcium gluconate or I.V. calcium chloride replaces calcium levels. Because hypocalcemia may not be corrected by calcium therapy alone, expect to give magnesium supplements as well. Also, vitamin D supplements may be ordered to facilitate calcium's absorption in the gastrointestinal tract.

52. A, C, E, F. Too much magnesium causes vasodilation and irregular heart muscle contractions, which decrease the blood pressure and slow the heart rate. It may also cause nausea and vomiting, facial flushing, and feelings of warmth.

53. A. Hypokalemia may be caused by severe vomiting and diarrhea in acute pancreatitis that results in potassium loss.

54. C. Chloride regulates osmotic pressure between compartments and forms hydrochloric acid in the stomach.

55. D. Water weight is highest during infancy, constituting up to 75% of total body weight. It begins declining with age due to the amount of increased body fat. In an older adult, body water content is 45% to 55% of body weight.

56. D. Lactated Ringer's solution is the infusion of choice for acute volume expansion. It contains a small amount of potassium along with lactate, a form of lactic acid that's metabolized by the liver to form bicarbonate, which helps buffer the blood against the effects of acidosis.

57. B. Metabolic alkalosis causes an increase in bicarbonate level, resulting in a nonrespiratory loss of acid.

58. B. Malnutrition, diarrhea, and diuretic use commonly cause hypomagnesemia. Loss of potassium and phosphorus from skeletal muscles typically results in muscle weakness, cramps, and arrhythmias.

59. D. Tap water enemas can cause a fluid volume deficit, which consequently decreases sodium and potassium levels. This can lead to water intoxication, a potentially life-threatening condition.

60. C. Bases, acids, and salts dissociate into ions when in a watery solution.

Glossary

absorption: taking up of a substance by cells or tissues

acid: substance that donates hydrogen ions

acid-base balance: mechanism by which the body's acids and bases are kept in balance

acidosis: condition resulting from the accumulation of acid or the loss of base

adenosine triphosphate (ATP): vital phosphorus-containing compound that represents stored energy in the cells; needed to carry out the body's functions

aldosterone: adrenocortical hormone that regulates sodium, potassium, and fluid balance

alkalosis: condition resulting from the accumulation of base or the loss of acid

anion: negatively charged ion, of which proteins, chloride, bicarbonate, and phosphorus are among the body's most plentiful

anion gap: measurement of the difference between the amount of sodium and the amount of bicarbonate and chloride in the blood

antidiuretic hormone (ADH): hormone made by the hypothalamus and released by the pituitary gland that decreases the production of urine by increasing the reabsorption of water by the renal tubules

anuria: absence of urine formation or output of less than 100 ml of urine in 24 hours

base: substance that accepts hydrogen ions

buffer: substance that, when combined with acids or bases, minimizes changes in pH

calcification: deposit of calcium phosphate in soft tissues that can occur with prolonged high serum phosphorus levels; can lead to organ dysfunction

calcium: positively charged ion involved in the structure and function of bones, impulse transmission, the blood clotting process, and the normal function of heart and skeletal muscles

carboxyhemoglobin: molecule of carbon monoxide and hemoglobin that prevents the normal transfer of oxygen and carbon dioxide; can result in asphyxiation or death

cation: positively charged ion, of which sodium, potassium, calcium, magnesium, and hydrogen are the body's most plentiful

cation-exchange resin: medication used to lower serum potassium levels by exchanging sodium ions for potassium ions in the gastrointestinal tract

chloride: most abundant anion in extracellular fluid; maintains serum osmolality and fluid, electrolyte, and acid-base balance

Chvostek's sign: abnormal spasm of facial muscles that may indicate hypocalcemia or tetany; tested by lightly tapping the facial nerve (upper cheek, below the zygomatic bone)

colloid: large molecule, such as albumin, that normally doesn't cross the capillary membrane

colloid osmotic pressure: pressure exerted by colloids in the vasculature

compensation: process by which one system (renal or respiratory) attempts to correct an acid-base disturbance in the other system

crystalloid: solute, such as sodium or glucose, that crosses the capillary membrane in solution

diuretics: class of medications acting at various points along the nephron to increase urine output, resulting in the loss of water and electrolytes

electrolyte: solute that separates in a solvent into electrically charged particles called *ions*

factor VIII (cryoprecipitate): antihemophilic factor recovered from fresh frozen plasma; instrumental in blood clotting

glomerular filtration rate (GFR): rate at which the glomeruli in the kidneys filter blood; normally occurs at a rate of 125 ml/minute

hydrostatic pressure: pressure exerted by fluid in the blood vessels

hypercapnia: partial pressure of carbon dioxide in arterial blood that's greater than 45 mm Hg

hyperchloremic metabolic acidosis: condition resulting from a deficit in bicarbonate ions and an increase in chloride ions, which causes a decrease in pH

hypervolemia: excess of fluid and solutes in extracellular fluid; can be caused by increased fluid intake, fluid shifts in the body, or renal failure

hypocapnia: partial pressure of carbon dioxide in arterial blood that's less than 35 mm Hg

hypochloremic metabolic alkalosis: condition caused by a deficit in chloride and a subsequent increase in bicarbonate that ultimately causes an increase in pH

hypotonic: solution that has fewer solutes than another solution

hypovolemia: condition marked by the loss of fluid and solutes from extracellular fluid that, if left untreated, can progress to hypovolemic shock

hypovolemic shock: potentially life-threatening condition in which a decreased blood volume leads to low cardiac output and poor tissue perfusion

hypoxemia: oxygen deficit in arterial blood (lower than 80 mm Hg)

hypoxia: oxygen deficit in the tissues

interstitial fluid: fluid surrounding cells that, with plasma, makes up extracellular fluid

isotonic solution: solution that has the same concentration of solutes as another solution

magnesium: cation located primarily in intracellular fluid that promotes efficient energy use, aids protein synthesis, regulates nerve and muscle impulses, and promotes cardiovascular function

metabolic acidosis: condition in which excess acid or reduced bicarbonate in the blood drops the arterial blood pH below 7.35

metabolic alkalosis: condition in which excess bicarbonate or reduced acid in the blood increases the arterial blood pH above 7.45

oliguria: low urine output; less than 400 ml/24 hours

osmolality: concentration of a solution; expressed in milliosmols per kilogram of solution

osmolarity: concentration of a solution; expressed in milliosmols per liter of solution

osmotic pressure: pressure exerted by a solute in solution on a semipermeable membrane

osmoreceptors: special sensing cells in the hypothalamus that respond to changes in the osmolality of blood

osteodystrophy: defective bone development; can occur within the face of prolonged elevated serum phosphorus levels

osteomalacia: softening of bone tissues due to demineralization; commonly accompanies chronic hypocalcemia

pH: measurement of the percentage of hydrogen ions in a solution; normal pH is 7.35 to 7.45 of arterial blood

phosphorus: anion located primarily in intracellular fluid; involved in maintaining bone and cell structure, maintaining storage of energy in cells, and aiding oxygen delivery to tissue

potassium: major intracellular cation involved in skeletal muscle contraction, fluid distribution, osmotic pressure, and acid-base balance as well as heartbeat regulation

pulmonary edema: abnormal fluid accumulation in the lungs; life-threatening condition

reabsorption: taking in, or absorbing, a substance again

renin: enzyme that's released by the kidneys into the blood; it triggers a series of reactions that produce angiotensin, a potent vasoconstrictor

resorption: loss of a substance through physiologic or pathologic means such as loss of calcium from bone

respiratory acidosis: acid-base disturbance caused by failure of the lungs to eliminate sufficient carbon dioxide; partial pressure of arterial carbon dioxide above 45 mm Hg and pH below 7.35

respiratory alkalosis: acid-base imbalance that occurs when the lungs eliminate more carbon dioxide than normal; partial pressure of arterial carbon dioxide below 35 mm Hg and pH above 7.45

rhabdomyolysis: disorder in which skeletal muscle is destroyed; causes intracellular contents to spill into extracellular fluid

sodium: major cation of extracellular fluid involved in regulating extracellular fluid volume, transmitting nerve impulses, and maintaining acid-base balance

tetany: condition caused by abnormal calcium metabolism; characterized by painful muscle spasms, cramps, and sharp flexion of the wrist and ankle joints

third-space fluid shift: movement of fluid out of the intravascular space into another body space such as the abdominal cavity

Trousseau's sign: carpal (wrist) spasm elicited by applying a blood pressure cuff to the upper arm and inflating it to a pressure 20 mm Hg above the patient's systolic blood pressure; indicates the presence of hypocalcemia

uremia: excess of urea and other nitrogenous wastes in the blood

uremic frost: powdery deposits of urea and uric acid salts on the skin, especially the face; caused by the excretion of nitrogenous compounds in sweat

water intoxication: condition in which excess water in the cells results in cellular swelling

Selected References

Dudek, S. G. (2013). *Nutrition essentials for nursing practice* (7th ed.). Philadelphia, PA: Lippincott Williams & Wilkins.

Gahart, B. L., & Nazareno, A. R. (2014). *Intravenous medications: A handbook for nurses and health professionals* (30th ed.). St. Louis, MO: Elsevier.

Hogan, M. A. (2012). *Pearson reviews & rationales: Fluids, electrolytes, & acid-base balance with nursing reviews and rationale* (3rd ed.). Saddle River, NJ: Pearson Education.

Ignatavicius, D. D., & Workman, L. (2012). *Medical-surgical nursing: Patient-centered collaborative care* (7th ed.). Philadelphia, PA: Saunders.

I.V. therapy made incredibly easy (5th ed.). (2012). Philadelphia, PA: Lippincott Williams & Wilkins.

Longo, D., Fauci, A., Kasper, D., Hauser, S., Jameson, J., & Loscalzo, J. (2012). *Harrison's principles of internal medicine* (18th ed.). New York, NY: McGraw-Hill.

Portable fluids and electrolytes. (2008). Philadelphia, PA: Lippincott Williams & Wilkins.

Smeltzer, S., & Bare, B. (2014). *Brunner & Suddarth's textbook of medical-surgical nursing* (13th ed.). Philadelphia, PA: Lippincott Williams & Wilkins.

Weinstein, S. (2014). *Plumer's principles & practice of intravenous therapy* (9th ed.). Philadelphia, PA: Lippincott Williams & Wilkins.

Weisberg, L. (2008). Management of severe hyperkalemia *Critical Care Medicine, 36*(12), 3246–3251.

Index

Note: i refers to an illustration; t refers to a table.

Note: i refers to an illustration; t refers to a table.

Note: i refers to an illustration; t refers to a table.

Note: i refers to an illustration; t refers to a table.